HOSPITAL ACQUIRED INFECTIONS

HOSPITAL ACQUIRED INFECTIONS

Power Strategies for Clinical Practice

Dr V. Muralidhar M.D. (Anaesth)
Senior Consultant
Anaesthesiology and Intensive Care
Indraprastha Apollo Hospitals
New Delhi

Dr Sumathi Muralidhar M.D. (Micro)
Microbiologist
Regional STD Teaching, Training & Research Centre
Vardhaman Mahavir Medical College
Safdarjang Hospital
New Delhi

Anshan

First published in the UK by

Anshan Limited
In 2007

6 Newlands Road,
Tunbridge Wells,
Kent.
TN4 9AT. UK

Tel: +44 (0) 1892 557767
Fax: +44 (0) 1892 530358

E-mail: info@anshan.co.uk
Web Site: www.anshan.co.uk

ISBN-10: 1 905740 55 7
ISBN-13: 978 1 905740 55 0

British Library Cataloguing in Publishing Data
A catalogue record for this book is available from the British Library

Printed and bound in India by Sanat Printers, Kundli, Haryana.

We dedicate this book to our parents for making us what we are today, and to all those patients whose lot we hope to improve.

CONTENTS

ABBREVIATIONS

OF IMPORTANT ORGANIZATIONS

AAMI	Association for the Advancements of Medical Instrumentation
ACDP	Advisory Committee on Dangerous Pathogens
AIA	American Institute of Architects
AORN	Association of Operating Room Nurses
APHA	American Public Health Association
APIC	Association for Practitioners in Infection Control
APSIC	Asia Pacific Society of Infection Control
ASCN	American Society for Clinical Nutrition
ASHP	American Society for Health System Pharmacists
ASM	American Society for Microbiology
ASPEN	American Society for Parenteral and Enteral Nutrition
ATS	American Thoracic Society
BSI	British Standards Institution
BTS	British Thoracic Society
CDC	Centre for Disease Control and Prevention
CEN	Committee European Nationalité
CIDS	Canadian Infectious Diseases Society
COSHH	Control of Substances Hazardous to Health
CPCB	Central Pollution Control Board

CSCCM	Council of Society of Critical Care Medicine
CTS	Canadian Thoracic Society
EPA	Environmental Protection Agency
EPIC	European Prevalence of infection in Intensive Care
ERS	European Respiratory Society
ESICM	European Society of Intensive Care Medicine
FDA	Food and Drug Administration
HACCP	Hazard Analysis Critical Control Point
HICPAC	Hospital Infection Control Practices Advisory Committee
HIS	Hospital Infection Society of India
IDSA	Infectious Diseases Society of America
ISO	International Standards Organization
JCAHO	Joint Commission for Accreditation of Healthcare Organizations
NCI	National Cancer Institute
NHS	National Health Scheme
NICD	National Institute of Communicable Diseases
NIOSH	National Institute of Occupational Safety and Health
NNIS	National Nosocomial Infection Surveillance
NSF	National Sanitation Foundation
ORNAC	Operating Room Nurses Association of Canada
OSHA	Occupational Safety and Health Agency
SENIC	Study of the Efficacy of Nosocomial Infection Control
SHEA	Society for Healthcare Epidemiology for America
SIS	Surgical Infections Society
USPHS	US Public Health Services

ACKNOWLEDGEMENTS

This book is the result of a joint dream we had three years ago. Our dream would have remained just that—a dream—but for the commendable support and help from several people, each an expert in his/her own field, whom we would like to collectively address as 'friends'.

We wish to express a veritable rain-shower of appreciation for the timely help, suggestions and criticisms offered by all our experts listed in Chapter 22.

We thank all organizations that have permitted us to use material from their websites. Every effort has been made to acknowledge the authors and the sources of the published material. However, if there has been an accidental oversight, corrections will be made in the next edition.

Our heartfelt and sincere gratitude to Mr Srikanth Vellore, a truly gifted young man, who has poured his time and talent into this book, by giving us the cover concept and all the wonderful diagrams/figures.

The staff at Viva Books merit our gratitude for their dedication and patience. We are also thankful to Mr Rajesh Sood for the clerical support rendered.

Finally, our gratitude must encompass our family members who have backed us through thick and thin in this venture. Here, our boys, Vivek and Prashanth, need a special word of thanks for allowing us to spend for the book, time that was rightfully theirs.

Forewords

Dr Ashok Rattan
Medical Microbiologist and Laboratory Director
Caribbean Epidemiology Centre (CAREC), PAHO/WHO
16–18 Jamaica Boulevard
Federation Park, St. Clair.
Port of Spain, Trinidad

Robert J. Kim-Farley, MD, MPH
Professor
Department of Epidemiology
School of Public Health
University of California, Los Angeles

We have an exciting future in modern healthcare. Advances have markedly prolonged the human lifespan, but accompanied by this increased life expectancy is the increasing challenge of controlling healthcare associated infections. Standardized practices for infection control arose in England in the early nineteenth century with the introduction of segregation of small pox and fever patients. Modern infection control is also grounded in the work of Ignaz Semmelweis, who in 1840s demonstrated the importance of hand hygiene for controlling transmission of infections in hospitals. In 1985, the Center for Disease Control and Prevention (CDC)'s Study on the Efficacy of Nosocomial Infection Control (SENIC) reported that hospitals with four key infection-control components—an effective hospital epidemiologist, one infection-control nurse for every 250 beds, active surveillance mechanism and ongoing control efforts—reduced nosocomial infection rates by approximately one-third.

Infection control is a cost-effective intervention and it is multi-dimensional. Many of our successes in controlling nosocomial infections have come from improving the design of invasive devices. Non-invasive monitoring devices and minimally invasive surgical techniques that avoid the high risk associated with bypassing normal host defense barriers have contributed significantly to this decrease. All infection control measures, however, have to pass the test of the 4 Ps—Are the recommendations Plausible (e.g. is it likely to work)? Are they Practical (e.g. are they affordable)? Are they Politically acceptable (e.g. will the administration agree)? and Will Personnel follow them (e.g. can they and will they)?

Over the next decade hospitals will become more like ICUs and more routine care will be delivered on an outpatient basis. Newer microbiologic techniques as well as application of molecular epidemiologic analysis will help us better understand the factors that lead to emergence of antibiotic resistances, single-use and non-invasive devices would further contribute to decrease of risks and management practices will become more demanding but user friendly. Dr V. Muralidhar, who has long and in depth experience in ICU and Dr Sumathi Muralidhar, an excellent clinical microbiologist, have written this beautifully illustrated and easy-to-follow book, which because of its contents and lucidity of presentation would become a must read for any serious practitioner of medicine.

Dr Ashok Rattan

Medical Microbiologist and Laboratory Director

CARIBBEAN EPIDEMIOLOGY CENTRE
Pan American Health Organization

Pan American Sanitary Bureau, Regional Office of the
World Health Organization
16–18 Jamaica Boulevard
Federation Park, St. Clair.
Port of Spain, Trinidad

Healthcare-associated infections, including hospital-acquired infections (HAIs), or nosocomial infections, are a major public health problem in both developing as well as developed countries. Worldwide, studies have shown an average of some 8.7 per cent of hospitalized patients have HAIs. Even in the United States alone, HAIs account for an estimated 2 million infections; some 90,000 deaths; and 4.5 billion dollars in excess health care costs each year.

The authors of this book, Drs. Muralidhar and Sumathi Muralidhar, with their distinguished background and complementary experiences as an intensive care specialist and microbiologist, respectively, provide the information and guidance on infection control and prevention critical to those working at all levels of the healthcare system, including: tertiary hospitals, secondary hospitals, primary health centers, nursing homes, clinics, laboratories, pain clinics, nursing homes, physiotherapy units and camps.

In addition to being a significant cause of death, HAIs may lead to disabling conditions, emotional stress and high economic costs due to increased lengths of hospital stays, additional drug costs and lost work.

The authors address, in a comprehensive manner, the current situation; the causes of HAIs; the means for their prevention, control and monitoring; and clinical practice guidelines that will be helpful for all levels of healthcare staff.

I truly hope that this book is widely read so that the needed awareness, partnerships and action will result in curbing the alarmingly high rates of HAIs in our healthcare systems. Each of us, playing our own role and using the evidence-based approaches highlighted in this book, can combat HAIs and help create the systems, supports, and procedures to ensure our hospitals and healthcare facilities treat and cure diseases, and are not their cause.

PROF ROBERT J. KIM-FARLEY

Professor
Department of Epidemiology
School of Public Health
University of California
Los Angeles U.S.A.

PREFACE

The activist is not the man who says the river is dirty. The activist is the man who cleans up the river.

—Ross Perot

Hospital-acquired infections (HAI) pose a significant health problem to patients, practitioners, organizations and countries. When we address this problem, there is often a feeling of despair and powerlessness, similar to the feeling one gets when looking at a dirty, polluted river. Our response varies from asking, 'Why doesn't someone take care of the problem?', to a feeling of detachment hoping that the problem is distant and is not going to affect us. The implications are serious—it affects everyone and everyone is responsible for correcting the problem. All of us, involved directly or indirectly in clinical practice, need to be activists in combating HAI!

We Can No Longer Say That We Are Not Responsible!

Increasing awareness amongst patients, demand for quality healthcare by the public, fear of litigation and stringent requirements for accreditation have all made it imperative for those involved in clinical practice at various levels in the healthcare set-up to adopt a proactive approach to the management of HAI.

Understanding Powerful Strategies and New Perspectives

The idea of this book was conceived to equip practitioners with powerful strategies and perspectives complementary to their clinical practice. Once the basic processes are understood, one can fine-tune them to their institutions and personalized needs, taking their clinical practice to a higher level.

Helping Decision-Making

This book also attempts to inspire, influence and empower those involved in clinical practice to make informed decisions, regarding manpower, materials and processes related to HAI control.

Terminologies—'Let's Talk the Same Language'

We are all used to looking at different areas concerning hospital acquired infections as separate, watertight compartments like the blind men trying to describe an elephant in their own ways. The effectiveness of combating HAI, a clinical risk, is dependent on many complex entities in a system—clinical, managerial, epidemiological, microbiological, etc. One not only needs inputs from all these areas, but also a coordinated approach. We need to talk the same language, think of the problem in its entirety, work together to solve the problem and try to look at the larger picture giving due emphasis to various aspects in equal measure.

The Silver Lining!

The book offers hope to every practitioner by empowering him/her with evidence based strategies to handle HAI with confidence. This optimism is aptly reflected in the design of the cover page—Thumbs Up!

V. Muralidhar
Sumathi Muralidhar

Chapter 1

Introduction to HAI

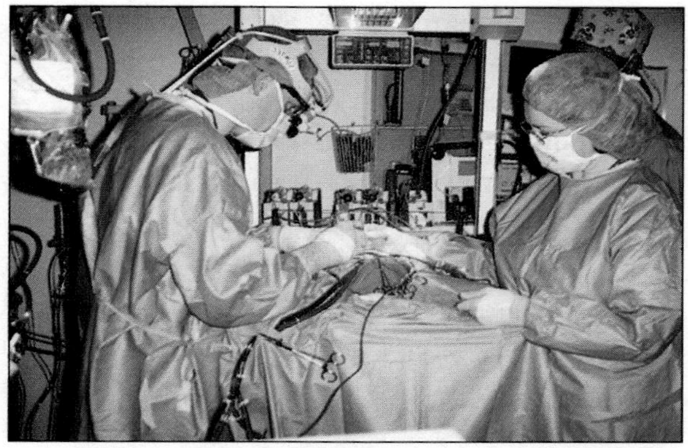

I do not want two diseases—one God made and one, the doctor made.

—Napoleon Bonaparte

Highlights

Definitions Galore!

HAI—Down the Ages

The Modern Era of Infection Control

The Hospital Environment

Opportunistic Infections as HAI

Community Acquired Infections as HAI

Global Dimensions of HAI

Why Control Hospital Acquired Infections?

INTRODUCTION

Significant progress has been made in preventing and managing Hospital Acquired Infections (HAI) since the problem was recognized over a century ago. However, these infections continue to be a major source of morbidity and mortality, affecting more than two million patients annually even in advanced countries like the USA, and an unknown, possibly higher, number in the developing countries.[1] The practice of modern medicine is fraught with several risks unique to the hospital set-up, which need to be addressed meticulously. (Photo 1.1)

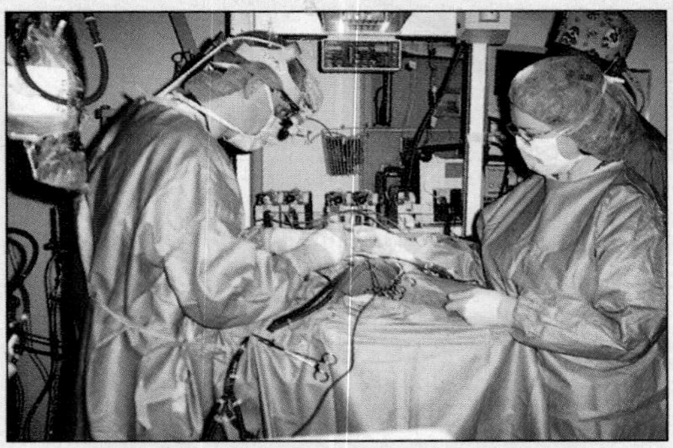

Photo 1.1: The practice of modern medicine is fraught with risk of HAI. An extra corporeal membrane oxygenator (ECMO) being started in a neonatal ICU

DEFINITIONS GALORE!

The terms **'Hospital Infection', 'Hospital Acquired Infection (HAI)'** and **'Nosocomial Infection'** are often used synonymously by many authorities. The definition, however, is a lengthy one and includes infections occurring in both the patient receiving care, as well as those occurring in the Health Care Worker (HCW) offering the care. The Center for Disease Control and Prevention (CDC) (Atlanta, Georgia, USA), has given certain definitions of nosocomial infections.[2] Accordingly, nosocomial infections may be localized or systemic, they may be due to an infectious agent or its toxin, and they may or may not manifest during the patient's stay in the hospital. If it is a nosocomial infection, it should not be present or incubating at the time of admission to the hospital. Also, colonization or inflammation is not nosocomial infection.[3, 4]

An infection is not considered a nosocomial infection if it is associated with a complication or extension of an infection that is already present on admission (of course, if a change in pathogen can be proven, then it can be labelled as nosocomial). Again, an infection in a neonate that is proven to be acquired transplacentally and evident within 48 hours of birth is not a nosocomial infection.[5]

Thus, **Hospital Acquired Infection** can be defined as 'an infection that is acquired by or originates in a patient while in a hospital or other healthcare facility and refers to a new disorder associated with being in a hospital, unrelated to the patient's primary condition for which admitted. In other words, it was not present or incubating when admitted, nor was it the residue of an infection acquired during a previous admission. It also includes those infections acquired in the hospital but appearing after discharge. Infections occurring among the Health Care Workers of the facility also come within the purview of HAI.' [6]

There is yet another term to add to the gamut of existing ones—**'Hospital Associated Infection'**. This is a newer term and seems most appropriate because it is sometimes not possible to say whether an infection was acquired by the patient in hospital or before he/she came into the hospital.[7]

Since the hospital is not the only institution offering healthcare facilities, it is now felt that other centres, like private nursing homes and dispensaries which offer healthcare services should also be included and addressed in infection-control practices. Thus, the latest term to come into practice is **Healthcare facility Associated Infections (HAI)**. In the course of this book, we shall continue to use the older term Hospital Acquired Infections, or HAI, for convenience and familiarity.

HAI—DOWN THE AGES

The concept of isolating patients with obviously infectious diseases has been recognized since ancient times, and the spread of infection that might ensue from the introduction of such patients into hospitals has been known to our forefathers for centuries. Yet, authentic records or reasoning are lacking. HAI, as we know it, had its humble beginnings only as late as the eighteenth century. When Louis Pasteur, the Father of Microbiology, disproved the theory of spontaneous generation of living forms, he began a trend in the discovery of microorganisms causing diseases, which were discovered in quick succession during the next few decades. (Photo 1.2)

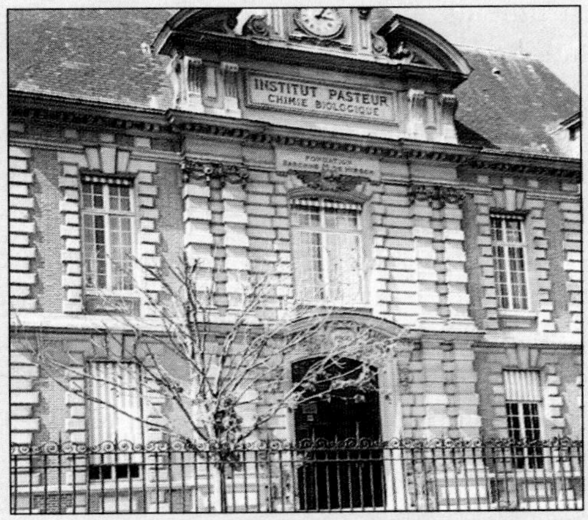

Photo 1.2: Pasteur Institute, Paris

Early nineteenth century saw the segregation of 'fever hospitals' from 'general hospitals', which followed as a result of the enormous amount of mortality and morbidity in hospitals due to sepsis, especially in orthopaedics, obstetric, gynaecological and paediatric cases. Ignaz Semmelweiss (1861) pioneered the concept of asepsis with his observations on puerperal sepsis: that it was associated with medical staff and students who attended to patients and also performed autopsies, without washing their hands. A dramatic reduction in infection rates was achieved by the introduction of the simple technique of hand-washing with chlorinated lime.

Around the same time, Florence Nightingale, after her experience of hospital sepsis at Scutari, made a much-quoted remark in her book, *Notes on Hospitals,* (1863) as follows: 'It may seem a strange principle to enunciate as the very first requirement in a hospital that it should do the sick no harm…the actual mortality in hospitals, especially in those of large crowded cities, is very much higher than any calculation founded on the mortality of the same class of diseases among patients treated out of hospital… .' She established important principles of nursing, hospital design and hygiene.

The contributions of Lord Lister, the Father of Antiseptic Surgery, compel a mention here. He observed a considerable improvement in the results of treatment of compound fractures and of surgical operations with the extensive use of carbolic acid to pack wounds, especially of compound fractures, to sterilize instruments and sutures, to decontaminate hands and as an air spray.

By the end of the nineteenth century, use of surgical gloves was introduced in the USA which marked the beginning of modern day operating techniques.

In the early part of the twentieth century, cubicle and barrier nursing were widely introduced and shown to be effective in preventing the spread of many childhood fevers. The first infection-control nurse was appointed in the UK in the early 1970s.[8]

The antibiotic era ushered in a confidence that infectious diseases would soon be conquered. But this myth was shattered almost as soon as it was conceived. Resistant strains took over the situation and the discovery of newer drugs could not keep pace with the rapidity with which resistant strains developed. The medical fraternity continues to battle with this situation even today. (Fig. 1.1)

The mid-twentieth century was a period when many of the established methods of infection control were laid down: clean air for operating theatres, aseptic procedures for wound dressing, isolation procedures, establishment of antibiotic policies, Hospital Infection Control Committees, etc.[9]

THE MODERN ERA OF INFECTION CONTROL

The period between 1950 and 1980 saw several organizations with significant activity in areas relevant to infection control grow and emerge into well-known providers of guidelines and standards. These organizations had the foresight to recognize that clinical practice standards and guidelines play a crucial role in

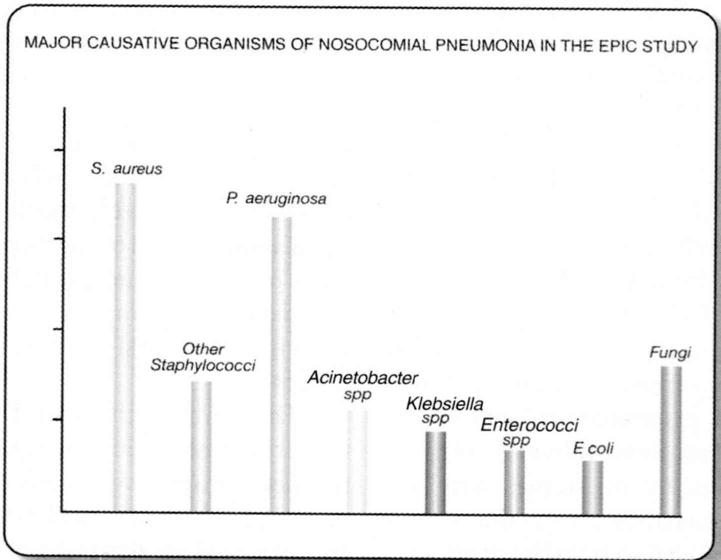

Figure 1.1: Source of data: Spencer RC. Predominant pathogens found in the European Prevalence of Infection in Intensive Care Study (EPIC). Eur J Clin Microbial Infect Dis 1996 15;281-285

medical practice. Foremost among these was the Center for Disease Control and prevention (CDC) located in Atlanta, Georgia (USA), which published a manual on isolation techniques for use in hospitals. Other such organizations include Hospital Infection Control Practices Advisory Committee (HICPAC), which published the monograph *Infection Control in the Hospital* in 1968; the American College of Surgeons; the American Academy of Paediatrics's Redbook Committee; the American Public Health Association (APHA), which published the manual *Control of Communicable Diseases;* the Association of Operating Room Nurses (AORN) and the Joint Commission for Accreditation of Healthcare Organizations (JCAHO).

The late 1980s saw the Society for Hospital Epidemiology (now called Society for Healthcare Epidemiology for America, SHEA) bring out a series of position papers on various aspects of infection control, including recommendations on the handling of medical waste. At the same time, the Association for Practitioners in Infection Control (APIC) developed and released four major guidelines related to disinfectants, hand-washing, endoscopy and long-term care. Soon there were more associations that became very active as developers of infection-control guidelines. These were: American Society for Microbiology (ASM), Surgical Infections Society (SIS), Occupational Health and Safety Agency (OSHA), the Environmental Protection Agency (EPA) and the Food and Drug Administration (FDA).

With the advent of HIV/AIDS in the 1980s, several organizations around the world have re-recognized the hazards and risks in the healthcare set-up. This has prompted a strong political support in several countries. Thus, in 1987, CDC published 'Recommendations for Prevention of HIV Transmission in Health care Settings' and in 1989, 'Universal Precautions for Prevention of Transmission of Human Immunodeficiency Virus, Hepatitis B virus and other blood-borne pathogens in healthcare settings'.

In spite of all these developments, today, we have reached a stage where we are still faced not only with newer problems but also older problems reappearing in newer forms. Drug-resistant organisms like MRSA, VRE, *Clostridium difficile*, *Staphylococcus epidermidis* and MDR tuberculosis are all posing major threats to infection-control measures and require revision of policies and protocols. Hence, the need to integrate infection control in the hospital with the wider community is being re-emphasized.[10, 11]

A quantum jump has been the introduction of quality management into the healthcare industry in the 1990s. Concepts of quality management were first introduced by Shewhart and later refined by Deming and Juran leading to a revolution in the Japanese car industry. These were later adopted by the American industry. The acceptance of these quality improvement principles by the healthcare organization was supported by organizations such as the Joint Commission on Accreditation of Hospitals, which made it mandatory for hospitals and doctors to participate in quality improvement in the USA. This has now been accepted all over Europe, although the accrediting bodies may be different. In this, a significant step has been the change from Quality Assurance (QA) to Continuous Quality Improvement (CQI), where the responsibility is placed on the system for identification and correction of problems. It is the 'system' and not the 'individual' (bad apple) that is responsible for a problem or problem processes. These principles are being increasingly applied to hospital infection control. (Fig. 1.2)

THE HOSPITAL ENVIRONMENT

The hospital provides a unique environment for the transmission of HAI. The reasons for this are multiple: **the biotic environment**—it facilitates transmission of microorganisms to and from patients, doctors, healthcare workers, visitors and the environment; **the inanimate objects—**the transmission may occur by fomites, water supply, droplets, air, food or direct contact; **iatrogenic causes**—the increase in invasive procedures, use of antibiotics, immuno-suppressants, transfusion services, transplant of organs and the like have contributed to an increase in HAI.

HAI can occur in primary, secondary or tertiary healthcare settings. One must also remember that HAI can occur in laboratories, animal facilities, dental clinics, blood banks and pain clinics.

OPPORTUNISTIC INFECTIONS AS HAI

Opportunistic infections are those that are caused by microorganisms which are not ordinarily pathogenic, but utilize the 'opportunity' to cause an infection when conditions are favourable in the host. This happens when the host immune status is lowered due to some cause. E.g. fungal infections occur more commonly in diabetics and terminally-ill patients. Opportunistic infections can occur as well in the hospital set-up as in the community. Those occurring in the hospitals can be labelled as HAI.

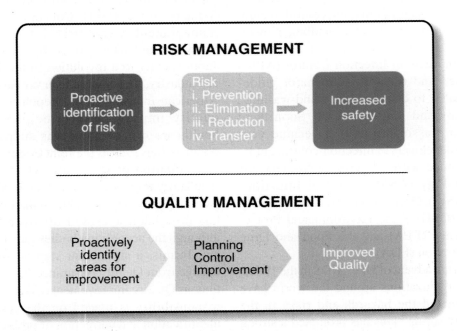

Figure 1.2: Introduction of quality and risk management concepts from industry to the field of medicine

COMMUNITY ACQUIRED INFECTIONS AS HAI

These are caused by microorganisms which are prevalent in the community outside the healthcare set-up. Yet, when a patient with a community acquired infection is admitted to the hospital, he is capable of transmitting the infection to other patients and HCWs, thus making the community acquired infection a hospital acquired one. E.g. HIV/AIDS, SARS.

GLOBAL DIMENSIONS OF HAI

Newer infections in the jet age have shown that infections may not be limited to a single country or continent. They have the potential to spread quickly and require equally quick measures which can limit their dissemination or spread. Control measures for these infections should include awareness, utilization of facilities at a global level, network for notification and rapid mobilization of resources.[12, 13, 14]

DRUG RESISTANCE

Importantly, HAI are often caused by drug-resistant organisms, which pose a great threat to efforts at management. If these resistant microorganisms gain entry into the community, they could cause havoc and defeat the best of infection-control activities.

WHY CONTROL HOSPITAL ACQUIRED INFECTIONS?

Healthcare workers are constantly under pressure to devise ways and means of bringing down the incidence of HAI. The reasons for this are threefold.

Firstly, HAI have far-reaching ill-effects on the health of the community at large. Any increase in the incidence of HAI would mean the spill-over of these infections into the community, with its inherent grave repercussions. So, in order to decrease the spread of infections in the community, it is important to curtail the occurrence of infections in the hospital set-up. Thus, control of infection in the hospital set-up is of paramount importance not only for patients and healthcare workers within the hospital, but for the community at large.[15, 16, 17]

Secondly, it is a known fact that with the increase in incidence of HAI, the patients' hospital stay also increases, and with it, the cost of patient care. This can add up to considerable amounts and assume burdensome proportions. Hospital stay, and the costs therein, can be reduced to a significant extent with careful planning and efficient infection-control measures. Cost-benefit and cost-effective studies have shown that hospitals with effective infection-control programmes, including surveillance methods, can reduce infections by an average of 40 per cent.[18] Those programmes that excluded surveillance reduced infection rates by 6 per cent only. Those without effective programmes had an increase of nosocomial infections by 18 per cent. Up to 30 per cent of HAI can be prevented. The socio-economic burden imposed by HAI has been calculated in managed healthcare systems and is considerable (£3.6 billion). The estimated annual economic cost is more than US$4.5 billion. Nosocomial infections account for about 50 per cent of all major complications of hospitalization, the remaining being medication errors, patient falls, and other non-infectious adverse events. Less tangible costs include increased length of stay and drug costs, risk of litigation by patients and the overall running of the hospitals. Studies advocate that clinicians should partner with economists and policy analysts to expand and improve the economic evidence available to reduce hospital complications such as nosocomial infections and other adverse patient/staff outcomes and thereby reduce the costs.[19]

Thirdly, good infection-control measures, routine surveillance of infected patients and feedback of results have been shown to reduce infection rates. The Department of Health, UK, estimates that in UK an estimated 5,000 deaths per year might be directly attributable to HAI, and another 15,000 deaths having HAI as a substantial contributing factor. Cruse and Foord recorded a fall in surgical site infections by as much as 50 per cent as a result of surveillance and feedback to healthcare providers.[20, 21]

With up to ten per cent of hospital patients at any time suffering from an infection acquired following their admission to hospital, the suffering of patients and their families, even in less serious infections, is considerable.

REFERENCES

1) Black JG. Microbiology – Principles and Explorations. 4th edn. John Wiley & Sons, Inc. NY. 1999; 402-433.

2) Gaynes RP and Horan TC. Surveillance of nosocomial infections. Appendix A: CDC definitions of nosocomial infections. In: Mayhall GC (ed). Hospital Epidemiology and Infection Control. Baltimore: Williams & Wilkins, 1996; 1-14.

3) Garner J S, Jarvis W R, Emori T G et al. CDC definitions for nosocomial infections. Am J Infect Control, 1988; 16: 128-140.

4) Abrutyn E, Goldmann DA and Scheckler WE. Definitions of nosocomial infections. In: Saunders Infection Control Reference Service (ed). W B Saunders Company, 1998; 17-21.

5) Beck-Sague C, Villarino E and Giuiano D. Infectious diseases and death among nursing home residents: Results of surveillance in 13 nursing homes. Infect control and hosp epidemiol, 1994; 15: 494-496.

6) Girard R, Perraud M, Pruss A et al. In: Ducel G, Fabry J, Nicolle L, eds. Prevention of hospital -acquired infections – A practical guide. 2nd edn. WHO 2002; 47-54.

7) Ayliffe GAJ, Fraise AP, Geddes AM et al. Control of Hospital Infection – A Practical Handbook. 4th edn. Arnold Publications. 2000; 1-13.

8) Shaheen Mehtar. In: A guide to Infection Control in the Hospital. An official publication of the International Society for Infectious Diseases. BC Decker Inc., 1998; 1-4.

9) Speller DCE and Humphrey H. Hospital Acquired Infection. In: Collier L, Balows A and Sussman M, eds. Topley & Wilson's Microbiology and microbial infections, 9th edn. Vol 3, Arnold Publishers, 1998; 187-230.

10) Hierholzer WJ. Infection control guidelines. In: Abrutyn E, Goldmann DA and Scheckler WE (eds.) Saunders Infection Control Reference Service. WB Saunders Company, 1998; 3-5.

11) Wenzel RP. Nosocomial infections, diagnosis, and study on the efficacy of nosocomial infection control: economic implications for hospitals under the prospective payment system. Am J Med 1885; 78 (6) (suppl. 2): 3-7

12) Wenzel RP. Towards a global perspective of nosocomial infections. Eur J Clin Microbiol 1987; 6: 341-343.

13) Masterson RG. Worthwhile infection control information? J. Hosp. Infect. 1999; 42(4): 269-274

14) Emmerson AM, Spencer RC, Cookson BD et al. Diploma in infection control (Dip HIC). J of Hosp. Infect.1997; 37 (3): 175-180.

15) GAJ Ayliffe, AP Fraise, AM Geddes et al. Control of Hospital Infection – A Practical Handbook. 4th edn., Arnold Publications. 2000; 356-385.

16) Marnoch G. Introduction: the management agenda for doctors. In: Ham C, Heginbotham C, Series Eds. Doctors and Management in the National Health Service. Health Services Management, Open Unversity Press, Buckingham, 1996; 1-11.

17) Robbins SP and Coulter M. Management. 7th edn, Pearson Education Asia, 2002; 1-25.

18) Emori TG, Banerjee SN, Culver DH et al. Nosocomial infections in elderly patients in the United States. Am J Med, 1991; 91(3)(Suppl 2): 289S-293S

19) Stone PW, Larson E and Kawar LN. A systematic audit of economic evidence linking nosocomial infections and infection control interventions: 1990-2000. Am J Infect Control. 2002; 30(3): 145-52.

20) Cruse PJE and Foord R. A five year prospective study of 23,649 surgical wounds. Arch Surg. 1973;107:206-210.

21) Cruse PJE and Foord R. The epidemiology of wound infections – a 10 year prospective study of 62,939 wounds. Surg Clin North Am.1980;60:27-39.

Chapter 2

Clinician as a Manager

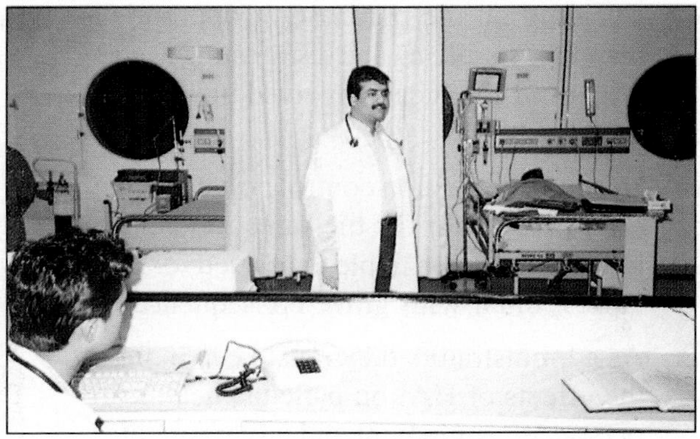

Doctors … (outside the administrative hierarchy) ... need to be convinced of the connections between clinical standards and organizational practice.

—Marnoch

Highlights

The Clinician as a Manager

Management, Medical Science and HAI—the Interface

Understanding Management

Management, Administration and Organization

The Process (steps) of Management

Control versus Improvement

Pyramidal Structure of Clinicians as Managers

A Clinician Manager—An Expanded Responsibility

INTRODUCTION

Clinicians are frequently involved in making important decisions such as:

a. Planning of a hospital, designing of OTs, ICUs, laboratories, etc.
b. Formulating antibiotic policies for the institution.
c. Deciding on the purchase of appropriate brands of sterilizing and disinfecting agents, drugs and chemicals involved in infection prevention.
d. Designing infection control policies. They are accountable for the infection-control policies and even liable to be sued for their lapses, often with grave consequences.
e. As administrators they must keep in mind the effects of HAI on patients, healthcare personnel, equipment and environment.
f. Implementation of various standardized procedures, as for sterilization and disinfection. They are also responsible for quality assurance and have to indulge in an ongoing process of monitoring agents and their use to achieve optimal benefits.[1] (Photo 2.1)

Therefore, anyone who is directly or indirectly affected by HAI has to be aware of the tremendous changes that have occurred in the managerial aspects of infection control. The success of every programme depends on the understanding and motivation levels because the maximum chance of transmission of HAI occurs at the patient–clinician interface (as when invasive procedures are carried out). Another problem is that, since healthcare workers are themselves victims of HAI, they need to ensure proper compliance and implementation of HAI control policies. Many a time, it is seen that a common problem such as HAI is not in their direct focus of interest. Clinicians in managerial positions are responsible for the control of nosocomial infections in their respective domains. But unless they understand how the system works and why things are done in a particular manner, it would be difficult to get them to comply with the instructions. They may not see their participation in clinical processes and evaluation, as part of the management process at all. Clinical practice not only needs an informed doctor but also an organized and effective system. A system is nothing but a collection of processes which is designed to carry out specific functions (like combating HAI in this case). Thus, combating HAI needs not only a deep knowledge and competence in clinical management but also an understanding of the managerial aspects taking into account work-related factors, team functioning and task details (protocols), all of which influence clinical practice.[2] The emphasis in this book is on a knowledge that is

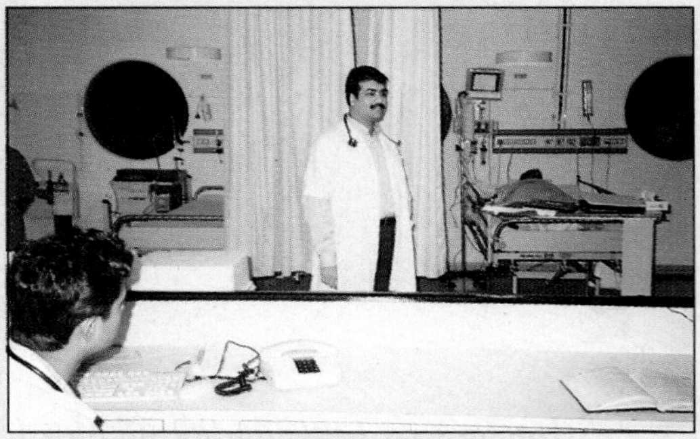

Photo 2.1: Doctors are involved in organizing, forecasting, commanding, coordinating and controlling in their specified areas, making them clinician-managers

complementary to clinical judgement and management, without which, clinical practice is incomplete and cannot exist. A few examples will highlight the essence of this message:

Example 1

Let us consider a gastroenterologist doing an endoscopy on his patient. He should be aware of the process in its entirety, and pay heed to aspects such as, whether the endoscope has been appropriately sterilized, the methods and duration of sterilization of endoscopes, whether his nurse is aware of 'Standard Precautions' etc. If he is unaware of all these aspects, and concentrates only on the procedure at hand, he may contribute to the occurrence of HAI.

Example 2

An intensivist looks after an intensive care/critical care unit. He is largely responsible for the prevention and treatment of nosocomial infections in very sick patients who are often already in an immunocompromised state and thus, most likely to acquire HAI. He thus needs to have a thorough knowledge of not only the treatment of infective disorders, but also about the principles of their transmission, their preventive measures and the managerial aspects of their control.

Example 3

A surgeon who desires an infection-free and uneventful post-operative status for his patient needs to perfect not only his surgical skills, but more importantly, the managerial aspects of HAI, like monitoring the processes which ensure that a patient is prevented from acquiring HAI, assuring quality of services from his team and decreasing the risks to his patients.

Example 4

A microbiologist is essentially an integral part of the infection-control committee, and is often called upon to lay down infection-control policies. These policies are often abstract and impossible to implement because there is very little written material dealing with the managerial aspects of HAI control. Hence, the microbiologist's approach is usually restricted to his/her knowledge of infective diseases, their causative organisms and modes of transmission. This alone is not sufficient in managing hospital infection-control programmes. They need to interface their activities with the clinician's needs and thus ought to have an overall picture of various managerial strategies and also be conversant with practical hospital epidemiology in places where an epidemiologist is unavailable.

Example 5

If a manager is called upon to organize the services in a hospital/nursing home, he should be informed about HAI and the modes of its occurrence. The infection-control committee (ICC), infection-control team (ICT) and the epidemiologist need to coordinate with the manager.

THE CLINICIAN AS A MANAGER

A manager is someone who works with and through other people by coordinating their work and activities in order to accomplish organizational goals.[3] In a very broad sense, 'anyone who can bring about a change is a manager'. Doctors are involved as managers in all the key roles such as forecasting, organizing, commanding, coordinating and controlling in their specified areas, and also hospital associated infections (HAI).[4, 5, 6] Every clinican is a manager, involved in healthcare delivery and thus needs to know and understand the managerial terms which are defined in the relevant sections of this book.

MANAGEMENT, MEDICAL SCIENCE AND HAI—THE INTERFACE

The failure of infection control in a healthcare setting is now largely being recognized as improper structuring, faulty processes and non-assessment of the outcome of processes.[7] Currently, there is an emphasis by the WHO and many governments, on improving the healthcare delivery by the application of modern management techniques.[3, 8] Management technologies of control can be understood as being intended to improve the behaviour of doctors with respect to the efficiency, economy and effectiveness of service delivery.[9] Management and its principles can remove several shortcomings in the existing methods of patient care. Management techniques are well established in business, industry, defence and other fields, where the managerial principles and methods of quality improvement were originally developed and successfully applied. They have now led to setting of standards or specifications for clinical care too.[3, 10] They provide an excellent basis for specifying and communicating optimal care processes and for evaluating actual clinical care. These concepts are further being extended to include combating HAI. Such a diverse use of management is referred to as the 'universality of management'.[8, 11]

UNDERSTANDING MANAGEMENT

Management is the process of coordinating work activities so that they are completed efficiently and effectively, with and through people.[3, 9] There are three contexts in which the term 'management' is used: 1) as a function, 2) as a set of activities, 3) as a team of people. All of the above are for the overall steering or directing of an organization to optimal performance.[7] But the term 'management' is also used in the context of therapy or treatment of a patient, which is not what is referred to in this chapter.

MANAGEMENT, ADMINISTRATION AND ORGANIZATION

The term 'management' is at times confused with 'administration' and even with 'organization. A simplified view is that 'administration', in a broad sense, means 'getting things done' or carrying out policies, e.g. government policies, and 'organization' refers to an orderly structure that has been systematized, while 'management' is 'the purposeful and effective use of resources—manpower, materials and money (finances)—for fulfilling a predetermined objective'.[12, 13, 14]

THE PROCESS (STEPS) OF MANAGEMENT

The process of management is a set of ongoing decisions and work activities that managers engage in, and the classical steps are: Plan, Organize, Lead and Control. The quality triology (planning, control, improvement) now includes 'improvement' as an additional step over the previous managerial processes.[15]

Managerial principles and perspectives are very relevant in the approach to the complex problem of HAI. To reduce HAI, one needs to plan by establishing goals, identifying problem areas, determining patient (customer) needs and developing services (product features) to meet those needs.

CONTROL VERSUS IMPROVEMENT

Control is a process which involves monitoring, comparing actual performance to the standard and taking action if necessary. It consists of observing actual performance, comparing this performance with some standard, and then taking action if the observed performance is significantly different from the standard.[5] This control process has a universal sequence of steps as follows:

1. Choosing what we want to regulate (e.g. catheter-related infections in the ICU)
2. Choosing a unit of measurement (e.g. percentage of infection)
3. Setting a goal for the control subject (e.g. infection percentage must be less than 2 per cent of catheters inserted)
4. Measuring the actual performance (e.g. the actual incidence)
5. Interpreting the difference between actual performance and the goal
6. Taking action on the difference observed

Now, the emphasis has shifted from 'quality control' to 'quality improvement' and hence the term 'infection control' sounds inadequate. The term 'control' in the quality triology is largely directed at meeting goals and preventing adverse change (Fig. 2.1). In other words, it aims at holding status quo. This is in contrast to the term 'improvement', which focuses on creating a change for the better, thereby changing the status quo.[16, 17] Yet the term 'control' enjoys a long-established popularity that is difficult to replace, for example, engineering controls, work practice controls, antibiotic controls, etc. But with the recent advent of total quality management, the end point to be achieved is 'quality'. This involves changes in the traditional managerial principles.[3]

The quality strategy was first introduced in the industry, where improvements in quality

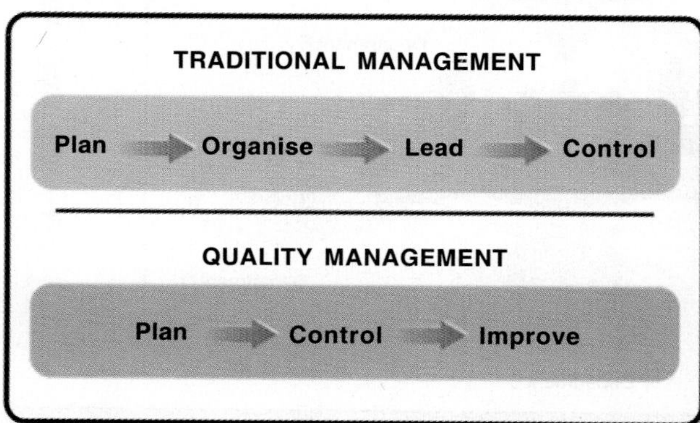

Figure 2.1: Traditional management versus quality management

were initially assessed by checking the 'product'. For example, let us consider a car in the car industry—the defective cars were first identified and then corrected. In course of time, quality was ensured by assessing the 'processes' involved in the production of the 'product', and thereby correcting the deficiencies in the 'processes', rather than the 'product' itself. The quality triology has now been applied extensively in the field of medicine and healthcare delivery. Though the outcomes and processes involved in the healthcare delivery are quite different from that seen in industry, there are several aspects of similarity, and hence they are applicable.[18]

Management Means

- Having clear-cut goals, strategies and objectives
- Adopting proper planning at various levels
- Collecting and organizing information to streamline the processes with an intent to evaluate, measure and control
- Purposeful handling of manpower, material and finances for fulfilling a predetermined objective

PYRAMIDAL STRUCTURE OF CLINICIANS AS MANAGERS

(FIGURE 2.2)

First-Line Managers

These managers are often called (in managerial parlance) supervisors, line managers, office managers, foremen, resident doctors and nurses. They are at the lowest rung of the

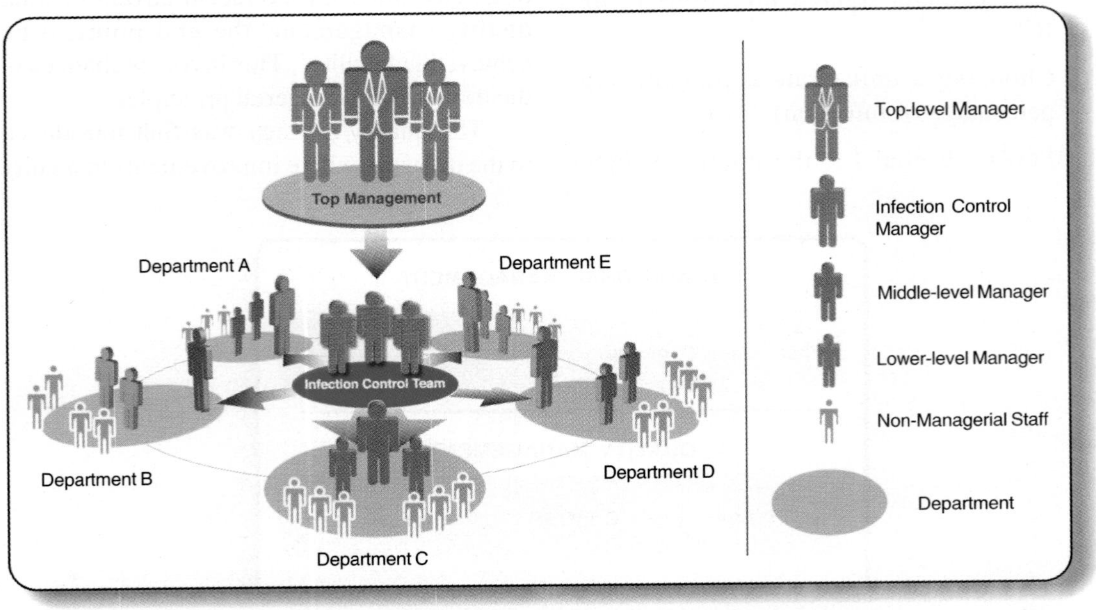

Figure 2.2: Integration of HAI activities (vertical and horizontal) in a hospital

ladder of managers.They form an important part of patient management and implementation of the policies of infection control. It is important for them to understand the 'why' and 'how' of infection-control policies for such policies to succeed. In the healthcare settings they are the key 'managers' wielding the final execution of policies. This group is in contact with the non-managerial staff.

Middle Managers

Includes all the levels of managers between the first-line managers and the top level of the organization. A middle manager is often called department head, project leader, plant manager or division manager. The middle level doctors and the heads of departments of various clinical areas, as also the nursing heads, fall into this category. They have the responsibility of managing their own domains and clinical areas and ensuring the implementation of infection-control policies and programmes.

Top Managers

They are present at the top or near the top of the organization. They are responsible for making organization-wide decisions and plans that affect the entire set-up. In the healthcare delivery set-up, the following could be categorized as the top management: people in charge of state health, the hospital administrators, heads of health institutions (president, vice-president, managing director, medical superintendent, director, etc.), hospital managers, CEOs of hospitals and nursing homes, nursing superintendents and the like.

Who are the managers in the following areas who could influence HAI-related policies?

1. Individual clinical areas:
   - intensive care
   - operating rooms
   - haemodialysis units
   - labour rooms
   - wards
   - solid organ transplant facility
2. Investigatory areas like spirometry, endoscopy, neurosciences, cath lab
3. Physiotherapy, hydrotherapy and pain clinics
4. Blood banks
5. Pharmacy
6. Wards
7. Laundry
8. Housekeeping
9. Food and catering
10. Autopsy/pathology units
11. Waste management set-up
12. Central Sterile Supply Department (CSSD)
13. Laboratories

A CLINICIAN MANAGER—AN EXPANDED RESPONSIBILITY

Traditionally, a clinician looks at the 'clinical process of care'. To him/her an improved process means better clinical management strategies. However, the focus should not be only on management of the patient. An expanded definition of improved processes should mean improved care, improved service, appropriateness, timeliness and improvement in various other aspects in the system.

A better outcome must not refer only to improved clinical outcomes. This must be expanded to mean patient satisfaction, health access, community needs, improved resources, management, networking and integration.

This book therefore helps a clinician to:

- Understand HAI-related terminology
- Understand strategies at various levels. Incorporate strategies into their own clinical areas
- Understand various spheres where they could exert their influence
- Plan HAI control policies of hospitals, nursing homes, operating suites, critical care units
- Make decisions in implementation of infection-control policies
- Purchase standard equipment, disinfectants and sterilants related to HAI controls
- Monitor HAI control processes
- Audit the processes and outcome
- Develop surveillance methodologies
- Develop standard operating procedures
- Understand relevance of accreditation and role of accreditation agencies
- Participate in national and international strategies
- Implement educational strategies
- Understand the consequences of improper implementation
- Develop a sense of accountability

REFERENCES

1) Civetta JM, Hudson-Civetta and Ball S. Decreasing catheter-related infection and hospital costs by continuous quality improvement. Crit Care Med. 1996; 24(11): 1660-1665.

2) Kirton OC, DeHaven B, Hudson-Cavetta J et al. Re-engineering ventilatory support to decrease days and improve resource uitlization. Ann Surg. 1996: 224(3): 396-404.

3) Marnoch G. Introduction: the management agenda for doctors. In: Ham C, Heginbotham C, Series Eds. Doctors and Management in the National Health Service. Health Services Management, Open Unversity Press, Buckingham, 1996; 1-11.

4) Kelleghan SI, Salemi C, Padilla S et al. An effective continuous quality improvement approach to prevention of ventilator-associated pneumonia. Am J Infect Control. 1993; 21(6): 322-330.

5) Joiner GA, Salisbury D and Bollin GE. Utilizing quality assurance as a tool for reducing risk of nosocomial ventilator-associated pneumonia. Am J Med Qual. 1996; 11(2): 100-103.

6) McGowan H, Mattson S, Silva K et al. Interdepartmental intervention and surveillance for ventilator-associated pneumonia in critical care patients; a continuous quality improvement activity. Am J Infect Control. 1994; 22(2): 111.

7) Barrett S. Infection control around the world (Editorial). J Hosp Infect, 2001; 47(1): 2.

8) Robbins SP and Contter M. Introduction to Management and organizations in management Ed. 1st Indian Reprint, Pearson Education Singapore. 2002; 2-25

9) Batra P and Mahendru D. Management ideas in action. Think Inc., 2001; 114.

10) Kelsey MC, National guidelines on infection control – the bottom rung of the ladder. J Hosp Infect. 2001; 47 (1): 1.

11) Gottlieb LK, Margolis CZ, Schoenbaum SC. Clinical practice guidelines at an HMO: development and implementation in a quality improvement model. Qual Rev Bull. 1990; 16: 80-86.

12) Lohr KN. Health, Healthcare and Quality of Care. In: Medicare a strategy for Quality Assurance Vol .II . Washington DC: National Academy Press. 1990; 19-44.

13) Donabedian A. Defining and measuring the quality of Healthcare. In: Wenzel RP, ed. Assessing Quality Healthcare – Perspectives for Clinicians. Baltimore: Williams & Wilkins, 1992; 41-64.

14) Jo Harris – Wehling. Defining Quality of Care. In: Lohr KN ed Medicare A Strategy for Quality Assurance (vol. II) Washington DC: National Academy Press,1990; 124- 139.

15) Berwick DM. Continuous improvement as an ideal in healthcare. N Engl J Med. 1989; 320(1): 53-56.

16) Wong A and Wenzel RP. Using Quality Improvement techniques for the prevention of Nosocomial Pneumonia.In: Jarvis WR ed. Nosocomial Pneumonia. New York: Marcel Dekker Inc. 2000; 187-201.

17) O' Leary DS. Accreditation in the quality improvement mold – a vision for tomorrow. Qual Rev Bull 1991; 27: 72-77.

18) Juran JM and Gryna FM. Manufacture. In: Quality Planning and Analysis. 3rd edn, New Delhi: Tata McGraw-Hill Publishing Company Limited. 1995; 343-376.

Chapter 3

Road Maps and Directions

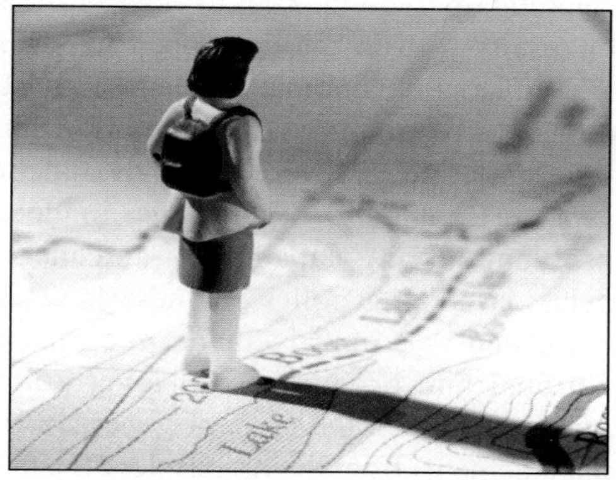

The great thing is not so much where we stand as in what direction we are moving.

—Oliver Wendall Holmes

Highlights

Leadership Issues

Establishing Direction for the HAI Control Programme

Strategies (The Road Maps)

Some Important Questions

INTRODUCTION

All developed countries practise infection control in some form, and though the aim of each country's infection-control programme is ultimately the same, viz., to reduce the incidence of Hospital Acquired Infections, there is a gross disparity in the actual results achieved. Developing countries have a lot of catching up to do in order to achieve the kind of results seen in the developed nations.[1] In addition to the economic problems, many governmental programmes (including HAI control programme) face several other dysfunctional aspects, like faulty operations, inadequate problem-solving capabilities and incorrect decision-making policies. These have to be identified and improvements facilitated by national and organizational level policies. Interventions (in the form of governance and management) from the highest levels can give a direction and motivate and inspire people to bring about a change in work culture, thus reducing the incidence of HAI, in all nations and organizations, be they rich or poor. So also, appropriate hospital practices can help in strengthening the governmental programmes in combating HAI.[2-6]

LEADERSHIP ISSUES

There are six key tasks that must be performed to bring about organizational change:

1. Establishing direction
2. Aligning people and processes
3. Motivating and inspiring people
4. Planning
5. Organizing
6. Controlling

The first three (establishing direction, aligning people and processes, motivating and inspiring people) are leadership tasks which are a part of governance and top management, intended to promote movement (progress) and take the organization forward (Table 3.1). The people involved with governance are often not involved in the day-to-day functioning of the organization but are concerned with providing effective leadership. The next three tasks (planning,

Table 3.1: Good leadership is a part of both governance and management.

Leadership	
Governance	**Management**
Parliament, ministry, board, trust Cabinet, Governing bodies	Management, bureaucracy CEO, heads of departments, clinician-managers, Nurse-managers, doctors

organizing and controlling) fall under the domain of management. (See chapter on clinician and manager.)[7-10]

1. Establishing Direction for the HAI Control Programme—Setting Goals and Objectives

Recognizing that HAI is a significant problem is a critical determinant to the success of a healthcare organization. Prioritizing HAI and setting goals helps acknowledge its presence and implications.

Setting goals is an important part of the process of planning because they provide the direction for all management decisions and form the criterion against which the actual work is measured. Setting up of goals and objectives, and achieving them at the end of a specified time frame, is the basis of this method. Infection-control goals and objectives are necessary for achieving the quality initiatives and improvements.[11-13] These give the programme the necessary impetus to surge ahead. For this, it is essential that planners at the highest levels are involved (national/ organizational/departmental) in prioritizing and enforcing issues.
In the year 2000 the HAI control programme received high priority in the national health programme (US) when it declared HAI control as one of the objectives to be achieved that year.[14] Goldman et al (1997) have pointed out that control of nosocomial antimicrobial-resistant bacteria should be a strategic priority for hospitals worldwide in combating HAI. They further advise that strategic goals should be formulated on the basis of multidisciplinary inputs from hospital personnel.[15] Processes and outcomes relevant to these strategic goals should be measured, and the relevant data used to design, implement and evaluate systemic measures to increase the appropriate use of infection-control practices.[16] At an organizational level, one of the tools of quality management, is the 'balanced score card'—a set of measurements and targets that are used to prioritize and quantify goals and objectives, and these have been used effectively by some to combat HAI.[11]

Definitions that are relevant

Goals: Goals are the desired outcomes for individuals, groups or entire organizations that may not necessarily be achieved.

Objective: A planned end point of all activities. It is either achieved or not achieved. Objectives must be SMART (Specific, Measurable, Agreed/Actionable, Realistic and Time bound)

Mission statement: Mission statement is the raison d'être (reason to be) of an organization, together with an explicit statement of the values or philosophy guiding its work. It is a compelling vision, the driving force of the organization. It describes an organization's identity, states the focus of the organization and shows benefit to customers, employees and owners alike. Mission statements need not highlight infection-control policies unless the organization is dedicated to infection control, e.g. UNAIDS, NACO. These mission statements and goals could be for the entire country's health programme, or it could be for an individual organization.

Governance: Act or manner of governing (Oxford dictionary)

Govern:

- Rule or control—a nation, subject, etc. with authority; conduct of affairs
- Influence or determine
- Be a standard or principle for; constitute a law for
- Check or control

Strategic goals

Strategic goals apply to all clinical and nonclinical areas in the organization including control of HAI. Some of the common strategic goals are:

1. Quality improvement
2. Risk management
3. Clinical performance

Goals specific to HAI control policies are given below:

1. To prevent patients and visitors from acquiring nosocomial infections in healthcare institutions
2. To protect healthcare workers from acquiring infections (inadvertently or otherwise) while carrying out their duties
3. To prevent the emergence and spread of drug-resistant organisms within hospitals
4. To ensure a safe environment outside the hospital by containing infection-generating processes
5. To lay down local operational protocols, develop systems and formulate policies as per accepted bodies
6. To ensure that quality of the systems are laid down by quality management techniques and appropriate surveillance programmes
7. To formulate specific strategies for specific infections, e.g. ventilator-associated pneumonia, catheter-related infections, UTI, etc.[17, 18, 19]
8. To monitor HAI
9. To train staff in prevention and control of HAI
10. To investigate outbreaks
11. To control outbreaks
12. To monitor staff health
13. To prevent staff-to-patient and patient-to-patient spread
14. To advise infection-control measures and isolation procedures

2. Aligning People and Processes to Combat HAI—Strategies and Strategic Planning

(Figure 3.1)

Governing bodies in any organization serve as a meeting ground for both practitioners and policy makers. All decisions taken jointly by them have a direct bearing on the patient–clinician interface. The main function of governance is to oversee and monitor key organizational processes and outcomes, and check whether the strategies proposed by the management are in alignment with the organizational mission, vision, goals and objectives. In the HAI control programme, there has to be an integration, both vertical (at primary, secondary and tertiary levels) and horizontal (see chapter on organization), for a successful execution of duties.[7, 10, 13] Aligning people is also concerned with selection of managers (who in turn determine structure and organization) and has a supportive role in nurturing individual efforts and providing the necessary

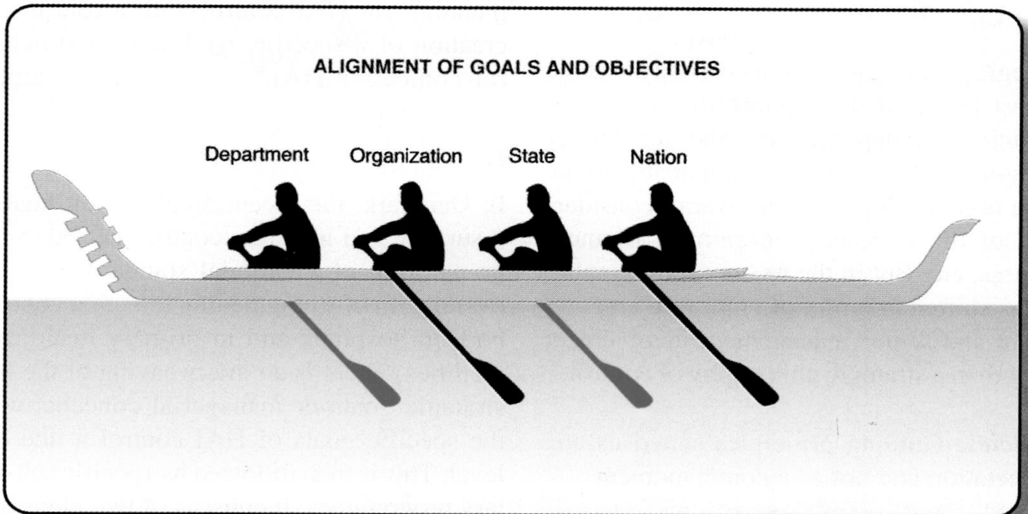

Figure 3.1: Direction, alignment and motivation (leadership) are required to achieve HAI-related goals and objectives

platform to extend those efforts throughout the organization.

It is important to develop systems that monitor (by using appropriate indicators—the dashboard concept) and ensure quality of clinical practice. This means development and use of the various performance management tools (see chapter on performance management and performance management map) which use laws, regulations, standards and guidelines, among other aspects, to guide, control and improve clinical activities that incorporate infection-control principles.

STRATEGIES (THE ROAD MAPS)

Strategies are the processes involved in translating goals to programmes. They are the all-encompassing road maps or directions given to the entire organization, without which there would be no outcome. To understand the connection between goals and the individual programmes, an analogy of a 'strategy stairway' can be used. Strategy formulation can be thought of as a stairway linking the core mission to its programmes and activities. The phrase 'strategy as a stairway' was coined by Robert Burakoff, an independent nonprofit strategy consultant.[20, 21] A number of organizations, both medical and non-medical, are using strategies to plan, be financially effective, efficient and viable. Using the same analogy, a programme such as the HAI control programme must flow from broad goals and an appropriate 'strategy platform', which includes : funding (financial), planning , organizational development and governance (managerial, administration), client and market development (relationships), programmes and service development (clinical and quality issues).

Strategic Planning

Strategic planning is planning carried out at the highest levels of the organization (national, institutional or departmental) and is generally a long-term plan (3–5 years) applicable to the entire organization, with an overall consideration of the various programmes, finance, business, etc. But in the recent times, emphasis has shifted to a mix of employee empowerment and senior management involvement rather than a strategic philosophy of control.[22]

> ***Policies:*** Guiding principles stated as an expectation and not as a commandment
>
> ***Strategy:*** Process of connecting lofty mission statements and goals to programmes
>
> ***Process:*** A series of steps and tasks that are required to deliver a given product or service[22-24]
>
> ***Planning:*** The process of defining goals, establishing strategies for achieving those goals, and developing methods to integrate and coordinate activities
>
> ***Plans:*** Documents outlining how goals are going to be achieved, including resource allocation, schedules and other necessary actions to accomplish the goals
>
> ***Programme:*** A sequence of activities designated to implement policies and accomplish objectives. A programme gives a step-by-step approach to guide the action necessary to reach a predetermined goal. Programmes must be closely integrated with objectives.

Example of Strategic Planning for HAI Control

There are a number of examples of strategic planning for HAI control with a role in the creation of a specific, well-defined structure for combating HAI.[9, 23] Two such examples are given below:

I.

In Denmark, the recent emphasis on quality assurance and infection control has led to the preparation of a national standard with the overall aim of strengthening infection control, both in hospitals and in primary healthcare facilities. There is an interweaving of the key strategic goals or managerial concepts with the specific goals of HAI control at the top level. This is then followed by specific subsidiary programmes. It consists of two elements: a main standard, which describes the requirements for the management system, and subsidiary standards, which describe the requirements for areas of infection control.[9, 10, 24]

The main standard consists of four processes and related elements: defining management responsibility, guidance on resources, guidance on infection-control measures and measurement, analysis and improvement. Together these four elements constitute an audit cycle (see chapter on Audit).

The subsidiary standards consist of all twelve major areas of infection control in clinical practice: hand hygiene, intravenous catheters, surveillance and investigation of outbreaks, surgical site infections, urinary continence aids, urinary catheters, textiles, purchase and maintenance of equipment, cleaning and quality control, food stuff and dental clinics.

The contents of the 12 subsidiary standards are based on the existing standards, while the main standard is largely innovative. The main purpose of the latter is to secure compliance with guidelines, which is usually the weak point of most organizations.

II.

In the United Kingdom, the National Health Scheme (NHS) provides guidelines and local operational protocols. These guidelines can be used as a benchmark for determining appropriate infection-prevention decisions as a part of the reflective practice to assess clinical effectiveness. They also provide a basis for clinical audit, evaluation and education, and facilitate ongoing quality improvements. These can be appropriately adapted and used by all hospital practitioners. This will, in addition, set the baseline for the development of more detailed protocols and ensure that all important standard principles for infection prevention are incorporated. Consequently, they are aimed at hospital managers, Hospital Infection Control (HIC) teams and individual healthcare practitioners. At an individual level, they are intended to influence the quality and clinical effectiveness of infection prevention decision-making.[25]

Examples of strategies (road maps) given in this book are the following:

1. Planning, organization, structure (interfacing and integrating)
2. Quality management
3. Risk management
4. Clinical performance management
5. Antibiotic policies
6. Epidemiologic strategies and strategies for specific programmes
7. Work practice controls
8. SOPs and process monitoring, sterilization and disinfection
9. Environmental management and engineering controls
10. Practice guidelines for individual diseases

Strategies are meant to

- Give direction and road maps
- Help decision making
- Help plan, evaluate and improve the system
- Give the clinician and managers at various levels, a framework in which they could fine-tune their infection-control activities within their organizations

3. Motivating and Inspiring People—Leadership

Infection control is a part of a safety culture which is basically built into the attitudes of people who work in an organization. When there is a direct involvement of the governing bodies and top managers, key organizational characteristics and cultures originate and get promoted (attitudes towards customer service, employees, social obligations, quality, safety and various other issues). The biggest challenge to leadership at various levels is to build a culture of safety—creating a vision, communicating ideas, convincing personnel of the urgency and necessity of the control programme, moving from a hierarchy to a networked community.[7-10] Making clinical practitioners understand and meet standards, such as those issued by the national professional regulatory bodies, is an integral part of this culture. In this case, the practitioners need to meet the infection-control standards.The infection-control programme is bound to fail if there is a lack of leadership in building a culture of combating HAI.

According to Killmann, Sexton and Serpa, 'culture is the invisible force behind the tangibles and observables in any organization, a social energy that moves people to act.

Culture is to an organization what personality is to the individual—a hidden, yet unifying theme that provides meaning, direction and mobilization. Organization charts and employee manuals are simply not enough to get members to work together.'[7]

SOME IMPORTANT QUESTIONS

Does your hospital/ nursing home have an HAI control programme?

Is combating HAI a part of your organizational goals and objectives?

Is HAI control included in your hospital's management agenda?

Are strategic goals such as 'quality management' a part of your hospital's planning process?

Are such strategic goals merged with individual and departmental programmes?

If the answer to any of the above questions is 'yes', then this book will help you realize your goals/ objectives.

If your answer to any of the above questions is 'no', even then this book will help you understand these terms.

REFERENCES

1) Barrett S. Infection control around the world (Editorial). J Hosp Infect, 2001; 47(1): 2.

2) Cabridain M. Managerial procedures and hospital practices; a case study of the development of a new medical discipline. Soc Sci Med. 1985; 20(2): 167-172

3) Simmons R, Phillips IF and Rahman M. Strengthening government health and family planning programmes: findings from an action research project in rural Bangladesh. Stud. Fam Plann 1984; 15(5): 212-221.

4) Hopkinson RB. Clinical Governance: putting it into practice in an acute trust. Clinical Manag. 1999; 8: 81-88

5) Wattis J and McGinnis P. Clinical Governance making it work. Clini Manag. 1999; 8: 12-18.

6) Masterson RG and Teare EL. Clinical Governance and infection Control in the United Kingdom. J of Hosp Infect. 2001; 47 (1): 25-31.

7) Ruchlin HS. The role of leadership in instilling a culture of safety: Lessons from Literature. J Healthcare manag. 2004; 49: 147-58

8) Allen RF. Four phases for bringing about cultural change. In: Kilmann RH, Saxton MJ, Serpa RA, eds. Gaining control of the corporate culture. San Francisco: Jossey-Bass. 1985; 332-350.

9) Bate P. Changing the culture of a hospital from hierarchy to networked community. Pub Admn. 2000; 78(3): 485 – 512.

10) Browman GP, Snider A and Ellis P. Negotiating for change. The healthcare manager as catalyst for evidence based practice: changing the healthcare environment and sharing experience. Healthcare Pap. 2003 3(3):10.

11) Mitra S. An introduction to TATA business excellence model (TBEM). Health Admin. Vol XI & XII . No 1 & 2. 2001; 9-13.

12) Piggot CS. The planning process. Ch 2. In: Business planning for healthcare management. 2nd ed. Open University Press; 12-33.

13) Pointer DD and Orlikoff JE. Functioning: Responsibilities. In: Getting to Great Principles of Healthcare Organization Governance. Jossey-Bass. A Wiley Company. 2002; 33–72.

14) Marone WJ. A Year 2000 Objectives for Preventing Nosocomial Infecions: How do we get there? Am J Med.1991; 91(Suppl 2): S39-S43.

15) Goldman DA, Weinstein RA, Wenzel RP et al. Strategies to prevent and control the emergence and spread of antimicrobial resistant micro organisms in hospitals. A challenge to hospital leadership. J Am Med Assoc. 1996; 275 (3): 234-40.

16) Clupper DR, Clupper JH and Peerson LW. Assess your quality of care quotient. Physician exe. 1997; 23 (6): 28-30.

17) Kelleghan SI, Salemi C, Padilla S et al. An effective continuous quality improvement approach to prevention of ventilator associated pneumonia. Am J Infect Control. 1993; 21(6): 322-330.

18) Joiner GA, Salisbury D and Bollin GE. Utilizing quality assurance as a tool for reducing risk of nosocomial ventilator-associated pneumonia. Am J Med Qual. 1996; 11(2): 100-103.

19) Civetta JM, Hudson-Civetta and Ball S. Decreasing catheter-related infection and hospital costs by continuous quality improvement. Crit Care Med. 1996; 24(11): 1660-1665.

20) Hosein IK, Hill DW, Jenkins LE et al. Clinical significance of emergence of bacterial resistance in the hospital enviromnment. J Appl Microbiol. 2002; (92 Suppl): 90s-97s.

21) Kasturi Rangan V. Lofty missions, Down-to-earth plans. Harvard Business Review. 2004; 8(3): 112-119.

22) Harris A. Risk management in practice: how are we managing? Clinical performance and healthcare. 2000; 8(3): 142-49.

23) Perez-Cuevas R, Guiscafre H, Munoz O et al. Improving physician prescribing patterns to treat rhinopharyngitis. Intervention strategies in two health systems in Mexico. Soc Sci Med.1996; 42 (8): 1185-1194.

24) Kolmos HJ. Role of the clinical microbiology laboratory in infection control – a Danish perspective. J Hosp Infect 2001; 48(suppl): S50 – S54.

25) Farrington M and Pascoe G. Risk management and infection control – time to get our priorities right in the United Kingdom. J of Hosp Infect. 2001; 47(1): 19-24.

Chapter 4

Aspects of Planning and Organization

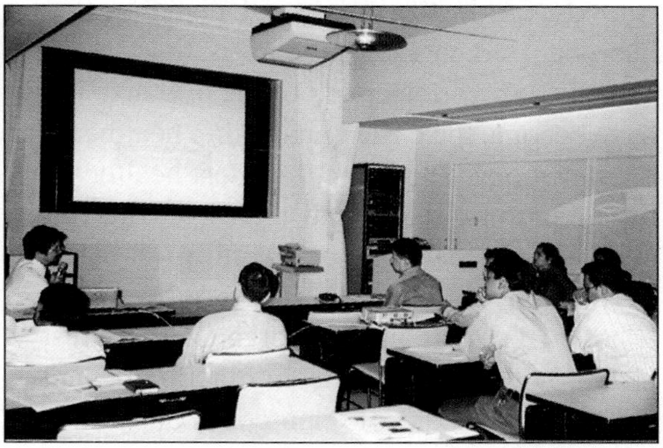

Team learning is vital because teams, not individuals, are the fundamental learning unit in modern organizations.

—Peter Senge

Highlights

Planning for Quality

Understanding Problems Related to HAI Control

Organizational Design and HAI

Fixing Staff Responsible for Infection Control: Primary, Secondary and Tertiary Levels

Defining the Roles (Job Description) in a Tertiary Care Hospital

INTRODUCTION

Hospital acquired infection rate is presently one of the top quality indicators looked at by the leadership of health organizations.[1] For any infection-control programme to succeed, it is imperative that the various areas of functioning move in a coordinated manner, with meticulous planning and execution. A significant change in the process of planning that has occurred in recent years is that 'work teams' from various parts of the organization have become the basic units within healthcare organizations. Therefore, for most healthcare organizations, integrated teamworking has become the focal point of organization-based performance and evaluation programmes[2] (Photo 4.1). A structure or organization must also provide a basis for team functioning and developing a sense of team cohesion. Teams should be conceptualized to include a vertical integration and a horizontal integration, based on a common purpose (HAI control in this case). And to realize the full benefit of a well-organized healthcare facility, every clinician's work should be integrated with other clinical disciplines (coordination across units) and non-clinical key support functions and activities, such as finance, human resources, information management and marketing. Thus, as Vincent et al put it[3], the effectiveness of combating a clinical risk (HAI) is dependent on many complex entities in a system, which include individual factors such as knowledge, skills and competence; regulatory structure; organizational standards, policies, goals, financial resources and constraints, administrative and managerial support; work environment and factors such as staffing levels, workload, design and availability of resources; team factors such as communication, supervision and education.

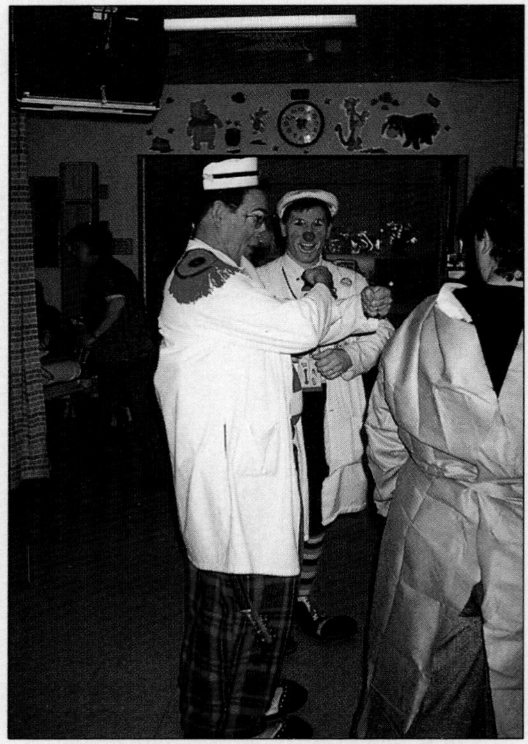

Photo 4.1: Team work: a team of clowns entertain children at Boston Children's Hospital, USA

PLANNING FOR QUALITY

In recent years, the heavy competition among healthcare organizations, increased litigation and public awareness have all made HAI control programme in any healthcare facility one of the key issues and a critical success factor.[4, 5] It could be considered an internal weakness and cause for external threat at times (litigation, media attention). This is evident from a SWOT analysis. The SWOT analysis is a process in management, which allows organizations to assess their Strengths, Weaknesses, Opportunities and Threats.[6]

Generally, health organizations use a combination of approaches for planning.

1. A Problem-Focused Approach

In this, there are four steps which include a) identifying quality problems; b) investigating and assessing each problem's magnitude, scope, consequences and cause; c) undertaking initiatives to correct the problem by making changes in the system, procedures and practices; d) monitoring the results and taking follow-up action.

Planning for specific clinical areas: taking into consideration special problems of specific areas and planning for specific infections. E.g. Catheter-related infections or nosocomial pneumonias. Tackling risks such as these must be a part of the planning process. Risk and clinical performance management should be built into the quality management programme.

2. The Continuous Total Approach

Continuous Quality Improvement (CQI) or Total Quality Management (TQM) again has four steps (a) understanding the nature of desired outcomes from the customers' perspective; (b) identifying, measuring and analysing variations in outcome; (c) studying the care process (typically with the assistance of employee teams) to isolate the causes of variations; (d) designing sustained initiatives to continuously improve the process so that the variations are reduced and outcomes are improved. (See chapter on quality improvement programme)

UNDERSTANDING PROBLEMS RELATED TO HAI CONTROL

The STEP Analysis (Social, Technological, Economic and Political)

The STEP analysis is a managerial tool for planning, and it emphasises the importance of social, technological, economic and political issues while planning HAI control services in a healthcare set-up.

Social and Political Considerations and HAI—A Combined Responsibility

The fight against HAI cannot be carried out in isolation by a single doctor, manager, organization, state or a nation. On the contrary, government agencies, academic centres, industrial and professional bodies each have unique strengths and talents that can be collectively brought to bear on the problem. For combating HAI at all levels of a health set-up, one has to combine management traditions, legislative requirements, resource and experience. The political and economic structures also affect development and enforcement of guidelines, standards, regulations and laws which are important aspects of planning, compliance and management of HAI control. The chapter on guidelines, standards, regulation and laws gives a detailed account of these in relation to HAI. In shaping healthcare policies, societies typically adopt one of the three broad strategies, which link their larger political economy and modes of exercising power: a) a marketplace strategy, b) a state-managerial strategy or c) a national participatory strategy. Because of their different arrangements of power, these strategies result in three very different approaches to responsibility for health and illness and this also applies to the problem of HAI.[7] In the recent years, there has been a global shift from a monopolistic market to an open market economy leading to competition and development of control and enforcement of universal standards for defining quality and performance (both internal and external accreditation agencies being involved).[8-10] Healthcare institutions have become responsive to consumer demands in terms of costs and quality of services. In addition to individual patients, insurance companies and employers have become the new consumers. Information on development of qualitative methodologies and documentation of quality processes and treatment are needed to standardize healthcare delivery and convince the above-mentioned agencies.[11]

Advocacy for HAI control

To bring about changes in the existing structure we need to look at it from a different perspective. As healthcare workers we need to understand the relation between politics, policies and political advocacy, in order to bring about changes in the system and policies. A system of 'organised advocacy' has been used to describe the collective activity of healthcare workers (professional bodies, nurses, doctors, etc.) to move the health and safety agenda.[12] Coalition building and media advocacy are also necessary for securing support for various issues. Learning about policy-related theories and strategies will enable effective working in a given political atmosphere. There are a number of programmes where advocacy and organized efforts have resulted in major policy changes[12]. Examples include:

I.

The threat of small-pox virus being used as a weapon of mass destruction, led the US government to initiate a programme to mass vaccinate against smallpox in 2002–2003. Several organizations expressed concern about the risks to safety of workers due to a lack of a safe design of needles. Constructive criticism by nursing and other healthcare organizations changed the government policy on small-pox vaccination. And this led to the modification of the programme—an example of how professional credibility and voice changed an existing programme, leading to safer practices.

II.

Another example of interaction of policy, politics and advocacy is the long-term efforts to implement the Needlestick Safety and Prevention Act of 2000, USA.

Also, a number of other successful efforts to bring about changes in staffing patterns, working time and other issues related to regulatory change, education, training, monitoring, implementation, legislative changes, voluntary initiatives, etc. (all related to HAI control) are seen in other reports.[12]

Economic Trends

Resource allocation for HAI-related programmes

HAI affects, on an average, about one in 10 patients in hospitals and is the cause of significant mortality and morbidity, especially in the developing countries. In a National Infection Surveillance System-based study in Iran, it was found that additional hospital stay attributed to nosocomial infection was increased by 6.62 days, while total incidence of nosocomial infections during the study period was 17.59%. Nosocomial infections, therefore, add considerable cost to the healthcare system.[13-15]

Administrative controls have been identified as an important defence against hazards to worker and patient safety. This involves resource allocation for various aspects of HAI control and for training of workers in these issues. Cost effective analysis, cost–benefit analysis, value engineering and various other budgeting processes have shown reduction of cost, and are beneficial.[16, 17]

Cost–benefit analysis

In this, the economic benefits of a programme are compared with the cost of the programme itself. Benefits are expressed in terms of monetary benefits to determine if the given programme is economically sound, and to select the best out of several alternative programmes. The scope of such a programme is limited in health planning because there is often a difficulty in expressing benefits in monetary terms. Healthcare policy is formulated by balancing quality, cost and scientific data and analyses, such that rational decisions are made.[18] In the present era of cost containment there are two types of costs that are important when we analyse the cost–benefit analysis:

I

The first is the cost associated with nosocomial infections directly in terms of loss of revenue to the hospital or the healthcare providers. Nosocomial infections represent a direct measurable cost to the hospital and care providers. In many cases they lead to operating deficits for hospitals and healthcare providers.[19]

In US hopsitals, nosocomial infections amount to 5–10 million dollars expense to the healthcare system. The significance in the other countries is at least equal if not more than that calculated in the US.[16, 17] These infections also prolong hospital stay and it was calculated in 1992 that the hospital stay in the US increased considerably, adding, on an average, $ 2100 to the patients' hospital bills. In countries which have a system of reimbursement from Medicare and Medicaid programmes, the reimbursement is based on a set fees according to the patients' diagnoses. Each diagnosis is classified into a particular group, called the diagnosis-related group (DRG). The recovery of the cost of treatment will fall short if the diagnosis does not include the nosocomial infection, for example, if the surgery is included without mentioning the post-operative surgical site infection. Correct coding of the 631 identified nosocomial infections would lead to a better recovery of the DRG. In countries where this kind of reimbursement is not an issue, there will be an underestimation of the problem as the nosocomial infections may not be recorded.[14]

The CDC estimates that these infections contribute to 0.7%–10 % of deaths and actually cause 0.1%–4.4% of all deaths occurring in hospitals. Based on the estimated costs of these nosocomial infections, they appear expensive to patients, insurees and health systems alike. In the present day of consumerism one must not forget the cost of litigation and compensation given to patients, relatives, visitors and healthcare personnel who get infected with HAI. There is also loss in terms of bad publicity and loss of business.

II

The second aspect of the cost calculation is the cost of the infection-control programme itself. The cost of the infection-control programme alone is difficult to calculate as this job is clubbed with other functions performed by the infection-control practitioners. Are infection-control programmes justifiable? Several authors and hospitals have shown a saving of two million dollars in one year due to the presence of an infection-control programme.[9-13]

Chaix and colleagues calculated the cost–benefit ratio for intensive care unit based on surveillance for *Methicillin-Resistant Staphylococcus aureus* (MRSA). This study shows the simplicity and applicability of cost–benefit analysis in infection control. The mean attributable cost of an MRSA infection was $ 9000, which included the cost of prevention and control(surveillance and isolation).[11]

Cost-effective analysis

(Figures 4.1, 4.2)

This is similar to cost–benefit analysis, but here the benefits are expressed in terms of results achieved (instead of monetary terms), e.g. number of lives saved or number of disease-free days. This is more promising in the field of health. Many healthcare practitioners argue against the use of cost-effective analyses, claiming that these assessments are not practical in day-to-day practice. Detsky and Naglie point out that the methods used to perform cost-effectiveness differ and that variable assumptions employed make it difficult to compare results.[18] In addition, cost effectiveness analyses require that the analyst projects events over time and into the future. Such projections are based on assumptions and the full effects of such events may not be known with certainty. Most people agree that analytical methods are more refined as cost–benefit methods and should continue to be used to assess the impact of the infection-control programmes and interventions (including surveillance). These calculations show the amount of money saved and the components of these analyses are then easily identified.

Value engineering: decreasing cost of commodities and raw materials

(Figures 4.3, 4.4)

Value engineering is a neologism advanced to

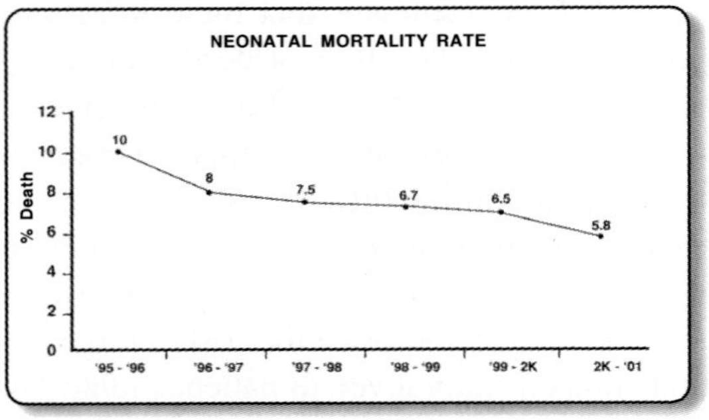

Figure 4.1: Fall in neonatal mortality rate with application of quality management.
(Reproduced with permission from Health Administrator vol. IX, X No. 1, 2; 2001)

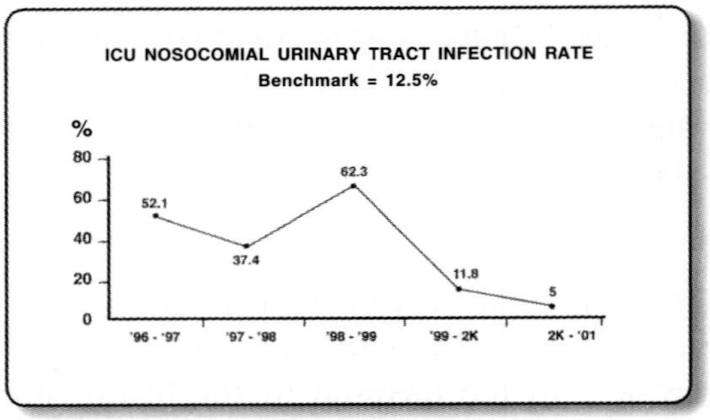

Figure 4.2: Fall in nosocomial urinary tract infection rate with application of quality management.
(Reproduced with permission from Health Administrator vol. IX, X No. 1, 2; 2001)

encourage physicians to look beyond widely-used concepts such as cost-effectiveness, to focus on enhancing the value of care by providing best outcomes at reasonable costs. The basic concept is to rationalize costs (of managing HAI) rather than rationing cost for achieving maximal benefit.[20] This concept has arisen because it has been found in various studies that perhaps 25% of care is inappropriate and there is a large variation in utilization of resources between healthcare organizations. Higher utilization does not necessarily mean improved health status or quality of healthcare. Better quality is not necessarily associated with higher cost, nor does spending less (by doing less) necessarily lead to lower quality. Thus, quality and cost are not tightly linked. A new term called value arose which meant quality/cost. Inputs into healthcare therefore must be rationalized and not rationed. Which means that one should add resources as long as there are positive results. After a particular amount of input, the benefits reach the top of the curve, and going beyond this merely results in negative benefit (e.g. complications, higher costs without patient benefit). The important concepts in this approach are: 1. Economic considerations in clinical decisions are neither unethical nor immoral; 2. The focus must be on costs and not charges (e.g. bills); 3. One must capture the indirect costs (patient's out-of-pocket losses); 4. The benefits and risks of alternative approaches must be identified. By adopting value engineering methods the cost of antibiotics and burn wound dressing savings of 49.35% and 50.07%, respectively, were achieved. Similarly, using indigenous substitute for the optical system of imported microscopes achieved a cost reduction by the approach of value engineering systematically.[21, 22]

Variance management

(Figure 4.5)

This is a tool to reduce variation in practice standards and expenditure. The two commonly practised management techniques that allow flexibility, autonomy and authority of the healthcare professionals are case management and utilization review.[3]

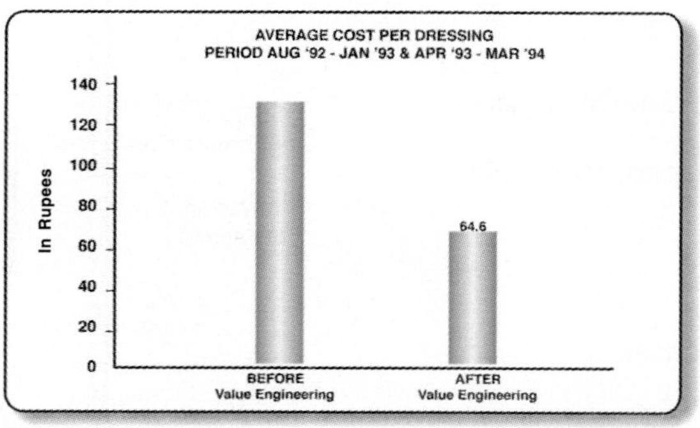

Figure 4.3: Reduction in cost of dressing after value engineering.
(Reproduced with permission from Health Administrator vol. IX, X No. 1, 2; 2001)

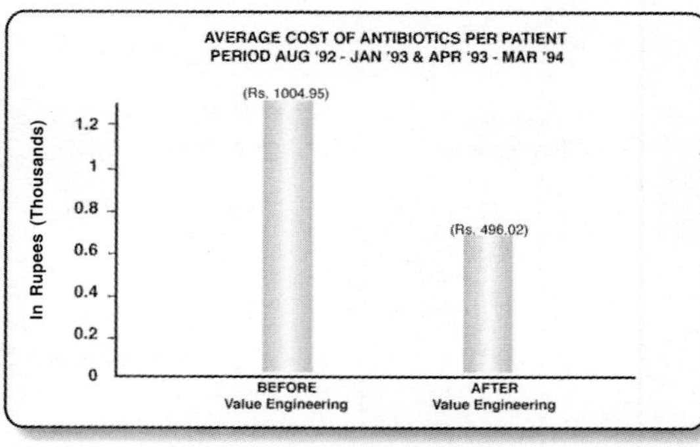

Figure 4.4: Reduction in cost of antibiotics after value engineering.
(Reproduced with permission from Health Administrator vol. IX, X No. 1, 2; 2001)

1. Case management

This technique tries to achieve cost control and desirable/appropriate outcomes by controlling the variance between optimum and actual care. This is carried out as follows:

- Patient is assigned a case manager on admission.
- Case manager monitors care given against standard protocols; coordinates with all care-givers (nurses, doctors, etc.).
- If there is variation between the two, case manager notifies those responsible for variation.
- Case manager follows the patient from entry to exit ensuring that the patient receives appropriate care.
- Thus, the protocols followed and the costs can be monitored from entry to exit.

2. Utilization review

- The resources used for the care of a particular patient are compared with an earlier benchmark (average). This identifies over- or under-utilization of resources associated with a particular outcome. The manager uses this data for optimizing future healthcare delivery.

Technological Changes: Emerging Media and Communication Channels

(Photo 4.2)

Increasingly, technological changes and innovations are revolutionizing HAI control. Education, training, surveillance, auditing, prescribing, diagnosis, treatment and medical information systems are all changing aspects of HAI control. Technology assessment is the systematic and scientific evaluation of cost-

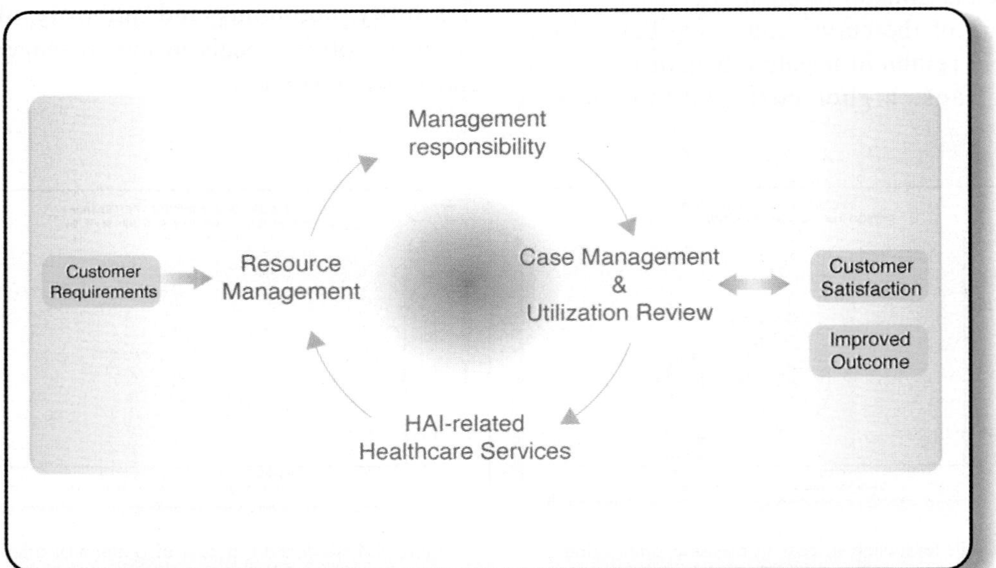

Figure 4.5: Variance management can decrease cost, variation and expenditure

and risk-effectiveness of both existing and new forms of treatment. Increased growth of the internet and its usage for education, training and awareness is also an advancement. However, the costs of procuring medical technology is always a constraint in most economies. Medical Information Systems are increasingly being used for HAI control. Any equipment or procedure used for the collection, recording, processing, storage, retrieval and display of clinical information comes within the purview of the medical information systems. The clinical record must contain the details of the diagnosis, treatment, condition at discharge and the post-discharge instructions to patients.[14] Other matters of concern in this context are: management of patient-related information with confidentiality and responsibility (e.g. HIV status must be respected). This is seen as a basic right of the patient. The clinical record of patients must be accessible only to those members of the staff who are authorized to maintain confidentiality, but at the same time take adequate measures for protection of other patients, medical and non-medical staff and visitors. Display material used to warn medical and paramedical staff (e.g. in patients with HIV or Hepatitis B) must not contain information about the infection. It should only warn the personnel that standard precautions have to be followed.

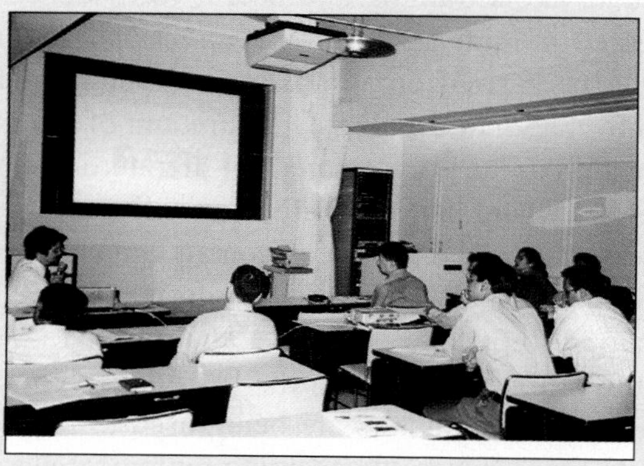

Photo 4.2: Technological advances have improved education, training, surveillance, auditing, diagnosis and treatment of HAI.

Any medical information specific to HAI is important for surveillance and hence advised to be coded as per the CDC codes. Information about HAI in in-patient facilities can be easily recorded and collected, but HAI occurring in out-patients and domiciliary patients are often difficult to document. The hospital must develop a system to process and utilize this information and divulge it to the concerned clinical and managerial staff for improvement. Advanced information systems are available now for surveillance of HAI. These facilities use automated systems that use antibiotic prescriptions, ICD-9 codes and various other codes available from various administrative databases. Specialized software can also be developed for audit and surveillance. These facilitate the infection-control activities and decrease the time spent on performing chart review. But none of these systems has been associated with cost savings.

Education and professional development in HAI

All hospital employees must know the objectives of the infection-control progamme which include:

- Monitoring HAI
- Training of staff in prevention and control of HAI
- Investigation of outbreaks
- Control of outbreaks

- Monitoring staff health
- Preventing staff-to-patient and patient-to-patient spread of HAI
- Advising infection-control measures and isolation

This would ensure their participation in various HAI control activities.

What should be taught?

All healthcare workers and also the persons specifically connected with infection-control committee have to be trained in HAI control measures. The APIC has identified eight educational standards that represent the knowledge base necessary for the effective practice of infection control:

1. Epidemiology and statistics
2. Microbiology
3. Infectious diseases
4. Sterilization, disinfection and sanitation
5. Patient-care practices
6. Education in HAI-control measures
7. Management skills
8. Employee health

This has been published as a curriculum for the training of an infection-control physician (ICP).

European educational guidelines related to HAI control have been given in the consensus recommendations of an international workshop organized by the European Society of Clinical Microbiology and Infectious Diseases (2004), and this includes core curriculum for medical training in infection control and healthcare epidemiology and certification to be established at the European level and implemented at the national level. The whole spectrum of healthcare services is covered (including ambulatory and long-term care facilities) in the curriculum.

Advances in telecommunications

Telecommunication has revolutionized education and data collection. Communication protocols include:

- Device–device communication
- Wireless communication
- Internet-based medical applications
- Hand-held medical devices
- Telemedicine

Professional development programmes

Education has to be a participatory learning experience aimed at the needs and likes of the practitioner. The bulk of learning should be at practice level including theoretical knowledge, skills training and access to evidence-based training. Education (patient and staff) can be carried out by using computers and information technology. The amount of information in the primary medical literature alone is overwhelming. MEDLINE, an online repository of medical abstracts, contains more than 8.6 million bibliographic entries from over 3800 current biomedical journals and adds 31,000 new entries each month. In recent years, advanced simulators are being used to facilitate preparedness for tackling biological warfare attacks and highly infectious organisms. Simulators are useful for learning where common computers are restricted in their capacities. These include psychomotor skills and attitude improvements. They can be used to learn facts, diagnostic techniques, therapeutic decision making and team activities (behaviour and attitudes). (See chapter on outbreaks and epidemics.)[23]

Members of quality-improvement committee should participate in teaching of nurses, orderlies (housekeeping), respiratory therapists, clinicians and microbiologists. Ensuring participation in educational activities is necessary to ensure compliance with such programmes. The other essential ingredients for a successful programme of professional development related to HAI control could include:

- Proof of attendance as a condition of employment
- A centralized record of all employees who have undergone training to be maintained in the quality-health or hospital epidemiology departments
- A written test before and after the training session as a measure of adequacy of training
- Feedback of results to be given with a refresher training included to keep abreast of the changing scenario

ORGANIZATIONAL DESIGN AND HAI

What Is an Organization?

An organization is a deliberate arrangement of people to accomplish a specific purpose. It involves the process of determining what tasks are to be done and by whom and coordination of activities. For HAI control this should include a) a (structure) chain of command in hospitals which is specific to HAI control, b) a chain of command at the primary, secondary and tertiary healthcare levels dedicated solely to HAI control, c) integration of quality, risk and performance management strategies specific to HAI control, and d) clinical integration across various disciplines and a structured HAI control programme.

> ***Organizations define tasks***
>
> What are the tasks to be done?
>
> Who is to do them?
>
> How are the tasks to be performed?
>
> When and where are decisions to be made?

Building Team Factors: Multidisciplinary Teams

Traditionally, the organizational design for managing HAI in a hospital is the Infection Control Committee (ICC). It means that a central committee is relegated the responsibility of initiating and implementing infection-control programmes and policies. As infection-control is growing in complexity, multidisciplinary infection-control teams are being formed as recommended by the consensus conference. Such teams are coordinated by faculty with specific knowledge of hospital epidemiology and specialists in preventive medicine, microbiology or infectious diseases.

Conventionally, the ICC plays a major role in quality assessment. But now there is a shift of emphasis from quality assessment to continuous quality improvement, a methodology that will require continued involvement by the ICC. In this, the first step is to form a multidisciplinary committee to address the problems of infection control in different areas. Depending on the area (operating room, intensive care unit, laboratory, etc.) they are dealing with, the committee should include members having a common purpose, with complementary skills and a commitment to each other's goals and successes. There should be cooperation between the HCW of these settings. The following points must be kept in mind:

1. Integrating HAI policies with clinical and non clinical areas
2. Elimination of departmental boundaries while focusing on the internal process of combating HAI at the organizational level
3. The focal point in the implementation is the greater importance placed on autonomy
4. Empowerment of the individual, with emphasis on the development of quality teams

Horizontal Integration

Coordination of HAI control activities across operating units and other departments that are at the same level in the process of delivering services (such as acute hospital care) is called **horizontal integration**.[24] The Society for Healthcare Epidemiology Panel Recommendations for Essential Activities (1999) recommends the following: Patients must have access to continuing services of trained professionals in infection control, prevention and epidemiology. HAI control activities must include acute care settings, one-day clinics, long-term care facilities and home-care settings. Transfers from one facility to another should be easily possible.

Vertical Integration at Various Levels

Designing a well-defined structure takes into consideration coordination and fixing the responsibility of personnel for HAI control activity. It is very important across operating units that are at different stages in the process of delivery of patient-care services, for example, primary, secondary and tertiary levels. This obviously requires meticulous planning, structuring and organizing at every level—national, state, institutional—and the details of these aspects have to be worked out; each functioning within the framework of its higher level. At each level, one has to keep in view the goals of the higher level and work in tandem with a common purpose to achieve a common goal. It is within this framework that infection-control workers in various organizations must develop their own methods and strategies and apply these techniques to their areas of work. The structure of global and national networks for surveillance and epidemiology are given in the chapter on surveillance.

Personnel Management and HAI

Personnel management involves leading, motivating, influencing, communicating and/or dealing with individuals or teams in the organization. Motivation of staff is extremely important in the compliance of infection-control policies and is possible with effective leadership and communication. Training with incentives and disincentives should be a part of personnel management. Employees in any organization have opinions, traditions, beliefs and practices concerning quality in relation to hospital infection control. This is a part of the quality culture and its understanding constitutes assessment of quality.

Leadership by Empowerment

Practitioners will need to take into account the fact that there are many individuals in their teams who are more than able to take on leadership roles. These individuals may be employees in organizations that they serve. Clinicians, nurses and paramedical HCWs need to be encouraged to take on roles that may sometimes lead them to direct the activity of their employers without fear of being resented for their contribution. This will be a new experience in some practices that have stuck to a hierarchical model with the boss firmly in command of his troops.

Formation of a quality circle greatly enhances the purpose of an ICC. A quality circle is a small group of employees from the same work area who voluntarily meet regularly to identify, analyse and resolve work-related problems. For example, a team looking into nosocomial pneumonia should ideally consist of representatives from respiratory therapy, nursing, intensive care, pulmonary critical care, infectious diseases, infection control, quality health, internal medicine and surgery. The committee should meet at least once a month and shoulder the responsibility of identifying opportunities for improvement in those areas. This not only improves the performance of the organization but also motivates and enriches the work-life of employees. To come up with local solutions for the management of HAI, one has to hone his skills of problem-solving and improve upon existing situations. This can best be accomplished with a multidisciplinary committee involved in that particular area. Brainstorming sessions can be added to bring in fresh ideas regarding cause and effect. Cause and effect diagrams (fish bone diagrams) help in identifying opportunities for improvement. From the various causes listed, the relative risk is identified and prioritized (pareto charts help in doing so) by reviewing existing policies and proposing new policies and procedures. To execute these policies, accountability of and approval from the committee are essential. Verbal communication, written communication, supervision and seeking help, team structure congruence, consistency and leadership are important for building teams.[3, 25]

Workload and HAI

Other factors important in personnel management are a conducive work environment, staffing levels, skill mix, workload and shift patterns; design, availability and maintenance of equipment; and administrative support. The consensus panel 1996 report published by the Society for Healthcare Epidemiology of America gave the following recommendations: Higher staffing levels of trained personnel; additional resources such as information technology, support for data management and communication; access to special laboratory services; education of HCW, employee health, compliance with guidelines, regulations and accreditation requirements and quality assurance promotion.[26]

In addition to staffing specifically for infection control within an organization, it is important to ensure optimum workloads among personnel such as nurses, housekeeping and junior doctors. This is important for two reasons: 1) to decrease the transmission of HAI and 2) to decrease health hazards to the personnel themselves. Inadequate staffing and training are both linked to an increase in HAI. Staffing levels are given by the respective bodies in their respective countries. In India, standards of basic minimum requirements for staffing in the ICU are given by the Infection Control Society of India. In other countries it is given by their respective national societies.[2, 4, 5, 27]

FIXING STAFF RESPONSIBLE FOR INFECTION CONTROL: PRIMARY, SECONDARY AND TERTIARY LEVELS

Responsibility for community acquired and HAI control activities is delegated to various personnel at primary, secondary and tertiary levels. This is well defined in some countries.[22] Details of laboratory network and responsibilities are discussed in the chapter on surveillance. The organizations and individuals listed below are a source of surveillance data, diagnosis, treatment, implementation of infection-control measures, taking preventive action, giving advice, practical assistance and training at various levels. **Examples of Organizations (individuals) responsible for infection-control in UK:**[22, 28, 29] Hospitals (medical microbiologist, infection-control doctor, infection-control nurse, genito-urinary medicine specialist); community trusts (health visitors, district nurses, school health nurses and doctors, TB nurse advisors); local authority departments: environmental health (environmental health officers); education (teachers); social services (social workers, home carers, residential home managers safety managers); local public health laboratory (medical microbiologist); public health laboratory service (medical microbiologist); communicable disease surveillance centre (consultant epidemiologist); primary care (general practitioners, practice nurses and other practice staff); private nursing homes and residential homes (managers, nursing staff); occupational health departments (occupational health doctors and nurses); day nurseries (managers, nursery nurses); general public (citizens, newspapers, radio, TV).

DEFINING THE ROLES (JOB DESCRIPTION) IN A TERTIARY CARE HOSPITAL

The key to HAI control is the role of the abovementioned infection-control personnel and committees to integrate vertically and horizontally all areas where HAI transmission occurs in a system—national or institutional.

Chain of command

The chain of command: staff responsible for administration and organization in tertiary care hospital.

Head of Hospital

Functions

To apply for authorization, implementation of government policies, formation of waste management/infection-control committee. The hospital administration or head should provide funds and resources for the infection-control programme, ensure a clean and safe environment, ensure availability of safe food and drinking water, ensure availability of sterile supplies and material and establish an infection-control committee and team.

Infection Control Committee (ICC)

Members are representative of medical, nursing, engineering, administrative, domestic, pharmacy, CSSD and microbiology departments. The committee formulates the policies for control of infection. Head of hospital will be the chairman of this committee. Infection Control Officer will be the secretary.

Functions

Policy-making regarding:

a. Provision of adequate building, equipment, isolation facilities, etc.

b. Ventilation of operation theatre, wards and units

c. Standardization of procedures for operation theatre, wards, house-keeping, waste disposal, kitchen, laundry and CSSD

d. Preparation of manuals for procedures like preoperative skin preparation, I/V infusions, catheterisation, lumbar puncture, wound dressing

e. Formulation of disinfection policy

f. Antibiotic policy for rational use of antibiotics in therapy and prophylaxis

Infection Control Team (ICT)

Members are: Infection Control Officer, Infection Control Nurse, incharge CSSD, incharge ICU.

Functions

a. Surveillance of infection to give baseline information about the level of endemic infection in the hospital

b. Monitoring of procedures (wound dressings, IV injections, etc.), sterilization and disinfection processes, bacteriological monitoring of critical environment and hazardous equipment

c. Training of staff in control of hospital infection

d. Investigation of outbreaks of infection: including detection of sources of infections with the help of typing procedures and epidemiological information

e. Controlling the outbreak by rectifying technical lapses if any

Infection Control Officer (ICO)

Usually a microbiologist

Functions

a. Secretary of Infection Control Committee (ICC) will be responsible to record minutes and arrange for meeting

b. Consultant member of ICC

c. Identification and reporting of pathogens and their antibiotic susceptibility patterns

d. Regular analysis and dissemination of antibiotic resistance data, emerging pathogens and unusual laboratory findings

e. Initiating surveillance of hospital infections and detection of outbreaks

f. Investigation of outbreaks

g. Training and education in infection-control procedures and practice

Infection Control Nurse (ICN)

A senior nursing sister must be appointed full time for this position.

One ICN for every 500 beds. Seconded to the department of microbiology under the management of ICO

Functions

a. Liaison between microbiology department and clinical departments for detection and control of hospital infection
b. Surveillance of infection and detection of outbreaks
c. Collection of specimens and preliminary processing; should be trained in basic microbiological techniques
d. Training and education of staff in infection-control procedures and practice under supervision of ICO
e. Creating awareness among patients and visitors about infection control

Waste Disposal Officer (WDO)

Directly responsible to head of the institution. Responsible for internal collection of waste, its transport and final disposal

Infection-Control Professional

(Recommended by SENIC1970 in USA)

The ICP is not available in many countries, but there have been recommendations by some of the important bodies to have this post to improve upon the traditional positions in the infection-control team.

The typical infection-control professional (ICP) with primary and full-time responsibility for preventing infections is a professional nurse, medical technologist, microbiologist, physician or epidemiologist.

The majority of ICPs work in acute care hospitals with about a fifth employed at non-acute inpatient institutions, long-term care, mental health and rehabilitation facilities. They balance work in a variety of healthcare, academic, or industry/consulting settings. ICPs are responsible for assisting healthcare institutions in providing a high level of patient care by preventing and reducing nosocomial infections through consistent day-to-day surveillance, implementation of control measures and personnel education.

ICPs investigate outbreaks of nosocomial infections, isolate sources of infection, implement corrective measures to limit the extent of infections, and help to ensure that similar episodes are not repeated. Through instruction and dissemination of information, ICPs train healthcare personnel on infection-control practices and techniques.

The typical ICP spends half his time performing surveillance of infection. Surveillance activity is an essential element of an infection-control programme as it provides data to identify infected patients and determine the sites of infection as well as the factors contributing to the infection.[30]

REFERENCES

1) Donahue JM and McGuire MB. The political economy of responsibility in health and illness. Soc Sci Med. 1995; 40 (1): 47-53
2) Barrett S. Infection control around the world (Editorial). J Hosp Infect, 2001; 47(1): 2.
3) Vincent C and Adams ST. The investigation and analysis of clinical incidents. In: Clinical Risk Management. Enhancing Patient Safety. 2nd edn. BMJ Books. 2001; 439-460.

4) Pavia M, Bianco A, Viggiani MA et al. Prevalence of hospital acquired infections in Italy. J Hosp Infect, 2000; 44(2): 135-139.

5) Rodriguez-Bano J, Pascual A. Hospital Infection Control in Spain. J Hosp Infect Control, 2001; 48(4): 258-260.

6) Pointer DD and Orlikoff JE. Functioning: Responsibilities. In: Getting to Great. Principles of Heath care organization governence. A Wiley Company. Jossey- Bass. 2002; 33-71.

7) Chaston I. Assessing strategic behaviour within the acute sector of the National Health Service. J Manag Med 1994; 8(5): 58-67.

8) Marone WJ. A Year 2000 Objectives for Preventing Nosocomial Infecions: How do we get there? Am J Med.1991; 91(Suppl 2): S39 -S43.

9) Pinner RW, Haley RW, Blumenstein BA, et al. High cost of nosocomial infections. Infect Control Hosp Epimemiol. 1982; 3:143-149.

10) Haley RW, Schaberg DR, Crossley KB, et al. Extra charges and prolongation of stay attributable to nosocomial infections: a prospective inter hospital comparison. Am J Med. 1981; 70 (1): 51-58.

11) Chaix C, Durand-Zaleski I, Alberti C et al. Control of endemic methicillin resistant *Staphylococcus aureus*: a cost-benefit analysis in an intensive care unit. J Am Med Assoc. 1999; 281(18): 1745-1751.

12) Foley M. Collective action in healthcare. In: Policy and Politics in Nursing and Healthcare. Mason DJ, Leavit JK, Chaffee MW (eds.) 4th edn. Saunders, St Louis, MO. 2002; 387-397.

13) Wenzel RP. Nosocomial infections, diagnosis, and study on the efficacy of nosocomial infection control: economic implications for hospitals under the prospective payment system. Am J Med 1985; 78 (6) (suppl.2): 3-7

14) Massanari RM, Wilkerson K, Streed SA et al. Reliability of reporting nosocomial infections in the discharge abstract and implications for receipt of revenues under prospective reimbursement. Am J Public Health. 1987; 77(5): 561-564.

15) Miller PJ, Farr BM and Gwaltney JMJ. Economic benefits of an effective infection control programme: case study and proposal. Rev Infect Dis. 1989; 11: 284-288.

16) Wenzel RP. The economics of nosocomial infections. J Hosp Infect 1995; 31 (2): 79-87.

17) Haley RW, Schaberg DR, Von Allmen SD et al. Estimating the extra charges and prolongation of hospitalization due to nosocomial infections: a comparison of methods. J Infect Dis. 1980; 141: 248-257.

18) Detsky AS and Naglie IG. A clinician's guide to cost-effectiveness. Ann Intern Med. 1990;113: 147-154.

19) Wilcox MH, Cunniffe JG, Trundle C et al. Financial burden of hospital-acquired *Clostridium difficile* infection. J Hosp Infect 1996; 34(1): 23-30

20) Bharat R. Value Engineering – a new concept in reducing cost of burn care. Health Administrator. Vol XI & XII . No 1 &2. 2001; 59-62.

21) Mishra M, Sinha TBK, Bandopadhyay SP et al. Indigenous substitute for the optical system of imported microscopes through value engineering. Health Administrator. Vol XI& XII. No 1 & 2. 2001; 63-67.

22) Naylor CD. What is appropriate care? New Engl J Med. 1998; 338:1918-1920.

23) Mohanty R, Sarosh RD and Saroj KK. Hospital information system in Medicare – An experience at Tata main hospital, Jamshedpur. Health Administrator. Vol XI & XII . No 1 & 2. 2001; 70-74.

24) Struelens MJ Professional organization of healthcare-associated infection control: time for action across the patient care system. Editorial review. In: Andiole VT, Finch RG.

Current Opinion in infectious Diseases (Indian edn). 2004; 1: 123-125.

25) Friedman C, Barnette M, Buck AS et al. Requirements for infrastructure and essential activities of infection control and epidemiology in out-of-hospitals settings: a consensus panel report. Association for professionals in infection control and epidemiology and society for healthcare epidemiology of America. Infect Control Hosp Epidemiol. 1999; 20(10): 695-705.

26) Haley RW, Culver DM, White JW et al. The efficacy of infection surveillance and control programs in preventing nosocomial infections in US hospitals. Am J of Epidemiol. 1985; 121(2):182-205.

27) Scheckler WE, Brimhall D, Buck AS et al. Requirements for infrastructure and essential activities of infection control and epidemiology in hospitals: a consensus panel report. Society for Healthcare Epidemiology of America. Am J Infect Control. 1998; 26: 47-60.

28) Health Canada Nosocomial and Occupational Infections Sections. Development of a resource model for infection prevention and control programs in acute, long term, and home settings: conference proceedings of the infection prevention and control alliance. Am J Infect Control. 2004; 32(1): 2-6.

29) Casey RC. An infection control link nurse network in the care home settings. Br J Nurs. 2004; 13: 166-170.

30) Schoch P, ESCMID sets its agenda for meeting the European challenges in clinical microbiology and infectious diseases. Eurosurveillance Weekly. 2004; 8 (14): 1.

Chapter 5

Understanding Quality and Its Measurement

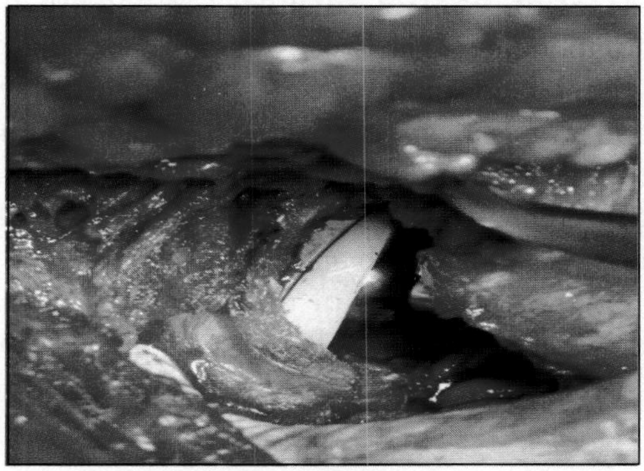

Quantity is what you can count. Quality is what you can count on.

—Anonymous

Highlights

Quality Management as an Organizational Philosophy and Strategy

Quality Improvement as an Obligation in Healthcare Delivery

Trying to Define Quality—Multifaceted as a Diamond

Performance

Concepts of Quality Assessment and Measurement

Terms Used in Quality Measurement

INTRODUCTION

It is easy to understand the differences in the quality of services provided in hotel industry because of the ranking the hotels get—three star, five star, seven star, etc. But can we delineate the quality differences in the services provided by the healthcare sector? What is quality? How do we improve quality of infection-control services? What are its components? The term 'quality', especially when used in the context of healthcare delivery, is a very abstract and ambigious one that needs understanding before one can comprehend its existence and work towards incorporating it into a system. (Photo 5.1)

The definitions of quality originated in the industry, and have later been applied to the healthcare institutions. One must realize, however, that it is not easy to compare production lines in the industry with that in the health sector, as, the delivery of healthcare service is infinitely more complex. In order to understand and implement quality improvement programmes, the clinician needs to comprehend what is required of him, translate it into action and merge it with his daily activities. This also applies to the control of HAI.

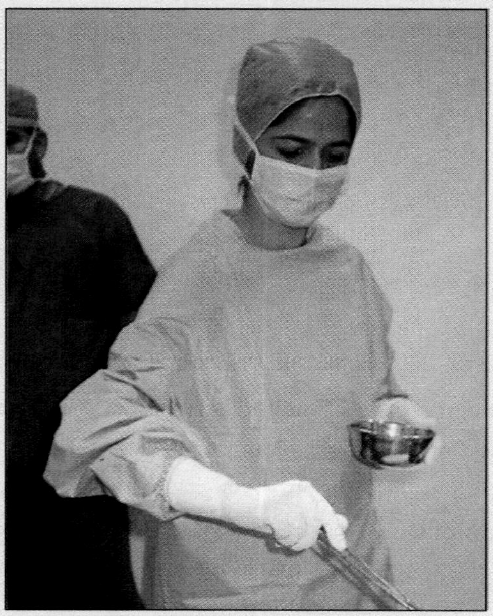

Photo 5.1: The term quality when used in the context of healthcare delivery, is ambiguous and needs to be understood before comprehending 'quality management'

QUALITY MANAGEMENT AS AN ORGANIZATIONAL PHILOSOPHY AND STRATEGY

Quality improvement is a philosophy and strategy by which an organization conducts itself. It dictates how resources are allocated to satisfy customer requirements (patients) and how improvement is brought about in the organization.Organizations should try to implement quality clinical care, and if a positive, consistent change has to be made in managing infection control, quality must be pursued tenaciously at all levels, be it national, organizational, departmental or individual.

QUALITY IMPROVEMENT AS AN OBLIGATION IN HEALTHCARE DELIVERY

The World Medical Association Declaration 1997 (see appendix) on quality improvement clearly states that doctors have a moral obligation to improve quality of services continuously. The quality of healthcare services is a reflection of patients' and society's preferences and values and implies that those have been taken into account in healthcare decisions and policy making.

Going one step further, quality management and audit became mandatory and a contractual obligation for doctors in many countries in the 1990s. For example, in the United Kingdom, under the Health and Safety Legislation, there is a requirement to report certain events to the health and safety executive for review. The act places under obligation all staff to report clinical and non-clinical incidents which are likely to have a bearing on the quality, safety or efficiency of care provided. However, quality assurance is still not mandatory in healthcare delivery systems of many countries.

TRYING TO DEFINE QUALITY—MULTIFACETED AS A DIAMOND

(PHOTO 5.2)

An english dictionary describes quality as 'high degree of goodness in a person or material'. Example of a definition incorporating only goodness and a single aspect of healthcare is as follows: 'The highest quality of medical care that best achieves legitimate medical and nonmedical goals.'[1] Is this possible and achievable? Is it practical to have the highest quality medical care? The problem with this definition is that it does not include all the dimensions of the quality of care. A definition including multiple facets would be: 'Quality of care is the degree (ranking) to which health services for individuals and populations (target population) increase the likelihood of desired outcomes (outcomes) and are consistent with current professional knowledge (conformation with standards).'[2]

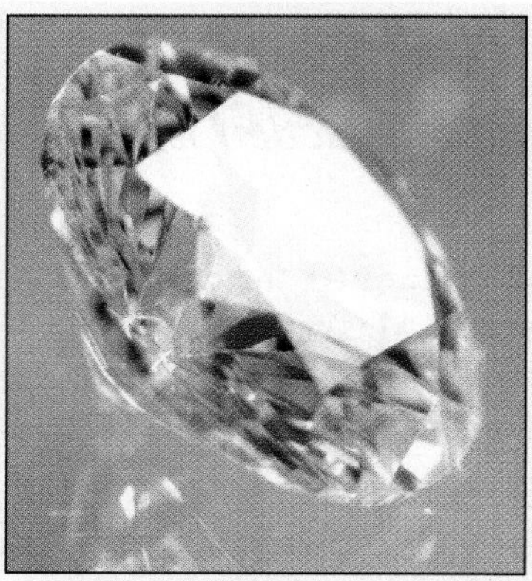

Photo 5.2: Quality is multifaceted as a diamond

Also, the concept of quality must take into consideration the other additional perspectives (facets) such as the following:

1. Providers' (Healthcare Institution's) Perspective

a. Conformity with standards concerned with care

The term quality is also used to define the degree of conformity with standards, with the best of medical knowledge and with accepted principles and practices. In other words, it is the degree of congruence between expectation and realization. This dimension of quality relates to the manner in which healthcare services are delivered, not the range of services available.[3] Quality means meeting the pre-determined requirements of the users for a particular substance or service. Palmer and Adams (1988) stated that 'quality of healthcare is measured by comparing data describing care received by patients to standards.' [4, 5, 6]

Often it is seen that several factors may affect patient outcomes, which are beyond a provider's control, including patient characteristics and circumstances. Such factors constrain what the healthcare process can achieve. In the light of these constraints quality may be best thought of as 'the delivery of healthcare services in such a fashion as to most efficiently, effectively and humanely return the patient to—or maintain the patient at—his highest level of functioning.'[3]

b. Minimizing variations of standards and processes in health services

Variations in healthcare from the standards can be identified and measured. But control through variation measurement has the potential to be rigid (it is rigid in most industries). In the healthcare set-up the flexibility may be decreased if adequate variances are not allowed or if the variances are unsuited to a particular patient. The two commonly practised management techniques that allow flexibility, autonomy and authority of the healthcare professional are case management and utilization review.[7, 8]

This can be assessed by taking the following into consideration:

- Access to healthcare services which should be preventive, diagnostic, therapeutic.
- Information given out to the patient.
- Continuity, management and coordination between various levels of care (primary, secondary and tertiary)
- Clinical staff—their knowledge, skill and efficiency

2. Consumers' (Patients') Perspective

Juran's method addresses customer needs and existing deficiencies in a system. Quality management involves establishing goals, identifying customers, determining customer needs and developing product features to meet those needs.[9] Deming, an American management theorist, defines quality as 'meeting customer requirements at a price they are willing to pay.' When all the above-discussed factors are made optimal and efficient, the outcome can be seen as a measure of patient satisfaction.

3. Buyers' (Insurance Company's) Perspective

The people who pay for the treatment (buyers) are concerned with cost effectiveness and constraints in professional care and resource. The expenditure related to HAI control activities underscores the constraints placed on professional performance by the state of technical, medical and scientific knowledge, implying that the state is dynamic, and that the healthcare provider is responsible for using the best knowledge base available (consistent with current professional knowledge). Quality of care and its improvement, along with reducing costs, has become a focal point in the healthcare agenda. Dimensions of financial constraints and accessibility within a single definition may create opposing pressures on the healthcare providers or policy makers.

Patient satisfaction is concerned with

- Cost of care (if the patient is paying): Cost of HAI is discussed in planning and organization (See chapter on planning and organization)
- Interpersonal skills of the provider: This is difficult to determine as HAI-related skills and knowledge are always given very little importance

- Symptom relief and functional improvement
- Good service: This is a function of positive perceptions. It includes, good intentions, sincere efforts, intelligent direction and skilful execution. Elements of the concept of consideration (anxiety, price plus loss of dignity, waiting time, etc.)
- Circumstances: Severity of illness and family circumstances must be taken into consideration
- Risk management and safety consideration. E.g. decreasing HAI and associated morbidity and mortality

4. Workers' Perspective

In the delivery of quality, Deming linked quality, productivity and the workers. Better quality also meant better working environment, better pay packets and more safety. Therefore, this looks at a completely different facet of quality. For example, controlling exposure of personnel to hazardous substances arising from work activity has been taken into account by Control of Substances Hazardous to Health (COSHH) regulations 1988 (US), and includes regulations for infective microorganisms and toxic substances.[9]

HAI-Related Components of Quality

Avedis Donabedian proposed an approach to solving problems with delivery of quality healthcare by focusing separately on the structure, process and outcome of the care administered (also called the Donabedian's triad)[4] (Fig. 5.1). This may be applied to any aspect of healthcare to split it up to its components and encompass a wide range of elements of care (health services). A similar approach can be used to understand the structure, processes and outcomes related to the control of HAI.[5] These three aspects are also useful for assessing quality: a) structure, b) process, c) outcome.

a. Structure

Structure refers to the characteristics of the setting in which care is provided. Quality of structural characteristics in combination with quality processes determine outcomes.

Examples of HAI-related structural characteristics:

1. Physical structure and design of different areas, e.g. operating room, ICU as per standards
2. Delivery system—distribution of hospital beds and physicians
3. Staffing in specific areas versus number of beds. (Adequate staffing is important in preventing HAI.)
4. Staff Qualifications—licensure and accreditation, training related to HAI

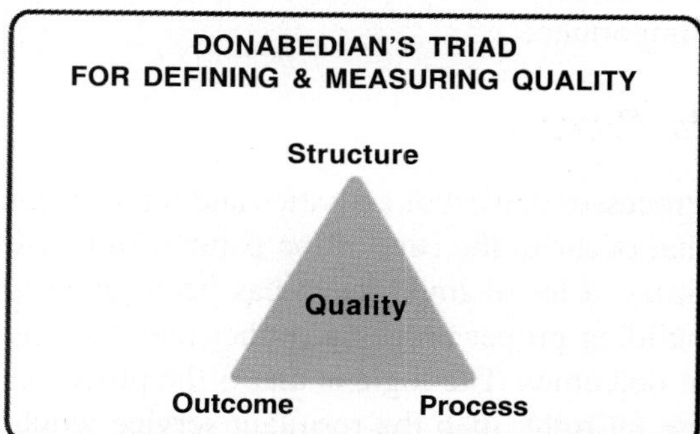

Figure 5.1: The Donabedian triad helps define the components of quality in healthcare delivery

5. Medical training and qualifications especially in relation to infection-control practices, e.g. operating room nurse needs to be adequately qualified and knowledgeable with infection-related practices
6. Resource inputs—amount of money allocated to HAI-control programmes
7. Written down policies: Practice guidelines, regulations, protocols, clearly defined responsibilities and SOPs related to HAI in different clinical/non-clinical areas
8. Facilities—licensing, accreditation
9. Equipment—diagnostic, surgical, disinfection and sterilization, urine pots, bedpans, thermometers, spatula, monitors, furniture, etc.
10. Access to support services (primary, secondary, tertiary) in case of HAI-related problems

> 'One purpose of the quality assurance system is to achieve a proper balance between the dimensions reflected in a given definition of quality, because dimensions of quality may well contradict each other.'
>
> All dimensions of quality must receive due importance.

b. Process

Processes consist of activities and interactions that occur in the care of the patient. In recent times, a lot of importance has been given to building proper processes rather than looking at outcomes. The logic is that if the processes are all right, then the resultant service would automatically be of a good quality. To understand further, an example would highlight this point. Let us look at a consumer product, e.g. soap. The quality of the product can be checked or the process of manufacture in the factory can be standardized and the processes can be checked. A good process would ensure a good quality product automatically. A bad product reflects on bad process. The same logic applies to the health industry.[10]

How care is provided should reflect appropriate use of the most current knowledge about scientific, clinical, technical, interpersonal, manual, cognitive, organizational and management elements of healthcare. Documentation is another aspect of quality which should be maintained at least to a minimum to enable continuity of care and peer evaluation. This means that data related to HAI must be appropriately stored for further evaluation. E.g. maintenance of records of processing equipment such as the steam sterilizers, ethylene oxide sterilizers and dry heat sterilizers.

HAI-Related Processes

- Referral
- Admission and readmissions
- Investigations
- Diagnoses
- General treatment
- Nursing care
- Drugs
- Screening and diagnostic procedures
- Disease prevention Techniques
- Quality of case notes (documentation/ lodging of HAI-related information)
- Communication (with other institutions in case of transfer of patient, all details of HAI)
- Discharge (should mention details of HAI)

- Control strategies
- Whether the quality of services is analysed: a system of internal review, external audit of process and outcome; standards and comparators
- Surveillance: whether quality indicators are built-in
- Whether the processes are validated, i.e. whether process monitoring is carried out. E.g. air microbiology tests of the sterile area of the SSD may be carried out at random, e.g. once a month
- HAI-related occupational health, etc.

c. Outcome

Leebov defines quality as 'doing the right things consistently to ensure the best possible clinical outcome for patients; satisfaction for all of the customers; retention of talented staff; and sound financial performance.' Unwanted outcomes indicate the importance of the link between process of healthcare and outcomes.[11]

Examples of HAI-related outcomes:

- Mortality due to HAI
- Infection rates among patients (wound infection rates, bacteremia, serious nosocomial infections rates such as the VAP, UTI, catheter-related infections)
- Infection rates among the staff
- Needle-stick injuries in staff
- Deep-seated infections
- Deaths from infectious causes
- Correct use of antibiotics
- Length of hospital stay
- Gross infection rate
- Drug utilization review: systematic analysis of the appropriateness and effectiveness of drugs used
- Symptom control
- Residual disability

Indirect Measures of Outcome

- Patient satisfaction
- Health status
- Recovery
- Improvement
- Iatrogenic illnesses (injuries)
- Rehospitalization

PERFORMANCE

Performance is defined as 'the processes a clinician applies while rendering clinical care and the outcomes resulting from applying those processes.' Therefore, measuring performance means measuring processes and outcomes. HAI-related processes and outcomes have been discussed in the section on 'Components of Quality.'

How Can Performance Be Measured?

There are four steps in measuring a process. These include:

1. Define the processes to be measured.
2. Identify the population of patients in whom the process is to be measured (the denominator).
3. Count the number of times a physician carries out the process in daily practice (the numerator).
4. Divide the numerator by the denominator.

The process measure is the ratio of the number of times the physician carried out the process (the numerator) divided by the number of times carrying out the process would be appropriate (the denominator). Or it may be expressed as a percentage of patients in whom the set criteria is achieved. If the level of performance is defined, it becomes the target to be achieved. (See Chapter 6.)

Important processes must be identified. What are the processes that matter? E.g. handwashing is of proven value.

Purpose of Performance Measurement

1. To improve quality of patient care: This is the most important purpose (prevent and manage HAI).
2. To hold healthcare workers accountable: This is not the primary purpose and is rarely done because the necessary tools for risk adjustment do not exist and the amount of scientific data required to have meaningful interpretation (scientific validity) is unavailable.
3. To identify high performers and learn from their methods (individuals and institutions).

What Should Be the Measure of Performance-Process or Outcome?

Emphasis should be placed on proactively correcting processes and bringing about reduction in variation, rather than reacting to, or correcting, outcome. The core of the planning process is the use of certain tools intended to gain valuable insights into performance (through process). One of the problems of performance measurement is that, before a process is incorporated into a performance measurement set, scientific evidence must exist documenting that compliance with the process improves patient outcome. Unfortunately, many widely accepted processes have not been scientifically validated to show that they lead to improved patient outcomes. Nevertheless, considerable progress has been made in this field.[12, 13]

Performance Measurement through Outcomes

Measuring outcomes is confusing and difficult because variables contribute to patient outcomes that are not under the control of the clinician. Measuring a performance is relevant only to the extent that the clinician has control over the variables being measured. To be meaningful, that number has to be corrected for a host of variables that were not under the clinician's control. That is, the outcome measure has to be 'risk adjusted'. In case of poor or adverse outcomes, risk adjustment models are not foolproof. Data on a large number of risk factors must be collected on every outcome requiring risk adjustments. This can be a considerable burden because data on ten or more risk factors may have to be collected for every outcome data element collected. A step further is the concept of performance management where a number of tools can be used to improve performance.[14, 15]

Tools for managing performance (individually and collectively) must be understood. (See chapter on managing clinical performance.)

CONCEPTS OF QUALITY ASSESSMENT AND MEASUREMENT

With the advent of quality management it became necessary to 'assess quality' and measures to ensure a 'quality' product or service. These concepts need to be applied to infection-control policies too in the healthcare systems, especially in the control of serious nosocomial infections.[16] Quality assessment is a broad term used to describe a company or organization-wide review (in this case, healthcare setting) of the status of quality. Assessment of quality comprises four elements:

1. Cost of poor quality
2. Standing in the market place
3. Quality culture in the organization (see definition of culture in the chapter 'Road Maps and Direction')
4. Operation of the organizational quality system[17-18]

THE TERMINOLOGY MAZE

Quality measurement became a mandatory and contractual obligation for doctors in many countries in the 1990s in order to achieve and maintain a high standard of healthcare delivery. There are a number of terms used in place of 'medical care evaluation' (permutations and combinations produce 96 phrases).[19]

I. Medical = health, clinical, professional

II. Care = standards, activity, quality, review, monitoring

III. Evaluation = assessment, assurance, audit

TERMS USED IN QUALITY MEASUREMENT

Quality Control

The term 'control' refers to the process employed in order to meet standards. This consists of observing actual performance, comparing the performance with some standard, and then taking action if the observed performance is significantly different from the standard.

In healthcare services, it generally refers to laboratory tests and deals with eliminating variation and errors in the testing processes. This may at the most be considered a part of, but not synonymous with quality assurance. Control, one of the triology of quality processes, is largely directed to meeting goals and preventing adverse change, i.e. holding status quo. The term quality control is now restricted to an activity under Internal Quality Control (IQC) and includes certain activities in laboratories, e.g. control of stains, media, reagents. etc.

Quality Assurance (QA)

(Figure 5.2)

The methodology of QA is essentially a surveillance system referring to activities of people in achieving static standards and intervening if the undesirable results are higher than accepted standards. The goal of QA is that it is aimed at achieving a static standard or threshold. The problem identification process in QA has a major disadvantage. Instead of identifying problem processes it deals with problem people.[20, 21]

ISO 8402-1986 defines quality assurance as related to a product or service: It includes all those planned or systematic actions neces-

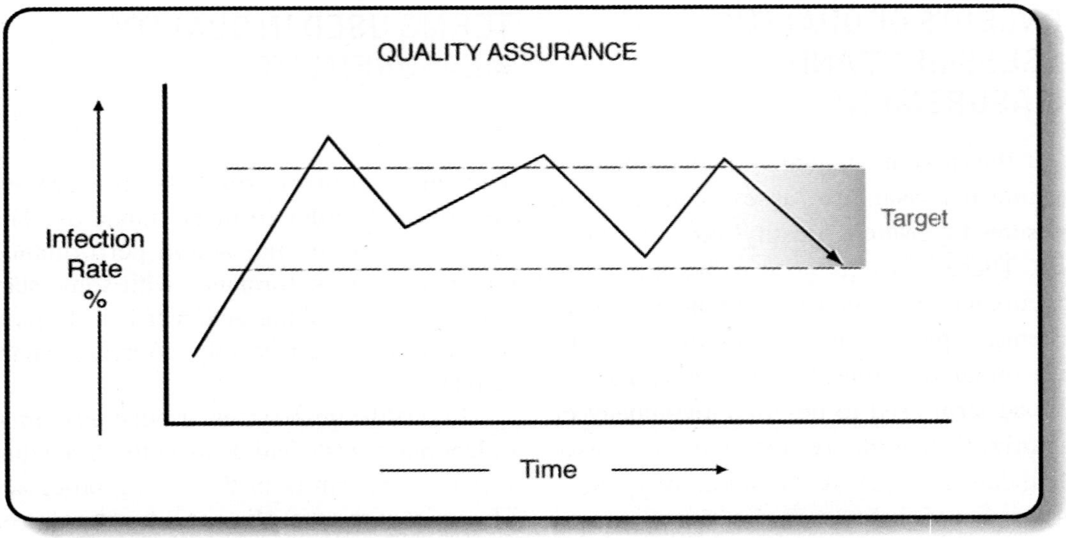

Figure 5.2: Quality assurance focuses on a 'status-quo' approach. The standards to be achieved are 'static'

sary to provide adequate confidence that a product or service will satisfy the requirements for quality. Quality assurance is a wide-ranging concept covering all matters that individually or collectively influence the quality of a product. It is a totality of arrangements made with the objective of ensuring that the product is of the quality required for its intended use. For example, in bacteriology and immunology, it spans a wide spectrum—from monitoring the performance of equipment and reagents to examining the clinical value of services and information. It combines IQC and external quality assessment (EQA). The aim of external quality assessment is to establish inter-hospital or inter-laboratory services. Both IQC and EQA are complementary in ensuring the reliability of the procedures, their results and the quality of the product.[22, 23]

Continuous Quality Improvement

(Figure 5.3)

A proactive method with the goal of identifying problem processes, with a never-ending attempt to better the processes, even if the quality is better than the accepted standard. Most importantly, this identifies problems in 'processes' rather than in 'people'. The goal is a continuous attempt at improvement.[21-24]

APPENDIX

Excerpts from World Medical Association Declaration with Guidelines for Continuous Quality Improvement in Healthcare

Adopted by the 49th World Medical Assem-

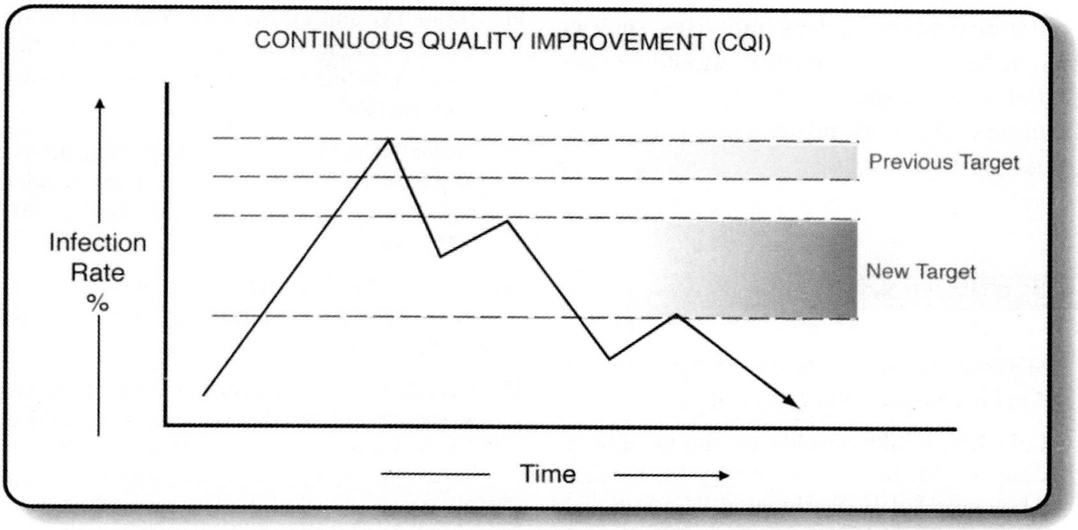

Figure 5.3: Continuous quality improvement is a constant effort to move from a previous to a new target (improve results)

bly, Hamburg, Germany, November 1997

(The World Medical Association, Inc. WMA policy. http://www.wma.net/e/policy/10-160_e.html)

Obligation for Quality Review

All physicians, other healthcare professionals (including health administrators) and institutions have to aspire to improve their work. Active participation by everyone in clinical audit and in quality review initiatives should be encouraged. Quality review evaluations can be used for independent external audit, with the aim of accreditation.

Standards for Good Quality Work

Those involved in work with patients need to specify the standards necessary for quality work and for the evaluation of the quality of the work. The resources and skill mix of staff within healthcare establishments should be adequate to attain the required standards of good quality work.

Recognition of Quality Review

All physicians should continuously evaluate the quality of their work and their level of ability by self-review methods. The quality of healthcare can be assessed by both internal and external methods. The agencies for both processes have to be widely approved, and the methods used must be generally accepted and based on research and sufficient knowledge.

Internal clinical peer review, observation of examination and of treatment methods, comparison with others, observation of the organization's ability to act and monitoring of the feedback from patients have to be continuous activities undertaken by every service provider.

External quality review initiatives, such as external peer review and audit, should be carried out with a frequency corresponding to the evolution of the field and always when there is special reason for it.

REFERENCES

1) Steffe GE. Quality Medical Care. A definition. J Am Med Assoc. 1998; 260(1): 56- 61.
2) Lohr KN. Health, Healthcare and Quality of Care. In: Medicare – A strategy for Quality Assurance Vol II. Washington DC: National Academy Press. 1990; 19-24.
3) Jo Harries – Wehling. Defining Quality of Care. In: Lohr KN ed. Medicare – A Strategy for Quality Assurance (Vol II). Washington DC National Academy Press. 1990; 124-139.
4) Donabedian A. Defining and measuring the quality of Healthcare. In: Wenzel RP, ed. Assessing Quality Healthcare. Perspective for clinicians. Baltimore : Williams & Wilkins. 1992; 41-64.
5) Donabedian A. Quality assessment and assurance: Unity of purpose, diversity of means. Inquiry. 1988; 25: 173-192.
6) Donabedian A. The quality of care: how can it be assessed? J Am Med Assoc 1988; 260(12): 1743-8.
7) Joiner GA, Salisbury D and Bollin GE. Utilizing quality assurance as a tool for reducing risk of nosocomial ventilator-associated pneumonia. Am J Med Qual 1996; 11(2): 100-103.
8) Marnoch G. Doctors and Management in the National Health Service. In: Ham C, Heginbotham C, Series eds. Health Services Management. Buckingham: Open University Press. 1996; 52-86.
9) Juran JM and Gryna FM. Manufacture In: Quality Planning and Analysis. 3rd edn, New Delhi: Tata McGraw-Hill Pubishing Company Limited. 1995; 343-376.
10) Fisher RB and Dearden CH. Improving the care of patients with major trauma in the accident and emergency department. Br Med J 1990; 300:1560-3.
11) Epstein AM. The outcomes movement – will it get us where we want to go? N Engl J Med 1990; 323: 266-9
12) Quaethoven P. Trends in Clinical Performance Measurement. Workshop on quality held on 23, September 2002 in Dresden. (http://www.epos.de/health/health-facility/dresden/trends.
13) Richards C, Emori TG, Peavy G et al. Promoting quality through measurement of performance and response: prevention success stories. Emerg Infect Dis. 2001; 7(2): 299-301.
14) Meehan TP, Chua-Reyes JM, Tate J et al. Process of care performance, patient characteristics, and outcomes in elderly patients hospitalized with community-acquired or nursing home-acquired pneumonia. Chest 2000; 117(5): 1378-85.
15) Schroeder SA. Outcome assessment 70 years late: are we ready? N Engl J Med 1987; 316(3): 160-1.
16) Berwick DM, Enthoven A and Bunker JP. Quality management in the NHS: the doctor's role-I. Br Med J. 1992; 304: 235-9.
17) Kumari S, Bhatia R and Heuck CC. Introduction in Quality Assurance in Bacteriology and Immunology, WHO Regional Publication, South- East Asia Series No.28. 1998; 1-9.
18) Lohr KN and Schroeder SA. A strategy for quality assurance in Medicare. N Engl J Med 1990; 322(10): 707-12
19) Prakash A. Definition and concept of Medical Audit. In:Medical Audit. Jaypee Brothers Medical Publishers. 2002; 17-24.

20) Berwick DM. Contiuous improvement as an ideal in healthcare. N Engl J Med. 1989; 320(1): 53-56.

21) Spencer EM, Mills AE, Rorty MV et al. Risk management and Quality Improvement Programmes. In: Organization Ethics in Health Care. New York: Oxford University Press. 2000; 171-185.

22) Kelleghan SI, Salemi C, Padilla S et al. An effective continuous quality improvement approach to the prevention of ventilator-associated pneumonia.Am J Infect Control. 1993; 21(6): 322-330.

23) McGowan H, Mattson S, Silva K et al. Interdepartmental intervention and surveillance for ventilator-associated pneumonia in critical care patients; a continuous quality improvement activity. Am J Infect Control. 1994; 22(2): 111.

24) O' Leary DS. Accreditation in the quality improvement mold – a vision for tomorrow. Quel Rev Bull. 1991; 27: 72-77.

Chapter 6

HAI and Continuous Quality Improvement—Implementation

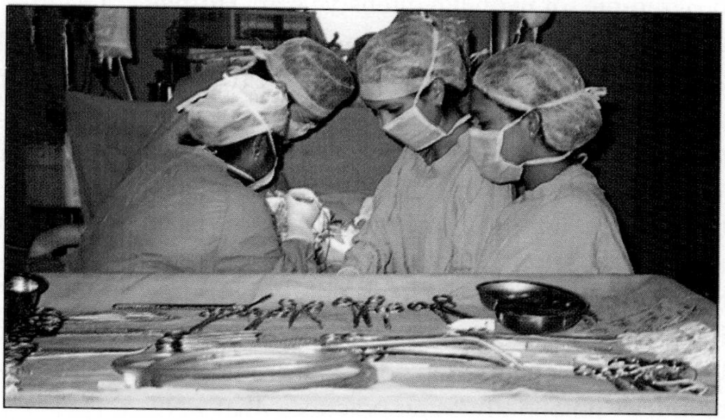

I know of no more encouraging a fact than the unquestionable ability of man to elevate his life by conscious endeavour.

—Henry David Thoreau

Highlights

Planning for Quality
Understanding Problems Related to HAI Control
Organizational Design and HAI
Fixing Staff Responsible for Infection Control: Primary, Secondary and Tertiary Levels
Defining the Roles (Job Description) in a Tertiary-Care Hospital

INTRODUCTION

The success of quality measurement and improvement has been shown in a number of studies. The use of quality improvement projects for making measurable improvements in quality with reduction in cost of care is being used in the area of hospital infection control. In a collaborative quality improvement programme for neonatal intensive care, Horbar et al have shown how a multidisciplinary model can be used.[1] A total of 76 neonatal ICUs participated in this study over a three-year period, forming multidisciplinary teams that worked under the direction of a trained facilitator. There was a drop in the infection rates in the ICUs from 22% to 16.6%. In this study the participants received instructions in quality improvement, reviewing performance data, identification of common goals and implementation of 'potentially better practices' that were developed through an analysis of the process of care and literature review. The conclusion was that this approach has the potential to improve outcomes in the neonatal ICUs. But before starting to evaluate the medical care provided by a hospital, certain conditions must be fulfilled.[2-4] (Photo 6.1)

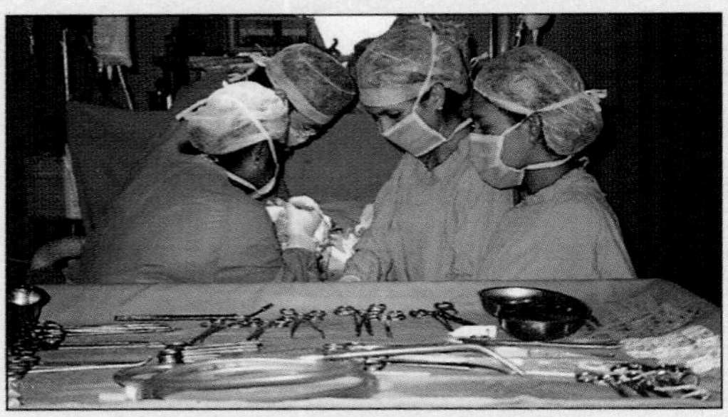

Photo 6.1: Hospital acquired infections can be brought down significantly by quality improvement techniques.

In another example, an 800-bed teaching hospital's rate of ventilator-associated nosocomial pneumonia in the surgical intensive care unit was 49.5 infections per 1,000 ventilator days. This was in excess of the 90th percentile.[5] Improving care, included changing tubing and cascades every 48 hours and Ambu bags every 24 hours, as well as increased clinical evaluation of patients was followed 12 months later by a decrease to 25.8 infections, well below the 90th percentile. Thus, the NNIS experience can be used as a source of guidance for assessing the effectiveness and utility of other indicator systems.[6]

ORGANIZING A QUALITY IMPROVEMENT PROGRAMME

Scope

Firstly, the scope of quality improvement process and evaluation should be delineated, which could be national, organizational, departmental or a specific programme related to HAI control. Whatever the scope, the principles remain the same.

Internal Audit

It is important to establish clearly as to who will evaluate the services provided, how often it should be done and whether qualitative or/and quantitative assessments have to be made. In order to facilitate evaluation by the medical audit committee, the clinical faculty and the infection-control committee should develop pre-determined acceptable norms with respect to common diagnoses handled under their specialities. Deviations from these norms can then be easily detected.

Clinical auditing may be a part of health promotion, improvement of the quality of practice, the improvement of clinical performance of doctors or as part of the annual internal audit.[7] Whatever the parameter, a definite and clear-cut goal must be set, which has a bearing upon the infection-control measures of the hospital and its promotion. Clinical auditing is done to improve patient care. It may be prospective or retrospective. A clinical audit is carried out by persons who are in the same area of work and who are also trained in auditing procedures. In the years to come, it is envisaged that clinical audit will be an important aspect of healthcare management.[8] An example of using national guidelines as audit criteria can be seen in the department of health, NHS, UK, where a system has developed based on national evidence-based guidelines for prevention of HAI.[9] In UK, the department of health guidelines provide local operational protocols, and these guidelines can be used as a benchmark for determining appropriate infection prevention decisions as a part of the reflective practice to assess clinical effectiveness. They also provide a basis for clinical audit, evaluation and education, and facilitate ongoing quality improvements. Consequently, they are aimed at hospital managers, HIC teams and individual healthcare practitioners. At an individual level, they are intended to influence the quality and clinical effectiveness of infection prevention decision-making. These guidelines can be used by practitioners, managers and others for the development of more detailed protocols and to ensure that all important standard principles for infection prevention are incorporated. The difference between these and the earlier guidelines is that they also become criteria for assessment of internal and external audit of these hospitals. Non-conformance to these standards and guidelines can lead to 1) action against the hospital (may lose licence/funding) 2) loss of accreditation 3) loss of public image 4) can also be used against erring individuals. Therefore, accountability must be built into the system.[10-15]

Accreditation (External Audit)

Accreditation involves an on-site survey of the hospital by a team of physicians, nurses and hospital administrators. During the survey, the team evaluates whether or not the hospital meets performance standards in a number of areas including patient safety and medical errors, pain management, medical staffing, infection control, laboratory practices and hospital management. There are different models which are followed by various health institutions, e.g. Malcolm Baldridge Model of Business Excellence, European Foundation for Quality Management EFQM Model, ISO 9000 and JCAHO. The ultimate aim of these agencies is to audit and improve quality.[16]

Role of Clinicians

Traditionally, an infection control committee plays a major role in quality assessment. The shift of emphasis from quality assurance to continuous quality improvement methodology will require the continued involvement of everyone. The first step is to form a multidisciplinary committee to address the problems of infection-control. Depending on the area (operating room, intensive care unit) they are dealing with, the committee should include members who have a common goal, have complementry skills and are committed to each other's goals and success.[17] For example, a team looking into nosocomial pneumonia should consist of representatives from respiratory therapy, nursing, intensive care nurse managers, pulmonary critical care, infectious diseases, infection control, quality health, internal medicine and surgery. The committee should meet at frequent (at least once a month) intervals. In other words, leadership and organization has been found to be effective when the persons involved are empowered to make changes (see chapter 4).

Clinicians must develop focused programmes for the prevention of nosocomial infections in their domains.[18] Quality improvement programmes must be embraced at the institutional level (involvement of top management) and clinicians at all levels. Only in this way can hospitals hope to successfully reduce their rates of nosocomial infections (e.g. VAP) and sustain or improve their efforts over time.[19]

PROCESS OF QUALITY IMPROVEMENT

The PDCA Cycle

(Figure 6.1, 6.2)

Deming, an American management theorist, described quality in terms of systems and processes within a set-up, believing that the system and management are the cause of any failure. He believed that everybody working in a system must be involved in the transformation to a better system and his approach was statistical in nature. One of the hallmarks of the Deming approach is the use of the PDCA (Plan-Do-Check-Act) cycle. The steps are essentially a restatement of a scientific method involving planning a project , execut-

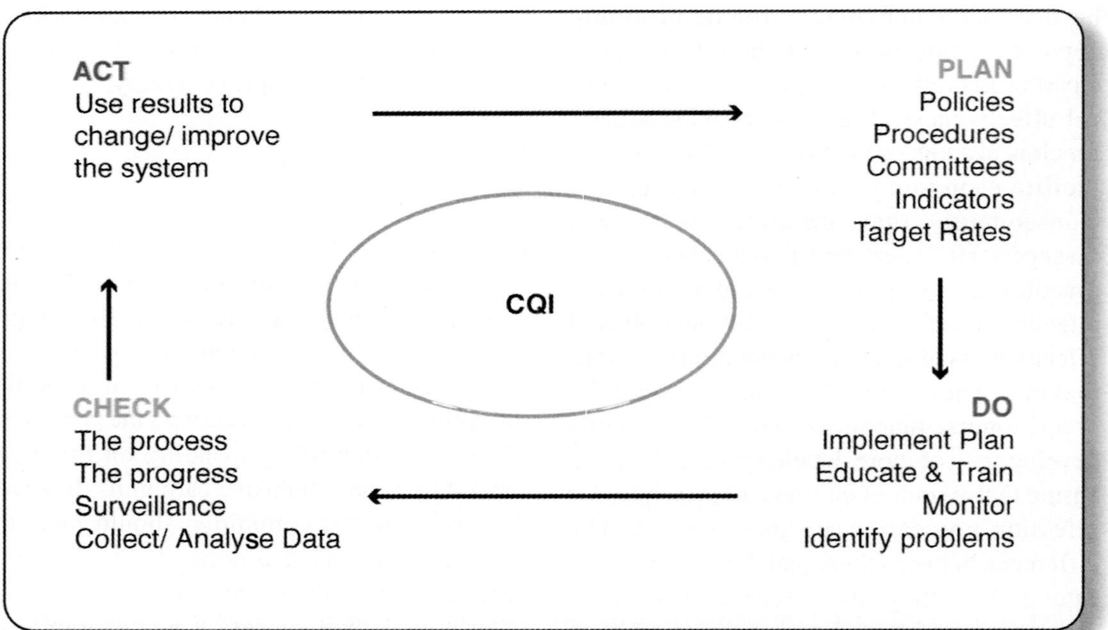

Figure 6.1: The PDCA cycle has four steps: Plan, Do, Check, Act

ing a project, examining the results and then using the results to readjust. One must cease dependence on inspection to achieve quality by building quality into the product, but at the same time minimizing the total cost. Improvise constantly and for ever, the system of production and service, to improve quality and productivity.

This may be carried out by using the Plan-Do-Check-Act (PDCA) cycle. Plan-Do-Check-Act Cycle (PDCA) is a process for quality improvement developed for quality control by Walter Shewhart and adapted for total quality management by W. Edwards Deming[20] (see Figs. 6.1, 6.2).

The continuous quality improvement process was formulated by the JCAHO as part of its agenda for change in accreditation programme for hospitals. It is an expansion of the PDCA with a ten-step procedure involving:

- The identification of responsibility
- Scope
- Priorities (which programme to tackle first)
- Verification of indicators
- Thresholds
- Analysis
- Planning
- Taking action
- Evaluation and
- Communication

Re-Engineering vs Quality Improvement

(Figures 6.3, 6.4)

Re-engineering is slightly different from CQI. This is defined as a fundamental process of rethinking and radical redesigning of processes to achieve dramatic improvement in performance. When it is adapted to healthcare delivery, the term clinical re-engineering is used. Intensive care activities where bench-

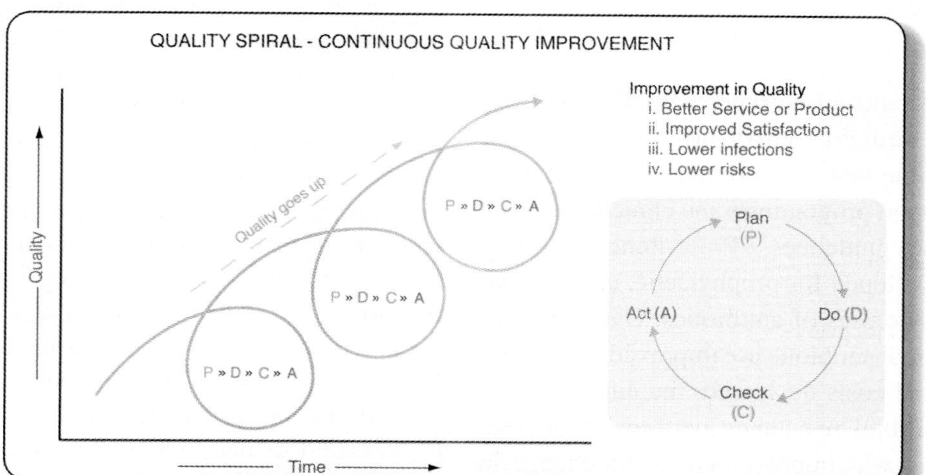

Figure 6.2: The quality spiral uses the PDCA cycle to improve constantly

marking and clinical re-engineering have been used to improve performance include ventilator weaning, catheter-related infections and antibiotic utilization, all of which can be found in literature.[21] A fine example of performance improvement using bench-marking and clinical re-engineering is their use in improving antibiotic utilization.

Benchmark: The overall performance or the performance in a specific case of an organization or individual that is judged to represent the best achievable standard for a product.

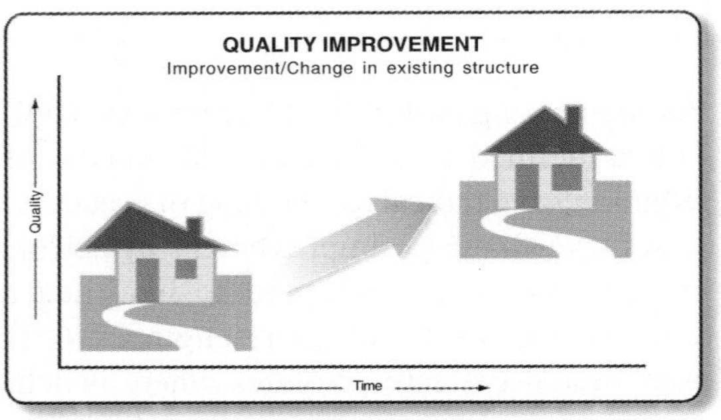

Figure 6.3: Quality improvement brings about changes in the existing structure

Pesotnik and co-workers have developed a comprehensive antibiotic management programme that used computer-assisted decision support programmes and clinician-derived consensus guidelines.[22] Prescribing guidelines were developed for prophylactic, empiric and therapeutic uses of antibiotics. Over a seven-year period, antibiotic use improved, antibiotic-associated costs decreased, the emergence of antimicrobial resistance patterns stabilized, and there was improvement or no change in outcomes and antibiotic complications.[23]

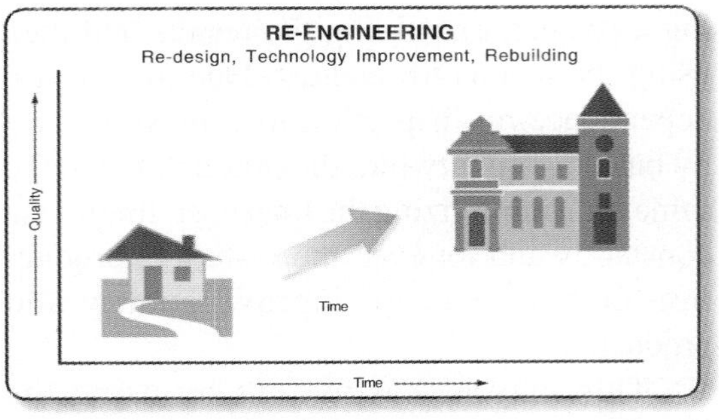

Figure 6.4: Re-engineering is a radical redesigning of the structure

PLAN - Do - Check - Act

Organizing Information for Planning

For quality improvement, information is the core basis of change. In other words, changing a system requires information. Information could be retrospective or prospective, clinical or non-clinical. Standards may be set for the first data collection, or it may be just to establish where one is heading in their infection-control activities. Some topics involve aspects of care, and it is advisable not to audit too many such aspects at the same time, because the audit then becomes unmanageable and complex.

Ideas, existing knowledge or data generated are the pieces of information used for planning, building structures and processes.The processes which are adopted should have in- built mechanisms for organized documentation, prospective collection and data evaluation. These are used for bringing about meaningful change. Records must contain details about the diagnosis and treatment of HAI. Any medical information specific to HAI is important for surveillance and hence advised to be coded as per CDC codes. Information on HAI can easily be collected in in-patient facilities, but information on out-patient and domiciliary patients is often difficult to document. Healthcare organizations must develop systems to store, record and utilize this information for improvement. Information about HAI is often undisclosed or unrecorded, fearing litigation. Information of epidemiological importance must be available to the HCW coming in contact with the patient (at the same time maintaining confidentiality) and the relevant information must be sent to appropriate bodies as per national and international guidelines.

Looking for Opportunities for Improvement

- Brainstorming sessions
- Reviewing existing policies
- Identifying the quality of current care: Data collection is done first to establish and identify the current position or quality of care.[24] Next, deficiencies are identified by comparing with existing standards.
- Identifying reasons for the inadequacy, if any

Data Collection

Medical information systems

Medical information systems include equipment or procedures (processes) for the collection, recording, processing, storage, retrieval and display of clinical or non-clinical information. Information can also be used for diagnosis, audit, surveillance or therapy. Advanced information systems are available for surveillance of HAI. These facilities use ICD-9 and various other codes available from various administrative databases. Automated systems for antibiotic prescribing are available. Special softwares are available for audit and surveillance to facilitate infection control activities and decrease the time spent on performing reviews.

Data collection personnel

One must understand that the infection-control data can be either a part of the area-specific audit or it may be done as a separate exercise or both. The data-collecting personnel should understand the why and how of collection (identify sources of data). Whoever collects the HAI-related data should be competent to make judgements on clinical subjects. Since this is a specialized job, people involved in the hospital infection control committee, nurses involved in the hospital infection programme, clinicians in their respective areas of work, physiotherapists, managers, hospital epidemiologists, microbiologists, laboratory health workers, etc. may be involved in this work.

Medical records

The importance of maintaining medical records is well known. Most hospitals around the globe practise it in some form or the other. The well-equipped and conscientious hospitals maintain computerized records in the form of data sheets and take daily printouts. This is an ideal method with a ready-reckoner data analysis especially for comparison of data between wards, departments, hospitals or even countries. Such data can also be linked across countries and continents through standardized software programmes like the WHO-NET or the infection-control computerized package—(WHO CARE). The above-mentioned methods, although desirable, are not always feasible. Hence, every hospital devises its own methods of record-keeping. Maintenance of records would not serve its intended purpose if the results/statistics are not made known to hospital authorities and personnel concerned, especially the hospital infection-control team.

Hence, a monthly, bi-monthly or a quarterly report must be submitted to the infection-control committee for scrutiny and appropriate action.

Organizing Data and Information

Newer ways of designing, improving and understanding processes and their pathways, redundancies, inefficiencies and misunderstandings are given below:

HAI-related data can be used for

- Diagnosis
- Treatment
- Surveillance
- Audit
- Quality improvement
- Epidemiological purposes
- Structure, Process and outcome monitoring
- Clinical records for medicolegal purposes
- Research
- Education

1. Flow charts

(Photo 6.2) (Figure 6.5)

Linking issues or problems in a logical sequence with a main objective of identifying the actual path a process follows. It is also made to identify who is responsible for the decisions.

2. Causal diagram or Fishbone diagram (the Ishikawa diagram)

(Figure 6.6)

Some institutions prefer to put them down as fish-bone charts (or the cause-and-effect chart) which depict all the causes of an outcome in a logical way to facilitate the identification of a problem. Studies show that such charts have a high user applicability because they are presented in a user-friendly design that allows the evaluator to map out causal relationship between primary goal and process factors that either facilitate or impede accomplishment of that goal. E.g. Used for quality improvement in the ICU for nosocomial pneumonia.[19] Fishbone chart is a depiction of relationships between outcome and effect and its contributors or causes.

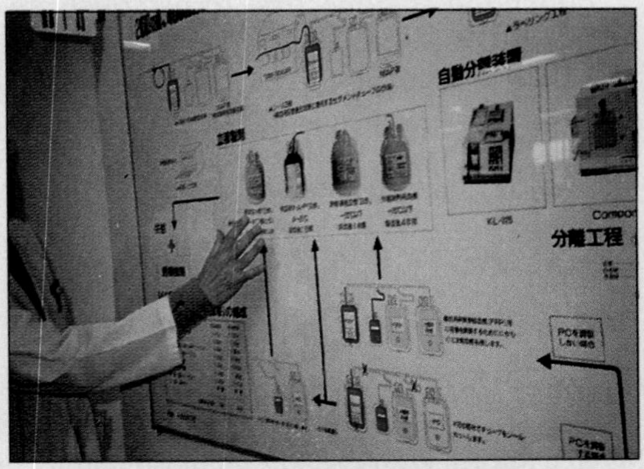

Photo 6.2: A simple flow diagram at a blood bank in Japan used to educate employees.

3. Force field analysis

In addition to identifying causal relationship, the forcefield diagram provides an estimate of the relative effect each process factor has on the outcome measure and the expected direction of the effect (i.e. positive or negative). Figure

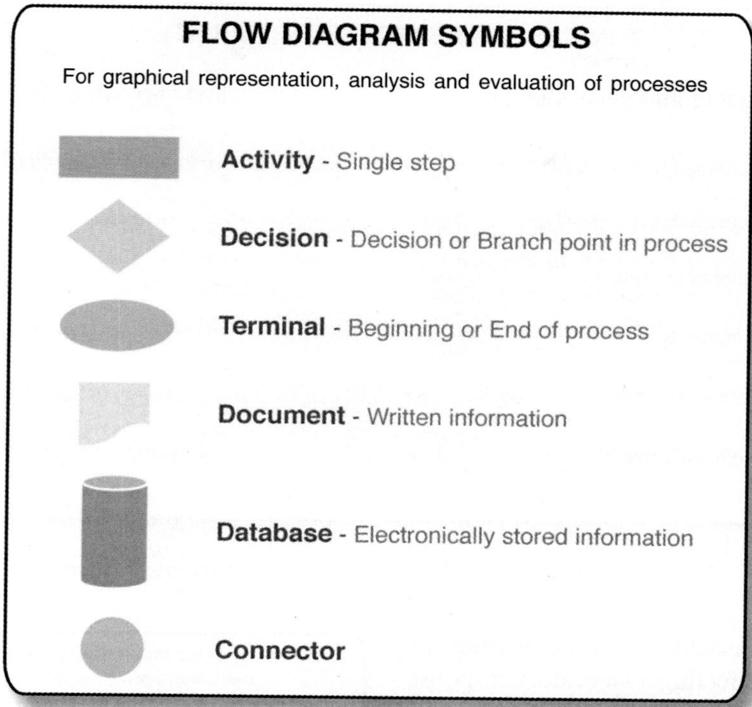

Figure 6.5: Commonly used flow diagram symbols to graphically portray a process

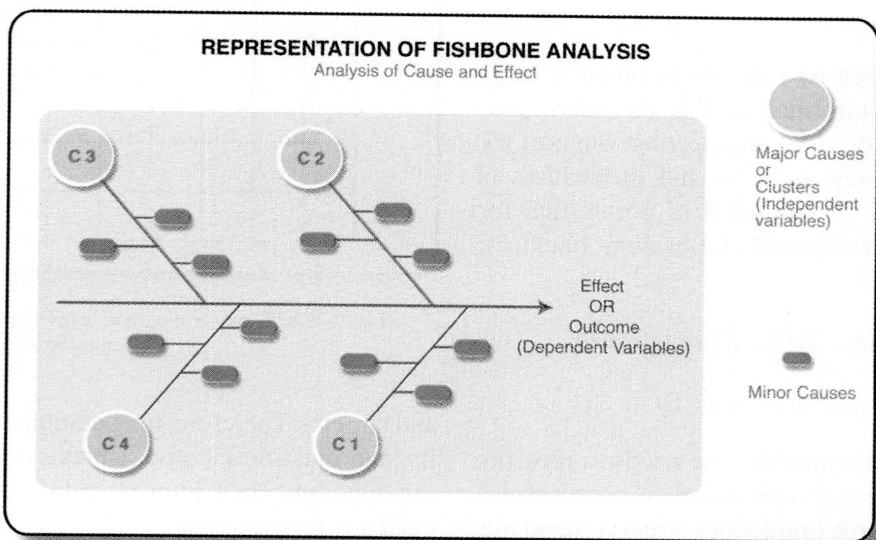

Figure 6.6: A depiction of relationships between causes and outcome: Fishbone diagram

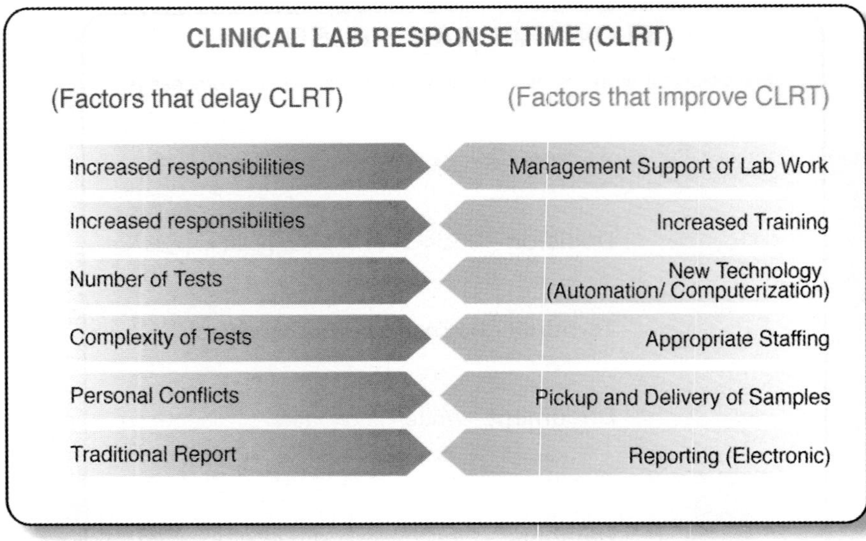

Figure 6.7: A force field analysis of a clinical laboratory response time

6.7 shows a forcefield diagram depicting the various factors affecting a laboratory response time. This is used to improve outcome.

4. Matrix diagram

(Figure 6.8)

These are used by planners to organize large amounts of information. E.g. the matrix diagram used for value engineering. Support for instituting new policies and procedures is obtained to get approval of committee for resources, personnel, laboratory backups, etc.[25]

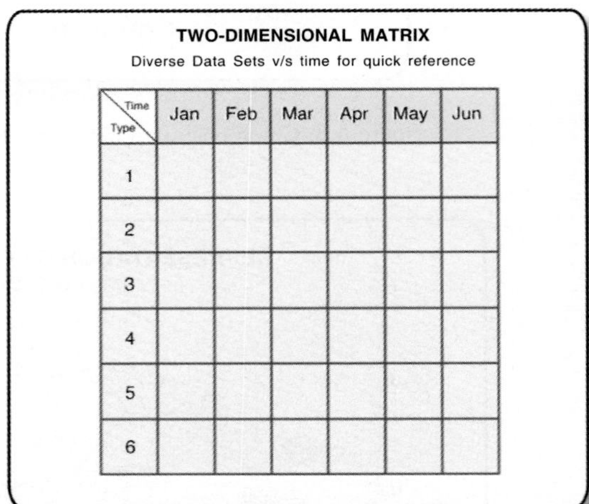

Figure 6.8: A matrix diagram helps organize large amounts of information

Plan - DO - Check - Act

Operationalizing Quality

To incorporate quality, one needs to measure clinical care activities and their conformance to set standards (guidelines, criteria, standards and targets). Therefore, to operationalize quality one must define and achieve certain parameters and then improvise in subsequent cycles.

Guidelines, Criteria, Standards and Targets

Guidelines

They can be defined as systematically developed statements to assist practitioner and patient decisions prospectively for specific clinical circumstances; in essence 'the right thing to do'.

Indicator

A measurable element of practice performance for which there is evidence or consensus that it can be used to assess quality, and hence change in quality, of care provided. They can measure activity (performance/process/activity indicator) or frequency with which an event occurred, such as influenza vaccinations.

Indicators can be of different types

a. Outcome indicators measure morbidity, mortality, health status, health-related quality of life and patient satisfaction.

b. Structural indicators give information on the organization such as personnel, finances, availability of appointments.

c. Process indicators describe actual medical care such as diagnosis, treatment, referral and prescribing. Since the focus is on quality improvement, the main emphasis is on process indicators, because improving the process has been described as the primary object of quality assessment/improvement.

Therefore, indicators are explicitly defined as measurable items which act as building blocks in the assessment of care. They shed light on the structure, process (inter-personal or clinical) and outcomes of care and are used to generate subsequent review criteria and standards which will help to operationalize quality indicators.They can infer a judgement on the quality of care provided (quality indicator).

Quality indicators

Clinical quality indicators are used to evaluate efficacy of efforts to prevent nosocomial infections. A clinical indicator may be defined as 'a quantitative measure that can be used as a guide to monitor and evaluate the quality of important patient care and support service activities.'

Quality indicators are not chosen randomly. They need to be developed and prioritized, because all processes are not equally important. Processes and outcomes which are chosen should be such that there is scientific evidence to prove that the specific process chosen for measurement makes a difference to the outcomes. Therefore, indicators must be developed by one of the three ways:

1. Systematically (evidenced-based)—by various techniques such as the Delphi technique or the RAND method.
2. Non-systematically (non-evidence-based)
3. Systematic (evidence-based) combined with consensus

Each clinical quality indicator has a threshold above which a detailed review is indicated.

A quicker method of selecting HAI-related indicators is to look at those recommended by important bodies such as the National Information Services and Systems (NISS) which provide standardized methods of data collection—indicators, device-associated rates and procedures for risk adjustment of data for improving quality and for inter-hospital comparison. Each clinical quality indicator has a threshold above which a detailed review is indicated and should be set up.[19, 24-26]

Indicators are discussed in various chapters

a. Chapter on clinical performance monitoring

b. Chapter on antibiotic policy

c. Chapter on practice guidelines– Definitions and indicators of major infections such as urinary tract infections, catheter related infections, nosocomial pneumonia, surgical skin infections

Some examples of indicators are given below[27]:

1. Hygiene practices

Objective: Monitoring of compliance with, and quality assessment of, hygienic practices

$$\text{Indicators} = \frac{\text{Numerator: Patient care procedures performed with appropriate hygiene precautions}}{\text{Denominator: Procedures requiring appropriate standard hygiene precautions/patient census/density of care of index}}$$

2. Antibiotic usage *(see chapter 19)*

Objective: Continuous monitoring and quality assessment of antibiotic utilization patterns

$$\text{Indicators} = \frac{\text{Numerator: Type of antimicrobial cures/doses and duration used for prophylaxis and treatment}}{\text{Denominator: Surgical interventions/documented infections (e.g. Bacteremia)/ patient admissions}}$$

Source of Data: Pharmacy records,operating room records, medical and nursing records, chart review, computerised patient records

3. Incidence of hospital infection

Objective: continuous monitoring of incidence of infection hospital-wide or selective cases

$$\text{Indicators} = \frac{\text{Numerator: Infection by site/ ward/procedure or device.}}{\text{Denominator: Patient admissions, hospital days/procedures/device-days}}$$

Source of Data: Laboratory and ward liaison, chart review,computerised record.

4. Prevalence of hospital infection

Objective: Periodic assessment of prevalence of infection, hospital-wide or in selective areas

$$\text{Indicators} = \frac{\text{Numerator: Infection by site/ ward/procedure or device}}{\text{Denominator: Patient census on the day of survey/procedures or device.}}$$

Source of Data: Laboratory and ward liaison, chart review, computerised record.

5. Outbreak warning

Objective: Detection and cluster analysis of transmissible organisms.

$$\text{Indicators} = \frac{\text{Numerator: Colonization/ or infection by specific microorganism}}{\text{Denominator: Patient admissions/ hospital days/procedure/ device-days}}$$

Source of Data: Laboratory-based study.

Infection-control indicator checklist by WHO (World Health Organization) [25]

Indicator 1: Sharps are handled safely to minimize the risk of sharps injury

Indicator 2: Instruments decontaminated fully

Indicator 3: Hands are washed appropriately to prevent cross infection[28]

Indicator 4 : Protective barrier is worn to prevent exposure to blood

Indicator 5: Waste disposed of safely

If Indicators Are Not Defined or Available

- Look for previous benchmark rates in your hospital or those set by bodies such as the NISS.
- If not available, conduct surveillance (active surveillance preferred) so that such baseline rates may be determined. Whole-house surveillance vs unit-based surveillance, reporting by laboratory or hospital staff of usual clusters is an additional means of data collection. Infection-control department or department of epidemiology usually conducts the surveillance.
- Inter-institutional rates cannot be compared without standardization of the case definition.

Indicators are used to indicate the quality of the structure, processes, outcomes and services. But there are a number of other aspects of care which need not be used as indicators but may be used as review criteria to assess or evaluate the care given (e.g. criteria-based audit).

A Review Criterion

A review criterion is a systematically developed statement relating to a single act of medical care that is so clearly defined, it is possible to say whether the element of care occurred or not retrospectively in order to assess the appropriateness of specific healthcare decisions, services and outcomes. Criteria are usually in the form of statements. E.g. all healthcare workers must wash hands before touching a patient. The three requirements of good criteria are 1) clinically relevant 2) clearly defined 3) easily measured. Criterion is the objective to be achieved. A criterion is an aspect of care which is usually a consensus opinion of a team of clinicians; (more than one criterion is criteria).

- All-or-none criteria
- A cut-off level criteria distinguishing between adequate or inadequate care.
- Other types of criteria may not be as straightforward—e.g. quality of life or cognitive function.
- Criteria can also be classified as objective/explicit and subjective/implicit where clinical judgement is used instead of measurable data.

Standard

The level of compliance with a criterion or indicator is called standard. A standard is expressed as a percentage of a criterion. It is important to stress that the standard a practice sets is what is right for the practice because practices differ so much.

Target standard

Target standard is set prospectively and stipulates a level of care that providers must strive to meet. The target is the proportion of patients in whom the criterion should be met. The target should be stated before the audit is undertaken. Unstated targets can lead to a vindication of the present practice, whether it be good or bad. The target must be realistic and attainable.

Achieved standard

Achieved standard is measured retrospectively and details whether a care provider met a predetermined standard.

Standard = criterion + performance

A standard is a statement of what the practice thinks it is achieving in the first audit cycle, and something to aim at in subsequent audit cycles.

Examples of—
Guideline

In the intensive care there is a link between raised blood sugar levels and increased nosocomial infections. If the blood sugar is raised, then the patient must have blood sugar controlled with monitoring at x time intervals.

Indicator

Patients with raised blood sugar above 150mg% should have their blood sugars measured every fourth hour.

Indicator numerator: Patients with blood sugar above 150mg% having had remeasured their sugars within four hours

Denominator: Patients with blood sugar of more than 150mg%.

Review criterion: If a patient's blood sugar was above 150mg % was it measured in four hours?

Standard: Target standard: 90% patients in ICU with blood sugar more than 150mg % should have their blood sugars measured in four hours.

Achieved standard: 80% patients in ICU with blood sugar more than 150mg % had their blood sugars measured in four hours.

Setting up clinical quality improvement (PDCA)

Select topic (structure, process, outcome)

a. Set indicators, criteria and standards

b. Assess practice—efficacy (A) effectiveness (B)

c. Compliance (A = B)

d. Non-compliance (A not equal to B)

e. Institute change

Efficacy: Optimal care under ideal conditions (not perfect care)

Effectiveness: usual care under present conditions (diagnosis, treatment, process, procedure, etc.)

Efficiency: Getting the maximum output with minimum input such as people, money and equipment (A measure of the degree to which the costs of resources used in a diagnosis, treatment or procedure)

Plan - Do - CHECK - Act

Surveillance

a. Once CQI is implemented, ongoing

surveillance provides the data with which to measure its effectiveness.

b. Process surveillance is a vital component of programme evaluation and is defined as 'consistent and quantitative monitoring of practices that directly or indirectly contribute to a health outcome and the use of those data to improve outcomes'.

c. Processess to be monitored are to be prioritized. In the case of preventive efforts it is important to examine the relative importance of risk factors to determine where effort must be directed. The outcome of the process to be targeted must be identified. E.g. compliance with handwashing, procedure followed for suctioning in ICU, frequency of suctioning, etc.

d. Statistical quality control is composed of process analysis, which is used to understand cause and effect, and process control, which, in turn, is used to determine whether the system is functioning normally.

e. Compliance with procedure and policy must be evaluated.

f. Quality improvement in process can only come about if there is a mechanism for use of collected data to impact upon clinical practice (audit).

g. The feedback is given to caregivers. Feedback may be in the form of infection rates, trend charts, etc.

h. Once CQI is implemented, ongoing surveillance provides the data with which to measure its effectiveness.

The above steps may be illustrated in a model called the Plan-Do-Check-Act (PDCA) cycle.

Audit—A Tool for Quality Improvement

Audit is a process that tells you whether you are actually doing what you are supposed to be doing. Research is a process which tries to find out what you should be doing to your patients. Therefore, collecting data for audit of hospital acquired infections must have specific targets and goals in each area of the hospital set-up. The sample estimation must be done from a statistical point of view. The sampling methods could be random, systematic, stratified or cluster.

The audit cycle

(Figure 6.9)

Audit is the process by which results are compared with the intended objectives. In other words, it is the assessment of how well a programme is functioning. Audit should always be considered during the planning and implementation stages of a programme or activity. Evaluation may be crucial in identifying the health benefits derived (i.e., the impact on morbidity, mortality, sequelae, patient satisfaction). Evaluation can be useful in identifying performance difficulties. Evaluation studies may also be carried out to generate information for other purposes, e.g., to attract attention to a problem, extension of control activities, training and patient management, etc. It is carried out by matching the procedures against approved standards, which are laid down on the basis of medical knowledge that provides us with the information about what should be done in order to achieve the best results.

The differences are subtle. Clinical audit is different from surveillance and research. It

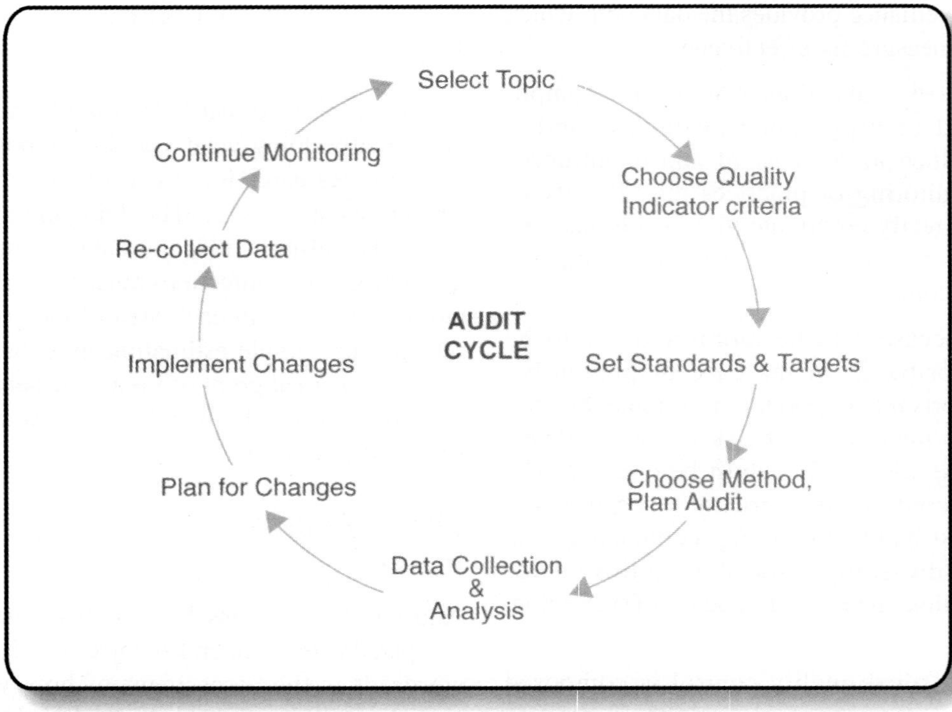

Figure 6.9: Steps of an audit cycle

is to evaluate and improve existing practices. This also requires an infrastructure for data collection. Sentinel case and criterion-based audit require high-quality medical record system and medical notes, through formats designed to assist the clerking of patients admitted with a particular problem for which the audit is being carried out or to provide a summary of their admission to hospital. Appropriate accumulated data has to be analysed and presented in an understandable manner. Unlike research data, the audit data is not intended to prove or disprove a hypothesis. Therefore, it requires only enough scientific rigour to convince the participants of the kind of changes brought about.

Audit should not be confused with

- Clinical research (which generates new knowledge having a general application influencing medical practice as a whole)
- Survey (Here the purpose is different)
- Surveillance
- Process monitoring
- Routine data collection (does not lead to improvements in delivery of healthcare)
- Industrial quality assurance (Human well being and the healthcare industry are infinitely more complex than production lines.)

There are also companies which specialize in the area of auditing and conduct the collection of data and help in the process of auditing. This is fast becoming a specialized job and a person needs to be trained in the process of planning and executing an audit. There are a number of areas which have been simplified by the use of computers and these include:

- Processing
- Preparing documents
- Storing data
- Manipulation of data

1. There are many types of software available for helping in data collection and auditing. These pieces of software specialize in specific areas of auditing. For example, ICU.
2. Clinical Audit may be carried out as a prospective or a retrospective procedure. The latter procedure is often performed to evaluate the effectiveness of infection-control procedures. Such an audit study was carried out in Sheffield, UK, and proved useful in many ways.[8, 12-15]

A criteria-based audit

The audit should be clinically important and relevant. One of the methods of prioritizing topics for audit is the use of Seedhouse Rings of Uncertainity. Criteria-based audit sees or notes departure from specified criteria (of structure, process or outcome).[15] The process of criterion-based audit is as follows:

- Define and agree on the standard (criteria in this case). E.g. protocols of management.
- Then measure the performance against the standard.
- Agree on changes to improve the performance against the standard.
- Repeat audit to ensure that the changes have had the desired and intended effect.

Criteria can be direct observation of clinical process

a. Surgical scrub
b. Diagnosis of nosocomial pneumonia (clinical, sampling, diagnostic criteria, laboratory response time etc.)

Quality assessment and auditing organizations

Parameters given below are from the quality assurance model of JCAHO.[16-17]

Normative weighted criteria

The following parameters related to HAI have been weighted as per their relative importance. They have been divided into structure, process and outcome criteria. The mentioned maximum weight that may be granted to a particular parameter is given.[17]

Structure Criteria

- Has a well-enunciated hospital infection-control committee incorporating a hospital administrator, microbiologist, clinician and a nursing administrator________ 5
- Has a functional hospital infection-control team incorporating microbiologist, nursing staff, house keeping staff and an epidemi ologist ________________ 5
- There exists a specific job description for each personnel of the above committee ________

____
____
______________________________ 5

- Physical facilities are conducive for prevention of hospital infection such as ward design, bed spacing, flooring, isolation rooms, drainage, etc.__________ 5
- House keeping services and biomedical waste management are appropriately incorporated into the hospital infection-control programme.__________
______________________________ 5
- Procedures and Policies

  Has well-enunciated principles of hospital infection control so as to eliminate sources of infection, and routes of spread. Has in place a system for surveillance of infection and investigations during outbreaks __________
  ____
  ____
  ______________________________ 5
- Existence of comprehensive standard operative procedures (SOPs) for hospital infection control programme including disinfection and sterilization of equipment, standard precautions, protective vaccinations (for hepatitis, tetanus and gas gangrene) use of disposables, housekeeping, disinfectants, handling of specimens, barrier and reverse barrier nursing. ____
  ______________________________ 5
- Has a functional antibiotic policy.______
  ____
  ______________________________ 5
- Has an interactive interdepartmental co-ordination with reference to hospital infection control programme including services such as housekeeping, CSSD and dietetics.__________
  ____
  ____
  ______________________________ 5

Process Criteria

- Scientific data collection and analysis related to hospital infection-control programme during surveillance and investigation of HAI. Comprehensive documentation exists. __________
  ______________________________ 5
- Scientific sample collection and laboratory investigation. Molecular methods are being utilized in laboratory investigations for HAI.__________ 5
- Internal and exernal audit for laboratory investigations. __________
  ______________________________ 5
- Awareness levels amongst various staff personnel regarding HAI.__________ 5
- Training and re-orientation programmes being conducted related to HAI. ____ 5
- Cost evaluation analysis for antibiotic usage, HAI etc. __________
  ____
  ______________________________ 5
- Activities aimed for achievement of CQI.
  ____
  ______________________________ 5

Outcome Criteria

- Hospital infection rate vis-a-vis incidence at local/national/international levels. 10
- Satisfactory internal and external laboratory audit.__________

______________________________ 5

- Staff and patient satisfaction. __________
____
______________________________ 5

Total credit points

The grading may be done as follows:

80–100	A++	(Outstanding)
70–80	A+	(Very good)
60–70	A	(Good)
50–60	B	(Average)
Below 50	C	(Below average)

The above-suggested credit parameter gradings may be modified appropriately for various health institutions.[17]

One has to keep in mind that quality is not a number and is a function of positive perceptions. It includes good intentions, sincere efforts, intelligent direction and skilful execution. All dimensions of quality must receive due weightage. The other important element in the area of service is the concept of consideration (elements of consideration include price plus the loss of dignity, waiting time, anxiety, etc.) The healthcare system in India is diversified and divergent with a drastic difference in the urban and rural areas. Thus the quality indicators must be appropriately defined.

Analysis and presentation of data

All accumulated data have to be analysed and presented in an understandable manner.

Primary statistical analysis in audit is deciding whether the observed quality is up to the standard. This involves a one-sample test of proportions. Deciding whether care has improved following an intervention involves a two-sample test on proportions. The other statistical methods concern ways in which data can be displayed so that they may be more easily understood. Because they are observational rather than experimental, audit data are subject to numerous biases and must be interpreted with care. Data must be available to the end-users so that they can take necessary action in their respective areas.

In an internal audit the internal audit committee analyses the data.

In a national audit the data is processed and audited at a national level.

In an external audit an external body conducts the audit and this is also used for the accreditation status of the hospital. The most important aspect is that the data must be used to bring about change.

Any pitfalls in the existing systems of healthcare have to be recorded, analysed and submitted for perusal. Necessary changes to be brought about must be clearly stated.

The audit cycle

(Figure 6.9)

The process of audit needs a certain amount of training and knowledge of the methods of auditing.[9-14, 26] Audit has to be carried out intermittently in a particular manner and this is a process of detection of the deficiencies and correcting and then finally checking if the changes made have really changed the healthcare delivery to patients. This completes the loop of the audit and the same subject could be re-audited again to improve it further. This constitutes an audit cycle.[9-14, 29]

Plan - Do - Check - ACT

Managing Change—Communication, Discussion, Motivation

Managing change is one of the most difficult aspects of administration. It may involve bringing about a change in roles, attitudes, goals, priorities, barriers, targets and criteria. Everyone concerned must be involved in the discussions. Issues must be thrashed out with clarity as to who or what needs to be changed, why the change is being brought about and what the benefits of the change are likely to be.

Staff Education

Employees in an organization have opinions, traditions, beliefs and practices concerning quality in relation to hospital infection control. This is a part of the company's quality culture. Understanding this culture should be a company-assessment of quality.

Administrative and clinical set-up determines the awareness, training and implementation of the CQI programme. Teaching should be done by the members of quality improvement committee. Members of the quality circle in clinical areas are targeted (doctors, nurses, orderlies, respiratory therapists and physicians). To provide incentives of compliance with programme, proof of attendance may be required as a condition of employment.

A centralised record of all employees who have undergone training should be maintained in the quality health or hospital epidemiology departments.To provide a measure of adequacy of training a written test could be given before and after the training session. Staff should evaluate the programme. Feedback of results should be given and a refresher training must be allowed to keep them up-to-date.

Implementation of Changes

After identifying the changes to be made, it is important to introduce the changes and sustain them.

This is a very difficult task. Commitment and motivation are crucial. In order to confirm that the change is sustained, it is necessary to audit again. When planning the next audit, it is advisable to break down each part into its components. Time has to be allocated for the various parts of the audit cycle. Any extra work that may have to be done is taken into account, for instance, one should normally audit against a practice protocol, but if there isn't one in existence, one may have to create an evidence-based protocol.

Second Audit

(Figure 6.10)

While discussing the changes that need to be made, one should set a date for the second audit, or further, data collection. There should be a realistic amount of time after the first data collection, to ensure that all the necessary changes have had the time and chance to take effect. A minimum amount of time is probably six months. A year is quite usual for a second data collection. If the changes have not resulted in improvement, one needs an alternative plan. It is necessary to assess if the right changes have been made and if everyone was committed to the change. Once the practice is performing satisfactorily, auditing may be done at a later date, or every few years, to see if the practice is maintaining its standard. To make sure that the set standards are achieved,

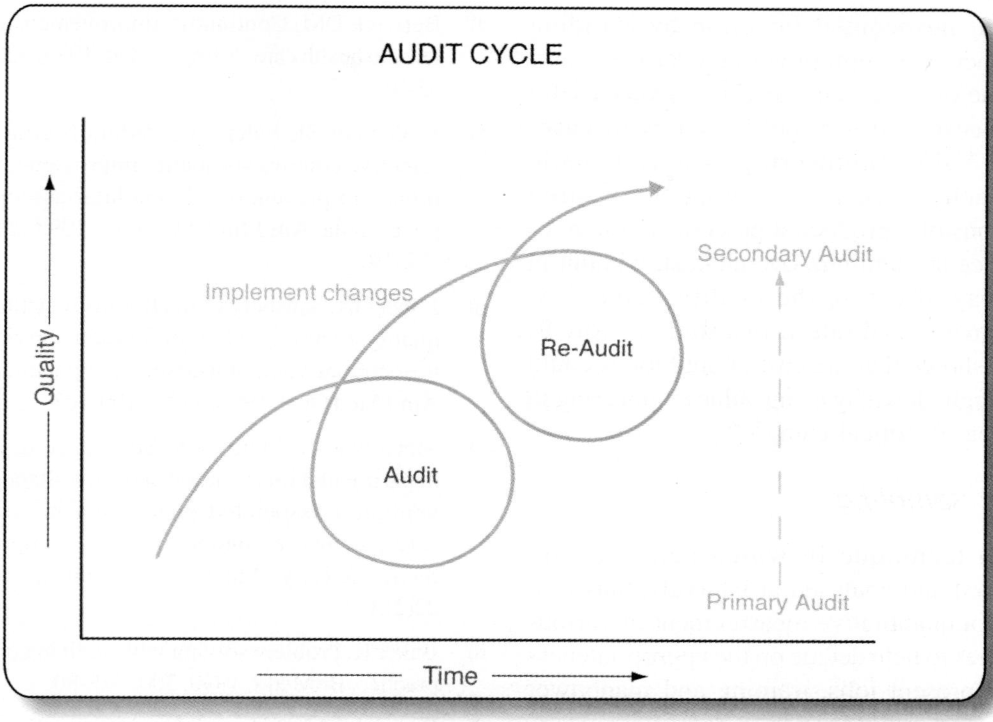

Figure 6.10: An audit cycle (Primary audit) needs to be followed up with a secondary audit

re-auditing must be done at appropriate intervals—maybe even every two or three years—just to make sure that the high standards set are being maintained consistently.[30, 31]

Improving Systems

Other methods of quantiative planning, information collection and improvement in systems—

Network analysis

This is a graphic plan of all the events and activities to be completed in order to reach an end objective. This technique has been used in various areas of management of HAI.

Programme Evaluation and Review Technique (PERT)

Construction of arrow diagrams representing a logical sequence of events to provide a basic discipline to the personnel involved in the project so as to avoid delays in the implementation of the plan. This is also called 'scheduling'. This is also used to solve complex problems such as that of nosocomial pneumonia.[6,7,18,19]

Critical Path Method (CPM)

This is to prevent delays in the longest path (critical path) of the network, which in turn would delay the entire project. This can be used to develop clinical pathways and indirectly prevent nosocomial infection by avoiding improper or inappropriate clinical pathways. The use of 'value engineering' is very useful to cut costs and is a tool in quality management. Value engineering is a systematic approach aimed at achieving the desired functions of a product, a process, a system or a service at minimum overall cost, without in any way affecting the quality, reliability, performance and safety. In a study by Ray B. it was shown that the cost of antibiotics could be brought down by using value engineering in the area of critical care.[25, 30]

Work sampling

It is a technique in which activities are observed and analysed at intervals, thus providing a quantitative measurement of various activities to help decide on the appropriateness of the present jobs, training and manpower needs.

REFERENCES

1) Horbar JD, Rogowiski J, Plesk et al. Collaborative quality improvement for neonatal intensive care. NIC/Q Project investigators of the Vermont Oxford network. Paediatrics. 2001; 107(1): 14-22.

2) Spencer EM, Mills AE, Rorty MV et al. Compliance, Risk management and Quality Improvement Programmes. In: Organization Ethics in Health Care. New York: Oxford University Press. 2000; 171-185.

3) Juran JM and Gryna FM. Manufacture In: Quality Planning and Analysis. 3rd edn, New Delhi: Tata McGraw-Hill Pubishing Company Limited. 1995; 343-376.

4) Berwick DM. Continuous improvement as an ideal in health care. N Engl J Med. 1989; 320(1): 53-56.

5) Kelleghan SI, Salemi C, Padilla S et al. An effective continuous quality improvement approach to prevention of ventilator-associated pneumonia. Am J Infect Control. 1993; 21(6): 322-330.

6) Joiner GA, Salisbury D and Bollin GE. Utilizing quality assurance as a tool for reducing risk of nosocomial ventilator-associated pneumonia. Am J Med Qual. 1996; 11(2): 100-103.

7) McGowan H, Mattson S, Silva K et al. Inter departmental intervention and surveillance for ventilator-associated pneumonia in critical care patients; a continuous quality improvement activity. Am J Infect Control. 1994; 22(2):111.

8) Baker R. Problem solving with audit in general practice. Br Med J. 1990; 300: 378-80.

9) Berwick DM, Enthoven A and Bunker JP. Quality management in the NHS: the doctor's role-I. Br Med J. 1992; 304: 235-9.

10) Bell D, Layton AJ and Gabbay J. Use of a guideline based questionnaire to audit hospital care of acute asthma. Br Med J. 1991; 302: 1440-3.

11) Crombie IK, Davies HTO, Abraham SCS et al. Methods of audit. In: The Audit Handbook. Improving Health Care through Clinical Audit. Chichester, England: John Wiley & Sons. 1993; 101-125.

12) Shaw CD. Aspects of audit:1. The background. BrMed J. 1980; I: 1256-8.

13) Gulliford MC, Petruckevitch A and Burney PGJ. Hospital case notes and medical audit: evaluation of non-response. Br Med J. 1991; 302: 1128-9.

14) Smith T. Medical audit: closing the feedback loop is vital. Br Med J. 1990; 300: 65.

15) Shaw CD. Criterion based audit. Br Med J. 1990; 300: 649-51.

16) O' Leary DS. Accreditation in the quality im provement mold – a vision for tomorrow. Quel Rev Bull. 1991; 27: 72-77.

17) Gupta SK and Kant S. Quality dimensions in hospital infection control. J of Acad Hosp Admn. 2002;14(2):1-5.

18) Kollef MH. Epidemiology and Risk factors for nosocomial pneumonia. Emphasis on prevention. Clin.chest.Med.1999; 20(3): 653-70.

19) Wong A and Wenzel RP. Using Quality Improvement techniques for the prevention of Nosocomial Pneumonia.In: Jarvis WR, ed. Nosocomial Pneumonia. New York: Marcel Dekker Inc. 2000; 187-201.

20) Juran JM and Gryna FM. Manufacture In: Quality Planning and Analysis. 3rd edn, New Delhi: Tata McGraw-Hill Pubishing Company Limited. 1995; 100-102.

21) Kirton OC, DeHaven B, Hudson-Civetta J et al: Re-engineering ventilatory support to decrease days and improve resource utilization. Ann Surg. 1996; 224(3): 396-404.

22) Pesotnik SL, Classen DC, Evan RS et al: Imple menting antibiotic practice guidelines through computer-assisted decision support: Clinical and financial outcomes. Ann Intern Med. 1996; 124(10): 884-890

23) Evans RS, Pesotnik SL, Cassen DC, et al: A computer-assisted management programme for antibiotics and other anti-infective agents. N Eng J Med. 1998; 338(4): 232-238.

24) Donabedian A. The quality of care: how it can be assessed? J Am Med Assoc. 1988; 260(12): 1743-8.

25) Ray B. Value engineering – a practical approach to managing cost in critical care. Health Administrator. Vol XI & XII No 1 & 2. 2001; 41-44.

26) Gaynes RP and Solomon S. Improving hospital-acquired infection rates: the CDC experience. Jt Comm J. Qual Improv. 1996; 22(7): 457-467.

27) Struelens MJ. Hospital Infection Control. In: Armstrong D, Cohen J, eds. Infectious Diseases. London: Mosby, 1999; 10.1-10.14

28) Guidelines for Preventing HIV,HBV and other infections in the Health Care Setting.Published by WHO Regional Office for South-East Asia, New Delhi, India.1996;61.

29) Macmillan L and Pringle M. Practice managers and practice management. Br Med J. 1992; 304: 1672-4.

30) Samaddar DP, Sampath Kumar, Sunder A et al . Value engineering in the ICU. Health Administrator. Vol XI & XII. No 1 & 2. 2001 45-58.

31) Crombie IK, Davies HTO, Abraham SCS et al. Overview of Audit. In: The Audit Handbook. Improving Health Care through Clinical Audit. Chichester, England: John Wiley & Sons. 1993; 25-46.

Chapter 7

Performance Management, Standards, Compliance

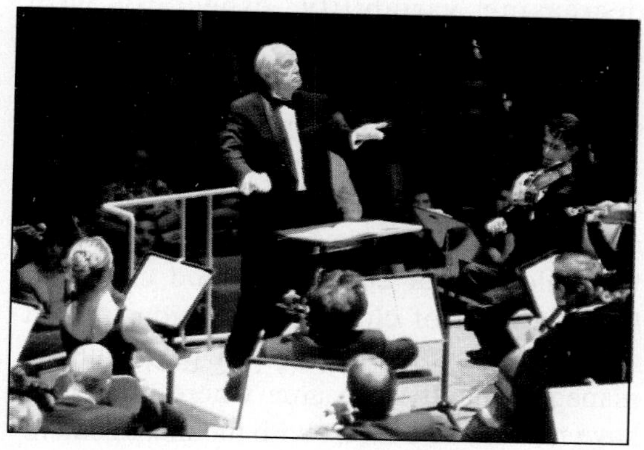

There is a difference between interest and commitment. When you are interested in doing something, you do it only when circumstances permit. When you are committed to it, you accept no excuses, only results.

—Art Turock

Highlights

Clinical Performance and Its Management

Performance Measurement and Clinical Performance Indicators

Standards of Care in Control of HAI

Performance Management Map

INTRODUCTION

Performance includes 'the processes a clinician applies while rendering clinical care and the outcomes resulting from applying those processes'. Therefore, measuring performance is measuring processes and outcomes. Performance management is a relatively new area, which aims at improving clinical care and decreasing variability, especially with regard to complex problems such as HAI. But in this chapter, we are particularly focusing on those aspects of management that can influence and improve the working of clinicians in the ultimate delivery of healthcare. This aspect of medical management dealing with technologies for controlling and changing the behaviour of clinicians, individually and collectively, is called clinical performance management. It is an area where clinicians have to work in concert with the management personnel and vice-versa, which means that clinical medicine can benefit from application of managerial techniques in its goal of improving healthcare delivery[1] (Photo 7.1). Clinical performance management and use of clinical performance indicators tell us how the system supports quality of clinical activity in a healthcare facility. Thus, performance management is a part of quality management.

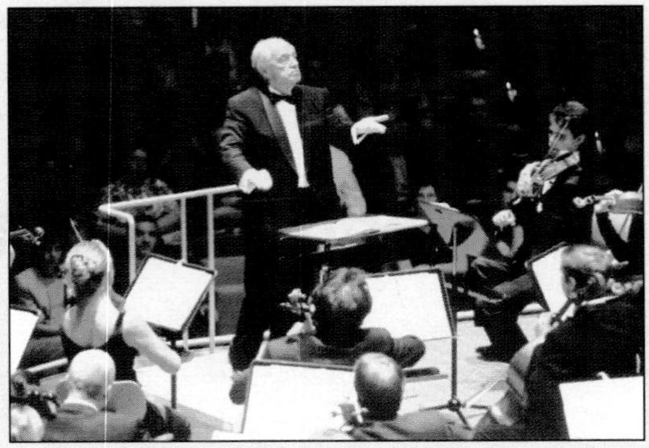

Photo 7.1: Performance management can be likened to a 'concert'. The conductor synchronises the performance of the musicians to achieve the best results.

CLINICAL PERFORMANCE AND ITS MANAGEMENT

Scenario I

Success of a surgical procedure is not only dependent on the short-term recovery, but also on prevention of infections which may surface after a period. It also depends on the performance of various personnel (not just the surgeon), their knowledge of procedures, and how they carry them out, individually and collectively, to bring about a favourable outcome. A study by Choux et al on the incidence of shunt infections offers excellent evidence of the importance of a team approach.[2]

They suggest a team approach (surgical protocol) and emphasize the importance of surgical preparation and technique in the preoperative period for an infection-free surgical experience. Some of the policies followed included:

- No shaving except in older children;
- In the operating room, shunt surgeries should be performed earlier in the day before other neurosurgical cases.
- Neonates should be operated upon before older children.
- Minimum number of persons in the theatre
- Using an iodine-impregnated adhesive plastic drape; opening the shunt only prior to insertion

- Using a no-touch technique to handle the shunt (Venes technique)[3]
- Only two incisions and a good quality skin closure
- Only one dose of antibiotic, which was enough to reduce the rate of infections from 7.75% to 1.04%.

This was superior to the practice of excessive use of antibiotics. HAI prevention and control forms a part of all clinical processes. Let us consider a surgical procedure being carried out in the operating room and try to enumerate the processes related to preventing HAI. These may include the following: skin preparation, precautions taken to protect HCWs, theatre-cleaning protocols, theatre attire, hand-washing and surgical scrub, facility design and engineering controls, sterility of equipment, process of prescribing antibiotics, anaesthesia, critical care, post-operative recovery, waste management, etc.[4]

This underscores the importance of the entire team working in cohesion and would only be effective if the performance of all those involved are of acceptable standards.

Scenario 2

Infection Control in the ICU: The ICU team includes a host of specialized employees of which physicians, respiratory therapists, nurses, environmental cleaning personnel and dieticians are all a part. Patients in the ICU are already compromised by several elements like disease processes, trauma, interruption of normal defence mechanisms (by mechanical ventilation, etc.), malnutrition due to the inability to eat, the inability to ambulate, etc. Hence, the clinical expertise of the ICU staff has a direct bearing on patient outcomes. All members need to work together to reduce the risk of a HAI to the lowest possible levels. How do we make them all synchronize and work in unison towards a common goal of achieving acceptable levels of performance?[4, 5]

PERFORMANCE MEASUREMENT AND CLINICAL PERFORMANCE INDICATORS

The definition of performance and its measurement are discussed in the chapter on quality assessment, measurement and operationalizing quality. Clinical performance management and use of clinical performance indicators tell us how the system supports quality.

Components of clinical performance measurement: Clinical and professional standards should be continuously imposed, and for this one needs to develop a performance measurement standard. This, in turn, can be accomplished by developing appropriate clinical performance indicators. These indicators can finally be incorporated into a clinical quality improvement practice.

Look for Implementation of Evidence-Based Practice in HAI Control

Evidence-based medicine—clinical management

The term 'Evidence-Based Medicine' (EBM) was coined in the early 1990s and was generally defined as 'the conscientious, explicit and judicious use of current best evidence in making decisions about the care of individual patients.'[6]

We are all familiar with the judicial system wherein verdicts are given and accepted based on clinching evidences. This need has also been felt in the medical profession. It is now considered more scientific to follow procedures and practices based on convincing proof that one is doing the right thing in the right way. Evidence-based medicine also makes for a more uniform form of clinical practice across institutions and nations improving clinical effectiveness.

Look for Improvement of Clinical Effectiveness

The process of clinical effectiveness has four steps as described by Swage, and these steps need to be practised for management of HAI.

1. Collect clinical evidence through primary research and scientific review.
2. Disseminate clinical guidelines that are based as much as possible on the evidence available.
3. Implement evidence-based and cost-effective practice through education, training and change management.
4. Assess the compliance to agreed practice guidelines and the evaluation of patient outcomes through quality monitoring processes.

Implement clinical effectiveness

- Decide on the question of evolving, defining, refining, prioritizing problems.
- Find the evidence.
- Create ideas of search strategy.
- Appraise the evidence.
- Spot new angles and roles (i.e. who has the skills).
- Agree to the best practice.
- Add clinical expertise: practical issues on application.
- Compare with the current practice.
- Identify the change needed.
- Agree amongst the group members.
- Carry out an action plan.
- Who is doing what, when, how—share the workload.
- Set review date.
- Accountability (Report to next meeting.)
- Keep notes of the action plan agreed.

Look for Evidence of the System Using Clinical Practice Guidelines

A clinical practice guideline constitutes a plan for managing a clinical problem based on evidence whenever possible and on consensus in the absense of evidence.[6] International and national guidelines can be locally adapted to ensure best practice in any clinical area. But it is necessary that adaptations are supported by evidence. In other words, pracitioners must be sure of the evidence base that they use when altering the national and international guidelines. Proposed guidelines and standards might be used as a point of reference in discussion between infection control team and managers about the arrangements needed to deliver a high quality infection service.[7] In addition, in some countries such as the UK, these guidelines are already providing quality assurance teams with a framework to monitor whether best practice is being achieved. The guidelines are also providing a framework for auditing. Thus, national evidence-based guidelines are intended to inform the development of detailed operational protocols at local levels and can be used to ensure that these incorporate the most important principles for prevention of hospital acquired infections. This has been addressed by the Infection Control Nurses Association and the Association of Domestic Managers, resulting in the adoption and publication of standards concerning hospital cleanliness, by the Department of Health.

Look for Clinical Care Pathways

Clinical care pathways (Synonyms: multidisciplinary pathways of care, protocols, integrated care pathways, critical care paths, anticipated path of recovery, pathways of care) must be made for improved clinical performance.

Definition: An integrated care pathway determines locally agreed, multidisciplinary practice, based on guidelines and evidence where available, for a specific patient/client group. It forms all or parts of the clinical record, documents the care given and facilitates the evaluation of outcomes for continuous quality improvement.[8-10] This is an adaptation of the critical path method of project planning (see chapter on developing systems in CQI implementation).

Example

Typically, a problem area which has wide variations in practice (such as diagnosis of nosocomial pneumonia) patterns is selected. The process is built from current clinical practice—noting difficulties in agreeing upon diagnostic criteria, sampling techniques, laboratory criteria, tests to be carried out and treatment strategies, collection of data as patients are treated, noting the outcomes and variations from the pathway, finally reviewing the pathway to make changes and improvements.[9, 10] Developing a clinical pathway has shown in many studies to improve outcome. There is a process of dynamic audit in this clinical practice involving a multidisciplinary care. In an intensive care unit, a multidisciplinary team can evolve a clinical care pathway, i.e. the various steps of prevention, diagnosis and management of HAI to avoid variation and delays. The steps of making a clinical care pathway have been given by Swage. Clinical pathways involved in HAI management are intradepartmental or interdisciplinary (multidisciplinary) and are institution specific.

Example

Development of clinical pathways leads to better coordination between the laboratories and wards e.g. investigation time, processing time, reporting time, etc.

Example

Better coordination between house-keeping staff, nursing staff and doctors (transport of patients with communicable HAI).

Steps of evolving clinical care pathways

Select important areas

Gather support for the project

Review practice

Define case type/client group

Agree on the time frame (e.g. admission to ward)

Agree on goals/outcome of care

Draw up the pathway

Train personnel
Pilot the pathway
Implement the pathway

Look for a System which can Manage Clinical Performance

Clinical governance sets out to ensure at the highest levels that systems to monitor quality of clinical practice are in place and are functioning properly. It ensures that clinical practitioners meet standards, such as those issued for national professional bodies. It puts into place a controls-assurance function for the systems of clinical quality management.

Look for Measures of Good Medical Practice

Maintaining good medical practice for HAI control

Participation in clinical audit, risk management procedures and learning the lessons from these to improve performance, are all indicators of good medical practice. There should be teaching, training, appraisal, assessment and adequate clinical supervision of juniors.

Relationship with patients

Look for informed consent of patients by the right person at the right time, confidentiality of patient information, adequate procedures being in place if performance concerns are raised about health professionals, evidence of learning from patient complaints and/or litigation.

Working with colleagues

Look for evidence of good teamwork.

Probity

Proper arrangements for research governance, proper arrangements for carrying out private practice.

Health

Look for access to occupational health services.

Good clinical care

Are the various steps of the process of clinical care (see chapter on process of clinical care) of HAI and evidence-based practice in place in your hospital?

Accreditation

Accreditation involves an on-site survey of the hospital by a team of physicians, nurses and hospital administrators. During the survey, the team evaluates whether or not the hospital meets performance standards in a number of areas, including patient safety and medical errors, pain management, medical staffing, infection control and hospital management. Depending on how well the hospital scores, the accreditation agency can award one of the different levels of accreditation.

STANDARDS OF CARE IN CONTROL OF HAI

The word 'standards' is used in the chapter on CQI implementation for quality measurement.

But now given below is the usage of the term 'standard' in a broader context. A 'standard' is described in the dictionary as something which is used as a basis for judging quality; it is the level of excellence you aim at, require or reach. Standard setting is a very important part of the process of quality improvement in control of HAI. Standards may be guidelines, regulations, laws or requirements for accreditation. Standards may be a group of guidelines or a subset of guidelines. Govermental policies, directives, regulations by important regulatory bodies all help in setting standards. To operationalize standard setting and implementation, we need to understand a number of concepts in the present day from the perspective of preventing litigation. The importance of various standards are as follows (decreasing importance):

Laws or court rulings related to HAI
↓
Regulations
↓
Manufacturing Standards (national)
↓
Guidelines

Standards of Care

Every clinician has a duty to exercise reasonable skill and care in the treatment of the patient. Standard of care is a level of care which one is obliged to provide. A 'standard of care in infection-control practice' has been established in some countries, which is applicable to a number of healthcare professionals. In the US, these include the practice of standard precautions, practice of transmission-based precautions, prevention of contact spread of infections by hand-washing practices, appropriate cleaning, disinfection and sterilization of medical devices and equipment and occupational (infective) hazard prevention to healthcare workers.

In addition, 'standards of professional conduct in infection control' have been framed in many countries. Failure to follow these standards constitutes unprofessional conduct. Therefore, if these standards are not met (failure to follow infection-control practices) and there is substantiation of the charges, then it can lead to disciplinary action, revocation of professional licence and/or professional liability. Regulations by OSHA (Occupational Safety and Health Administration) also enforce teaching and training of the standard precautions to all employees by the 'Blood Borne Pathogen Standard'.

Organizational Standards

Standards are very variable in practice and are dependant on a variety of factors, e.g. economic factors (see chapter on quality measurement). A group/organization/nation sets its own standards and then progresses to higher levels in subsequent quality cycles. The highest standards or the ideal situations are rarely met, but it is imperative that minimum standards are met. When the highest standards are not attainable, then the aim should be to attain at least a minimum set of standards at all times. A classical example is sterilization or high level disinfection for endoscopes. An organization may set very high standards for itself, far above the standards acceptable nationally. But important things to remember are that it should be acceptable to a peer group, it should be ethical and the organization must generate evidence to support the deviation from set standards. It should demonstrate cost benefit and cost effectiveness. Compliance means trying to fulfil the standards. Responsible organizations comply with standards of care. Regulations and laws help enforcing standards of care (controlling) and managing performance.[11, 12]

National and International Standardization Committees: (Manufacturing Standards)

Standards for manufacture (industrial specification), building and architecture and maintenance are laid down by organized national standard committees composed of nominated clinicians, experts from government agencies and manufacturers nominated by appropriate trade associations. In this context 'a standard is a document available to the public, drawn up with the cooperation and consensus or general approval of all interests affected by it, based on consolidated results of science, technology and experience, aimed at the promotion of community benefits and approved by a body recognized on the national, regional or international level'.

Examples of some of the standardization bodies include:

Indian Standards Institution (ISI)

British Standards Institution (BSI)

European Standards Committee (CEN)

International Standards Organization (ISO)

Standards laid down by these bodies are not legally enforceable, but as compared to guidelines, they are stronger. They also give a direction to the quality of practices followed in a particular country.

Statutes and Statutory Regulations (Regulatory Standards)

Regulations are rules or standards set up by government organizations or independent bodies and the health organizations are legally bound to accept these standards and enforce them. They help in regulating the basic standards in a particular country or state. In addition to regulations, they also provide guidelines. There are a number of regulatory organizations in the US and Europe. They focus on various aspects of infection control.

These are Acts of Parliaments, and subsidiary regulations are different in different countries. They form the basis of legal action (civil or criminal prosecution):

a. They are less detailed than guidelines or standards.

b. Guidelines or standards may be added to give specific detail to the regulations.

c. Not following these would not only incite legal action but can also lead to action by government and regulatory institutions.

Use of standard guidelines enable a consistent approach to be established, and monitored, but they are not legally enforceable. E.g. CDC guidelines focus on strategies for disinfection and sterilization of medical equipment in the USA. These guidelines do not recommend specific chemical germicides that are formulated for use on medical equipment or environmental surfaces in the healthcare setting. These are further converted into regulations by important regulatory bodies. Some examples include the following:

Employee Protection Agency (EPA) of the USA is a body that registers disinfectants and sterilants based on microbicidal efficacy data submitted by the manufacturer. EPA is responsible for the regulation of safety and efficacy claims for low and intermediate level disinfectants, and also the toxicity of active ingredients.

Occupational safety and health administration (OSHA) gives guidelines for proper usage and minimization of worker exposure to chemical disinfectants and sterilants. OSHA directs employers in the USA to establish work controls whenever there is potential for worker exposure. Guidelines to employers are given by the OSHA. These bodies not only ensure that updated guidelines are available but also monitor and enforce their implementation.

Association for Practitioners in Infection Control (APIC) assess healthcare professionals in their decisions involving selection and use of specific disinfectants.

There are also state and local bodies that are concerned with environmental issues such as hazardous waste disposal methods. The guidelines given by these bodies are now available on their respective websites. The regulatory bodies can be grouped into a) international and b) national bodies. The largest international society for ICPs is probably the Association for Practitioners in Infection Control and Epidemiology (APIC) based in the United States. APIC was founded in 1972, and currently represents some 12,000 members comprising nurses, medical technologists, microbiologists, epidemiologists, physicians and other healthcare personnel whose primary responsibility within their facilities is infection prevention and control.

In Europe, the European council passes regulations, and the CEN (Committe European Nationalite) sets the standards, and this is mandatory on the part of the various countries to legislate within a particular time frame and applies to the HAI-related issues.

Legal Standards

(Table 7.1)

An increasing number of cases are filed against healthcare workers and organizations when a patient develops HAI after invasive procedures. Added to this, even healthcare workers sue organizations when they acquire HAI during their course of duty. The doctor or an organization is not guilty of negligence if he has acted in accordance with a practice accepted as proper by a responsible body of opinion of medical men skilled in that particular art. A doctor or an organization is not negligent merely because there is a body of opinion that takes a contrary view. E.g. a doctor or an organization is not negligent if a practice is not adopted universally in the country. E.g. ultraclean air systems.[13]

Negligence is also looked for based on previous court judgements, existing regulations, standards or guidelines. A civil suit is filed when there is suspicion of negligence leading to morbidity/injury leading to various consequences short of death. A criminal suit can be filed in case of death. To prove negligence one has to establish that the healthcare worker/healthcare organization owed a duty of care (preventing HAI) towards the patient, e.g. waste management policies. A judgement or law or regulation may help form a standard. A breach of a duty of care leads to negligence when the patient suffers an HAI due to this. Negligence could also be due to lack of reasonable skill of a competent practitioner in that speciality. Therefore, it is important to define the set of skills and knowledge used in clinical practice for HAI prevention, diagnosis, man-

Table 7.1: Standards need to be understood and defined in relation to HAI. These standards may vary from country to country but common issues and steps to be taken to prevent negligence are given below.

Compliance with guidelines, regulations and laws related to HAI	
Issues	**Steps taken to prevent negligence**
Duty of care and standard of care towards preventing HAI in HCW, patients, visitors	Take steps to prevent HAI by complying with appropriate standards.
Guidelines related to HAI	Use evidence-based guidelines and standard procedures.
Deviation from accepted practice	When you deviate from accepted practice guidelines, you must have database/ evidence to support (e.g. can use higher standards).
Deviation from regulations and laws related to HAI	Do not deviate from regulations and laws.
Inherent risks of HAI if present, e.g. infection after surgery or invasive procedures	Must be explained and consent taken
Medical management of HAI	Follow accepted guidelines, tests, treatment, etc.
Error of judgement in treatment/diagnosis	May occur but not considered as negligence
Errors of omission. E.g. skin preparation before surgery	Considered as care undertaken without requisite caution. Treated as negligence.
Choice of treatment/Management, e.g. surgical treatment vs medical treatment	Consent to be taken
Prosthetics, implants	A) Follow manufacturer's orders, e.g. do not use after date of expiry. B) Do not use in case of damaged packaging. C) Ensure proper storage. D) Do not re-sterilize if it is a single-use item. E) Guarantee and warranty.
Statutory regulations, laws related to environment, waste mangement, blood transfusion, food and beverages, water purification	Comply.

Table 7.1: (Contd.)

Generally, in many countries, these laws are grouped into Consumer safety Environmental hygiene Medical devices Tests for disinfection Blood, toxic agents and diagnostic tests	Comply.
Occupational hazards due to chemicals, e.g. gluteraldehyde, ethylene oxide and other disinfectants, specific infections	Comply with regulations, laws.
Vicarious responsibility (responsibility of administration) 1. Errors in aseptic technique prior to surgical/ invasive procedures 2. Improper hospital hygiene (clean surroundings) 3. Improper sterilization and maintenance of sterility of various equipment 4. Hospital employees acquiring infection due to inadequate protection 5. When patients acquire infections in the hospital due to inadequate protection, from other patients or infected employees	The organization may be held responsible for negligence, e.g. faulty sterilization process. Therefore, must provide adequate, training, education for staff (doctors, technicians, nurses) Must take care to provide infection-control policies and execute them
In case of accidents and mishaps, e.g. spills, exposure to infections	Must take adequate care and prompt action if it has occurred

agement or treatment. A constant effort has to be made to avoid 1) outdated skills 2) not adopting safety measures that are known to be necessary (standard of care).

Some safety aspects to avoid negligence

- Maintain a hospital manual of policies related to HAI.
- Comply with laws, regulations, standards and guidelines.
- Take informed consent (inform about infection as a complication of procedures).
- Maintain proper records: It is important to ensure that all relevant comments and recommendations are written in the patient's records.
- Adopt risk management strategies
- Counsel the employees.

Consequences of being negligent in infection-control policies:

a. Sanctions against hospitals by appropriate authorities

b. Civil proceedings against hospital or healthcare workers for negligence

c. Criminal proceedings against hospitals or healthcare workers in case of death

d. Refusal of insurance companies to fund treatment in a particular private hospital

e. Health purchasers may obtain medical services from another hospital

Example of laws

1. Health and Safety at Work Act (1974), Control of Substances Hazardous to Health Regulations (COSHH) Act of Parliament (1988).
2. Legislation on blood and blood products in India—human blood is covered under the definition of 'drug' under section 3(b) of Drugs and Cosmetics Act 1940. It is imperative that blood banks be regulated under the provisions of the drugs and cosmetics act and rules thereunder. The Central Government has amended these rules from time to time and the latest amendment was made in 1999 to meet the directions of the Supreme Court.
3. Waste Management—Ministry of environment and forest, Government of India has issued a notification on biomedical waste management under the Environment (protection) Act, 1986. The defaulting hospitals, nursing homes, veterinary hospitals, animal houses, pathological labs and blood banks generating wastes are liable to be penalised as per provisions of the Environment (protection) Act 1998 and other pollution control acts.

PERFORMANCE MANAGEMENT MAP[14]

(FIGURE 7.1)

There are a number of strategies and standards, which have already been discussed and some of them will be discussed in the subsequent chapters. It is extremely confusing for a reader to understand how one should select them.What are the combinations of tools and strategies you would select for the country's HAI control programme?

a. Emphasis on changes based on self-learning and evaluation

b. Emphasis on control

c. Emphasis on strategies which have large inputs from the medical profession.

d. Emphasis on strategies which are management or profession driven.

A performance management map helps in selecting tools and strategies. This mix of strategies and tools varies with the organization, people, level of training, education, laws and existing managerial and administrative controls.

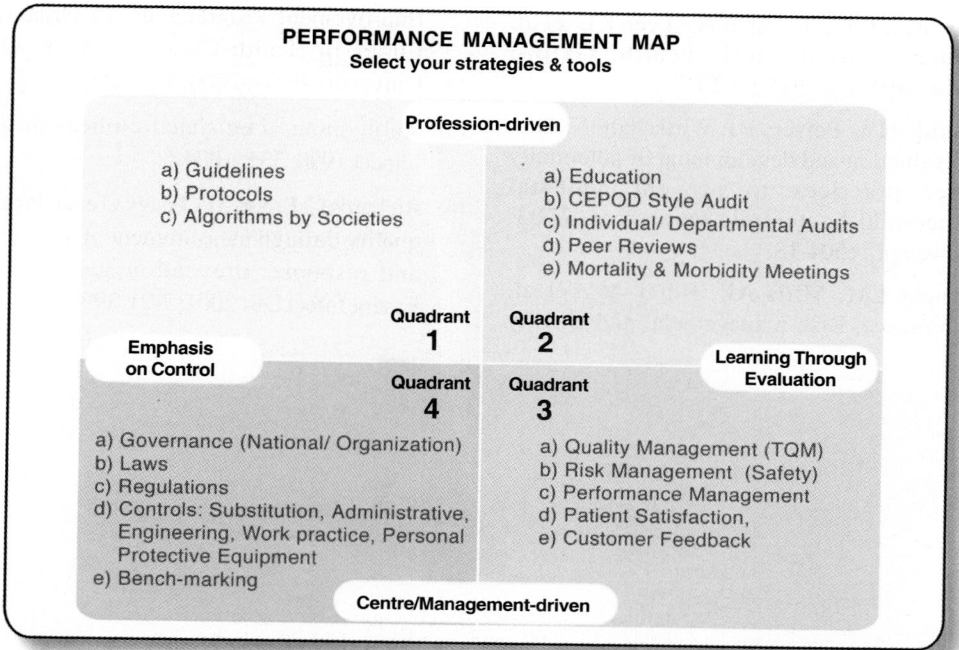

Figure 7.1: A performance management map helps select strategies and tools.

REFERENCES

1) Ignatavicius DD and Hausman KA. Development and implementation of Clinical Care Pathways. In: Clinical Care Pathways for Collaborative Practice. WB Saunders Company. Philadelphia 2002; 16-26.

2) Choux M, Genitori L, Lang D et al. Shunt Implantation: Reducing the incidence of shunt infection. J. Neurosurg. 1992; 77(6): 875-880.

3) Venes JL. Control of shunt infections: report of 150 consecutive cases. J. of Neurosurg. 1976; 45: 311-314.

4) O'Leary DS. The Joint Commission looks to the future. J Am Med Assoc 1987; 258(7): 951-52.

5) Marnoch G. Introduction: the management agenda for doctors. In: Ham C, Heginbotham C, Series eds. Doctors and Management in the National Health Service. Health Services Management, Open Unversity Press, Buckingham, 1996; 1-11.

6) Sackett D L ed. In: Evidence-based medicine: how to practice and teach Evidence based medicine, Churchill Livingstone. NY 1997; 2

7) Kilbride HW, Wirtschafter DD, Powers RJ et al. Implementation of evidence-based potentially better practices to decrease nosocomial infections. Pediatrics.2003; 111(4 suppl): 519-33.

8) Health Department, UK. J Hosp Infect. 2001;47 (suppl): S1-82.

9) Vincent C and Adams ST. The investigation and analysis of clinical incidents. In: Clinical Risk Management. Enhancing Patient Safety. 2nd edn. BMJ Books. 2001; 439-460.

10) Brownson R C, Baker E A, Leet T L et al. Evidence based public health. Oxford University Press. 2003; 3-43.

11) Kilbride HW, Powers RJ, Wirtschafter DD et al. Evaluation and development of potentially better practices to prevent neonatal nosocomial bacteremia.Pediatrics. 2003; 111(4suppl): e504-18.

12) Spencer EM, Mills AE, Rorty MV et al. Compliance, Risk management, and Quality Improvement Programmes. In Organization Ethics in Health Care.New York: Oxford University Press. 2000; 171-185.

13) Anonymous. Legislated clinical medicine. Lancet 1990; 335: 1004-6.

14) Richards C, Emori TG, Peavy G et al. Promoting quality through measurement of performance and response: prevention success stories. Emerg Infect Dis. 2001; 7(2): 299-301.

Chapter 8

Safety and Risk Management

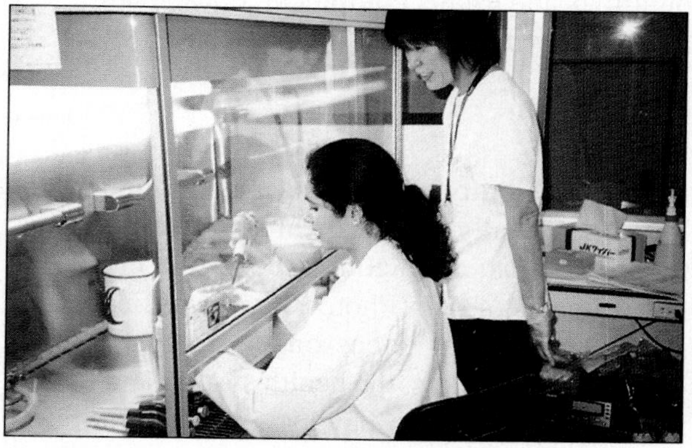

Medicine used to be simple, ineffective and relatively safe. Now it is complex, effective and potentially dangerous.

—Sir Cyril Chantler

Highlights

Understanding 'Errors' and Managing Risk

'The Six Sigma Factor'

The Processes of Risk Management

Some Common HAI-Related Risks—Risk Reduction

INTRODUCTION

We are all aware that a number of situations exist in our day-to-day practice where the patient or the healthcare worker runs the risk of getting infected. What is this risk? It relates to the probability that actual harm will result from a hazard and this may result from, and affect people (patients, visitors and staff), buildings and estate, equipment, consumables and the environment.[1]

Risk

It is the possibility of incurring a misfortune or loss. Historically, the medical profession has focused on patient factors as being the major determinants of risk (Photo 8.1). Increasingly, however, we must focus on the role of the healthcare providers, the health system and its infrastructure, as also having a major role in determining the risk and the outcome.

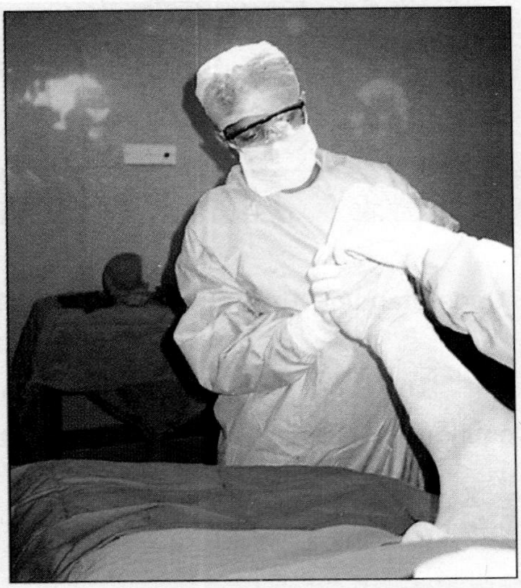

Photo 8.1: Risk management: A surgeon can decrease risk to a patient by using various means of control in routine clinical practices.

Hazard

A hazard is an inherent property of an object capable of causing harm to humans and the environment, e.g. corrosive chemical. Means of control is a process that eliminates or minimizes exposure to a hazard, e.g. protective gloves.

Risk Management

It is the process of carrying out decisions that will minimize the adverse effects or accidental losses upon persons or organizations. Implicit in this definition is the idea that risk management is concerned with the identification, evaluation and prevention of accidental losses (including losses from unforeseen lawsuits) that pose a significant threat to the smooth performance of an organization. They may even result in financial losses (e.g. litigation) to the organization, thus preventing it from fulfilling its mission. Risk management is a recently introduced managerial tool, in the area of infection control, with a proactive approach that identifies risks, assesses the potential severity and frequency of the risks, eliminates those that can be eliminated and minimizes the effect of those that cannot be eliminated.

Organizations, infection-control teams and management teams not only have to deal with risks from infectious causes, but also with non-clinical risks. Hence, management of risks posed by infections have to compete with risks due to other non-infective factors for financial and legal priorities. To convince managers and administrators to allocate resources for HAI control, clinicians have to collect data prospectively and prove priority over other risks and thus deal with them appropriately.[1]

UNDERSTANDING 'ERRORS' IN MANAGING RISK

(TABLE 8.1)

Reducing risks means much more than just reducing morbidity or mortality. A few decades ago, risk could only be assessed by outcome indicators such as mortality and morbidity. But, the problem here is that the damage has already occurred. By detecting and reporting faulty 'processes', one can reduce the chance of critical incidents, which would further reduce the chances of morbidity or mortality. This is a much more beneficial proposition.

> Errors in processes →Clinical or critical incidents →Morbidity (adverse event) →Mortality

Risk management is a concept wherein remedial measures are undertaken for medical errors within the healthcare set-up occurring due to system, organizational, human and technical lapses. Accidents result from multiple and unexpected errors. A key to minimizing errors and improving safety is a better understanding of their precursors and in doing so, collecting information on 'process errors' or 'critical incidents'. Progress can only be made if it is understood that the latent causes of 'errors' are still unidentified and we need to understand them (rather than identifying the persons to blame or 'bad apples') and learn to design systems better, to minimize future errors. This is the reason for which data is collected in the form of 'critical incidents' or 'process errors'.

Any occurrence which is not consistent with the routine care of patient or operation of

Table 8.1: Comparison of risk management strategies in the aviation and medical industries

The Aviation Industry	The Medical Industry
1. Looks at process errors	1. Does not look at process errors
2. Outcome analysis is considered too late	2. Mainly looks at outcome data
3. Checklists for critical processes Critical incident reporting widely followed	3. Checklists are often not mandatory Not all organizations and doctors report critical incidents
4. Serious attitude towards risks	4. Often the attitude is casual
5. Insurance claims taken into account during the planning stage	5. Insurance claims are not taken into account during the planning stage
6. Loss of reputation given a high priority	6. Often not the case
7. Customers' complaints taken seriously and focused upon	7. Patients' complaints not acted upon
8. Organized way of looking at risks	8. Non-organized way of risk management

the institution, or an occurrence that could have led (if not corrected and discovered in time) or did lead to an undesirable outcome ranging from increased length of stay to death, is termed a clinical or critical incident.[2]

Incident reporting is a process whereby a hospital worker is required to fill up a form when a patient has been harmed, or there has been the potential for harm. Unfortunately, few healthcare institutions meticulously maintain such a record.[3]

The primary purpose of incident reporting in clinical risk management is to reduce injuries to patients and staff. It permits the collection of incident data, which allows the analysis of trends that may identify organizational, system and environmental problems, all of which may increase the likelihood of human error.[4-5]

Types of HAI-related risks encountered in the clinical set-up

- Clinical risk—during diagnosis, treatment, transport, containment, triage, practice patterns, post-operative
- Laboratory risk/blood bank risk
- Employee risk
- Organizational risk
- Environmental risk

'THE SIX SIGMA FACTOR'

(PHOTO 8.2)

Some of the high risk organizations (HROs) (e.g., the airlines industry, nuclear installation units, aircraft carriers, etc.) perform extremely dangerous work under extreme pressure, where there is need to perform consistently with no scope for errors. How are they able to do this? This is possible because of the system's ability to bring down process errors by having checklists and taking serious cognizance of faulty processes and warnings, and stopping them from progressing into critical incidents or adverse events. An analogy has been drawn between these organizations and medical set-ups. The US Institute of Medicine recommends that the healthcare system in future should aim for a 'six sigma' reliability, which means fewer than 3.4 errors per million tasks. This is only possible with the support of organizational systems designed to prevent the consequences of unavoidable human error.[6]

All these, when applied to infection-control practices, would mean a reduction of process errors in relation to HAI control.

To Bring about a Remedial Change, One Has to Emphasize

- the need for reduction in errors
- a need for leadership and vision, to bring about a culture of risk management
- the need for better data systems and information on precursors to adverse outcomes (incident reporting, etc.)
- commitment and skills development among providers
- a need for better accountability[7]

Goals of Risk Management in HAI Control

1. To identify probable areas of actual and potential risks
2. To limit risk to patients, visitors, employees.

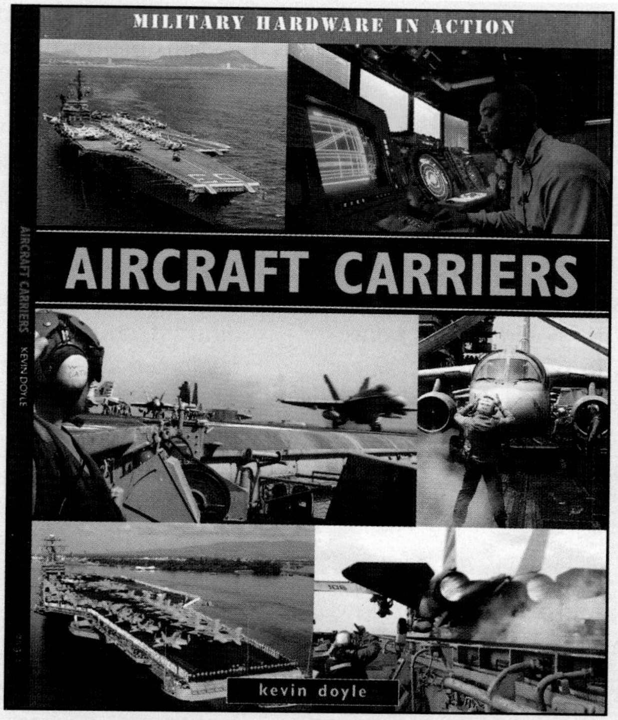

Photo 8.2: Risk management strategies are used in aircraft carriers where there is a need to perform consistently under extreme pressure with no scope for errors. Can the same be used in the medical industry?

3. To limit financial loss to the organization and employees
4. To limit damage to reputation, e.g. adverse publicity and loss of business due to HAI-related litigation
5. To prevent harm to patients irrespective of costs

Risk management is a proactive approach that could vary according to places and circumstances. For example, yellow fever or Crutzfeld Jacob disease may not be a serious risk in the Indian context, while tuberculosis is not as much of a problem in the western world as it is in India. The approach towards tackling risks would also vary according to the awareness, economic conditions, attitudes, statutory and legal practices of a country. The attitudes of the health managers and the political climate very often determine the action that will be taken after risk identification. Necessary action also needs to be taken against people posing the risk.

THE PROCESSES OF RISK MANAGEMENT CONSIST OF

1. Risk identification and assessment
2. Risk analysis

3. Risk control (risk prevention, risk avoidance, risk shifting)
4. Risk monitoring

1. Risk Identification and Assessment in HAI

Safety in clinical practice begins with risk identification and assessment. The magnitude of the risk has to be estimated and its consequences and hazards to personnel/equipment or the institution have to be weighed.

Role of the organization and management

(Table 8.2)

Every organization should consider the following points in managing risks:

1. The greatest risk is addressed first.
2. Senior management personnel must be committed to bringing about this change.
3. The committment must also extend to bringing about an 'infection-control culture' with the objective of reducing hospital acquired infections.
4. For this to work effectively, the infection-control culture should reach out to all the members of the staff and for them to be responsible for risk assessment at departmental levels.
5. If the chief executives can demonstrate that appropriate risk assessments have been carried out, supported by evidence of documentation and review, and that adequate policies and procedures are in place, then disciplinary action can be taken against staff who are shown to have neglected such policies and procedures.
6. Risks may be posed to patients (who can acquire infection), to healthcare workers (who can acquire infection or may develop complications due to exposure to chemicals, and other processes such as the ETO plant), or to the organization (litigation, loss of reputation).
7. Counselling can prevent a number of problems as in case of needle-stick injuries in healthcare workers. Counselling should also be available to doctors, nurses and healthcare workers who are faced with litigation. In hospitals across the USA, legal cells are available in hospitals for counselling when the healthcare worker is faced with litigation. They help them in understanding legal jargon and provide advice. It must be understood here that

Table 8.2: Differences in approaches between traditional infection-control team and risk management group

Non-proactive	Proactive
Top management not involved in management	Strategic goal for top management
More academic approach (laboratory, ward, surveillance, patient published literature)	Analysis of audits, staff opinions, health and safety legislation report

risk management is not restricted to reduction of the financial impact of litigation and insurance claims.[8]

How is risk assessed?

(Figure 8.1)

There are a number of sources from which a risk management group draws its information to organize its priorities.

Active internal surveillance, which includes department staff surveillance and audit visits, passive surveillance of incident reports, complaints and claims, clinical opinion of relevance, publications of health and safety legislation, reports of national and international risk management groups and, sometimes, even 'sentinel events' may be useful.

Sentinel or adverse event policy—these events include incidents like nosocomial infections, unplanned removal of invasive lines, medication errors, falls, pressure sores, skin deficiencies, physical restraints, neurologic compromise, respiratory arrest and delayed diagnosis/treatment.[9] A study carried out in Japan suggests that many hospitals could monitor the quality of the nursing services by using several sources to collect adverse events, and these sources include incident reports, logs, checklists, nurse interviews, medication error questionnaires, urine leucocyte tests, patient interviews and medical records.[10]

Apart from these direct issues of infection control, certain other indirect issues also have a bearing on risk reduction, such as food safety, building safety, plant and equipment

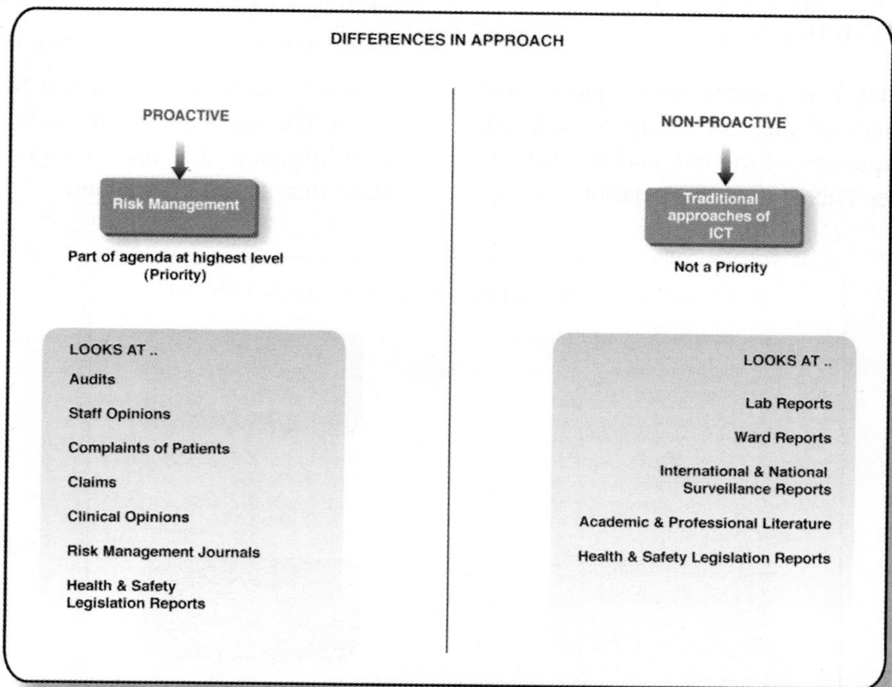

Figure 8.1: Traditional versus modern risk management strategies

safety, medical equipment safety and waste management.

Risk assessment is made

1. From the number of past incidents or hazards related to tasks
2. From a knowledge of natural morbidity and mortality rates
3. From statistics of human infectious dose if a microorganism is involved
4. From knowledge of the efficacy of immunization and treatment options available
5. From the clinical knowledge of transmission modes of important clinical infections (case management problems)[11]

2. & 3. Risk Analysis and Risk Control/ Elimination

The next step is to analyse the frequency and consequences of the risk being considered. The consequences of the risk can be assessed by analysis. This is done by persons who are specially trained in analysing and controlling risks, e.g. clinical risk, financial impact of the risk, potential litigation costs, damage to reputation or adverse publicity with loss of business and harm to patients irrespective of costs. Here, the risk management committee and risk manager are entrusted with the task of carrying out this function.[10, 12]

Risk management committee

(Figure 8.2)

Changing circumstances and requirements are identified by this committee. The responsibilities of risk management committee are

- to produce reports on how risk is being managed across all areas and to define the type, frequency, format and responsibilities of these reports
- maintenance of records of risk data
- to take action and document the action taken. The implication of this is that, in case of a litigation, it is insufficient to merely state that action was taken.

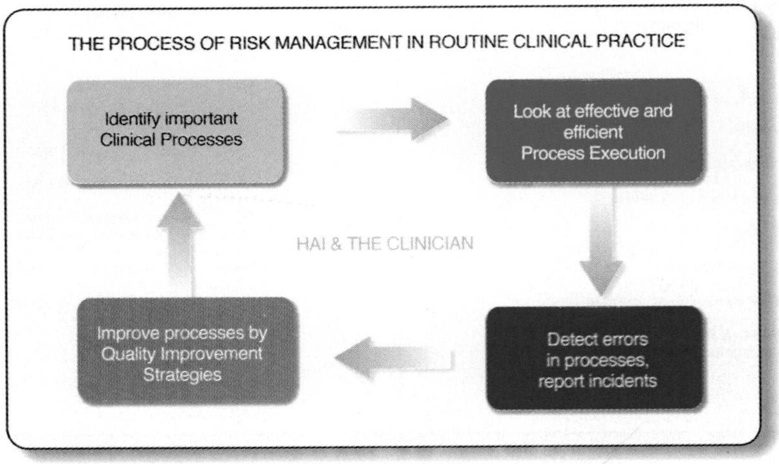

Figure 8.2: The process of risk management in routine clinical practice

Risk managers

Risk managers must be trained in risk management, as a separate managerial area, and they can work at various levels in bringing about change. An example of a national level risk management committee is seen in the UK, NHS trust hospitals, which work in concert with the clinical governance committee and audit committee.[9]

Organizational level

At an organizational level, a risk manager has the role of identifying potential losses and assessing them, choosing an appropriate technique to prevent situations which can lead to loss; he also has to implement the risk management programme. The duties also involve a number of other tasks such as:

- Workers' compensation for occupational diseases and employee injury
- Patient and visitor injuries
- Transportation accidents
- Exposure to hazardous wastes
- Fraud in the third-party reimbursement
- Embezzelment
- Breaches of contract
- Defamation charges
- Protection against medical malpractice for its medical staff
- Insurance (risk coverage)
- Financing
- Handling claims
- Education of the various hospital personnel involved in the risk management programme
- Recording of adverse events
- Preparing reports

Risk managers employ three strategies to protect a healthcare organization. These are sometimes called 'control function'.[13, 14]

1. Risk prevention (e.g. educational programmes)
2. Risk avoidance (e.g. drop certain healthcare services because of potential for law suits)
3. Risk shifting (transfering responsibility of offering certain healthcare services to another organization or group)

Organizational approach

An organizational approach is quite different from that of an infection-control committee with emphasis on:

- Patient satisfaction
- Customers' complaints
- Litigation/claims

The risk management function can be broken down into four steps:

a. Identification and analysis of loss exposures
b. Selection of the appropriate mechanism(s) to reduce or, if possible, eliminate the possibility of loss
c. Implementation of the chosen technique(s)
d. Monitoring and reviewing the results[14]

Systematic task appraisal for risks[6]

The risks involved in the performance of various tasks should be considered in a systematic manner, both in totality and by a break-up of the processes. For example, let us consider the processes in a laboratory (Photo 8.3); the collection, transportation and receipt of specimens through pre-examination handling, the actual testing process and any subsequent steps such as disposal of specimens and associated laboratory waste should all be examined for potential risks. The task of all ancillary staff not directly involved with specimens must also be assessed, together with the use of machinery, equipment and appliances.

Questions should then be answered:

1. How should the task be performed?
2. Who should do what?
3. What materials are to be used?
4. Where should the task be performed?
5. What can go wrong while carrying out these processes?

This is followed by the identification of hazard, which in turn is followed by defining safe methods.

An excellent example of the merits of such systematic appraisal methods can be seen in the following situation:

The average risk of transmission of blood-borne pathogens following a single percutaneous exposure has been estimated to be 33.3% for hepatitis B virus (HBV), 3.3% for Hepatitis C virus (HCV) and 0.31% for Human Immunodeficiency Virus (HIV). This has led to the development of Standard Precautions (a sharps policy), development of work practice controls (handling sharps) and engineering controls (new technology for prevention of pricks or needle-stick injuries).[3]

The frequency of the risk can be derived at by noting down the frequency of its occurrence and classifying them in the categories (Fig. 8.3).

- High risk (e.g. once a week)
- Medium risk (e.g. once a month)
- Low risk (e.g. less than once a month)

An informative matrix can then be derived, which will direct the management efforts and resources (prioritizing risks).

When a particular process is identified as carrying a definite risk, measures to bypass such a process or substitute it with another safer one need to be arrived at, and to eliminate its adverse effects on people, equipment or the institution.

Patients are also exposed to various risks of acquiring infections during their stay in the hospital. This risk can be effectively addressed and often eliminated by keeping hospital stay as brief as possible.[11, 15]

Some Examples of Risk Elimination/ Reduction

Risks can be eliminated by changing over to a different mode of therapy or using a different strategy.

Example 1

Using disposal technology instead of reusable items for intubation. In this regard, the various departments have to develop policies which are economically feasible and practical.

Example 2

Healthcare workers are vaccinated appropriately against certain infections, e.g. Hepatitis B.

Example 3

Healthcare workers who are immunocompromised or immunodeficient should be

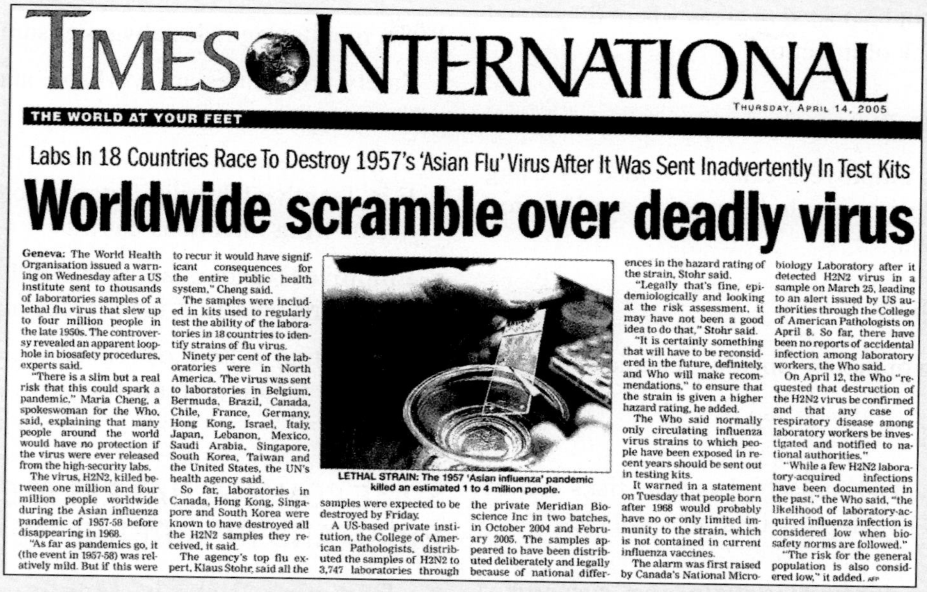

TIMES INTERNATIONAL

THE WORLD AT YOUR FEET

THURSDAY, APRIL 14, 2005

Labs In 18 Countries Race To Destroy 1957's 'Asian Flu' Virus After It Was Sent Inadvertently In Test Kits

Worldwide scramble over deadly virus

Geneva: The World Health Organisation issued a warning on Wednesday after a US institute sent to thousands of laboratories samples of a lethal flu virus that slew up to four million people in the late 1950s. The controversy revealed an apparent loophole in biosafety procedures, experts said.

"There is a slim but a real risk that this could spark a pandemic," Maria Cheng, a spokeswoman for the Who, said, explaining that many people around the world would have no protection if the virus were ever released from the high-security labs.

The virus, H2N2, killed between one million and four million people worldwide during the Asian influenza pandemic of 1957-58 before disappearing in 1968.

"As far as pandemics go, it (the event in 1957-58) was relatively mild. But if this were to recur it would have significant consequences for the entire public health system," Cheng said.

The samples were included in kits used to regularly test the ability of the laboratories in 18 countries to identify strains of flu virus.

Ninety per cent of the laboratories were in North America. The virus was sent to laboratories in Belgium, Bermuda, Brazil, Canada, Chile, France, Germany, Hong Kong, Israel, Italy, Japan, Lebanon, Mexico, Saudi Arabia, Singapore, South Korea, Taiwan and the United States, the UN's health agency said.

So far, laboratories in Canada, Hong Kong, Singapore and South Korea were known to have destroyed all the H2N2 samples they received, it said.

The agency's top flu expert, Klaus Stohr, said all the samples were expected to be destroyed by Friday.

A US-based private institution, the College of American Pathologists, distributed the samples of H2N2 to 3,747 laboratories through the private Meridian Bioscience Inc in two batches, in October 2004 and February 2005. The samples appeared to have been distributed deliberately and legally because of national differences in the hazard rating of the strain, Stohr said.

"Legally that's fine, epidemiologically and looking at the risk assessment, it may have not been a good idea to do that," Stohr said.

"It is certainly something that will have to be reconsidered in the future, definitely, and Who will make recommendations," to ensure that the strain is given a higher hazard rating, he added.

The Who said normally only circulating influenza virus strains to which people have been exposed in recent years should be sent out in testing kits.

It warned in a statement on Tuesday that people born after 1968 would probably have no or only limited immunity to the strain, which is not contained in current influenza vaccines.

The alarm was first raised by Canada's National Microbiology Laboratory after it detected H2N2 virus in a sample on March 25, leading to an alert issued by US authorities through the College of American Pathologists on April 8. So far, there have been no reports of accidental infection among laboratory workers, the Who said.

On April 12, the Who "requested that destruction of the H2N2 virus be confirmed and that any case of respiratory disease among laboratory workers be investigated and notified to national authorities."

"While a few H2N2 laboratory-acquired infections have been documented in the past," the Who said, "the likelihood of laboratory-acquired influenza infection is considered low when biosafety norms are followed."

"The risk for the general population is also considered low," it added. AFP

LETHAL STRAIN: The 1957 'Asian influenza' pandemic killed an estimated 1 to 4 million people.

Photo 8.3: Laboratories could be a risk to healthcare workers and to the community.

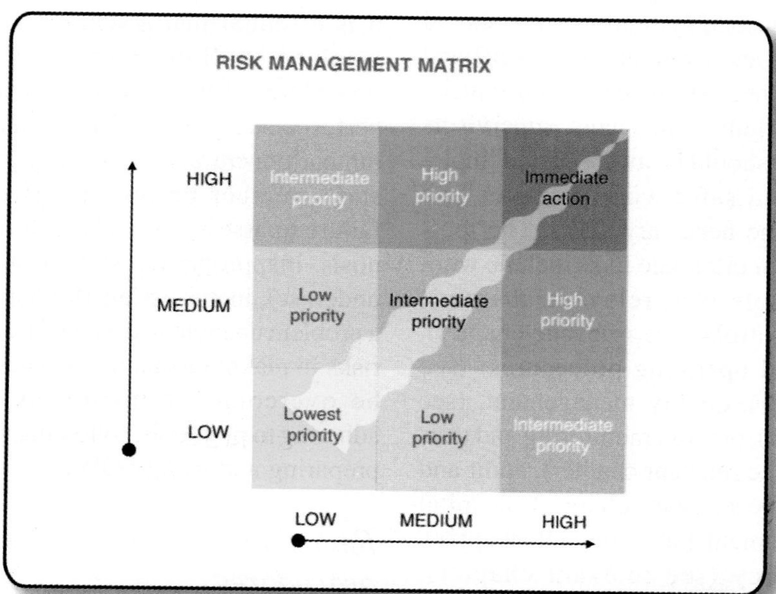

Figure 8.3: The risk management matrix can prioritize and quantify risks.

screened properly before employment and should not be posted in areas where they stand a high risk of infection.

Example 4

Risks to employees can be avoided by using better designed ethylene oxide sterilization equipment.

Example 5

Banning of mouth pipetting techniques.

Example 6

The financial impact of various risks can be reduced by adopting insurance policies.

Risk reduction: developing systems of work

Risks can now be managed by appropriate strategy. Documented systems of work should be agreed upon and available to all staff and must be implemented correctly and consistently. Staff, including managers, supervisors and employees, should be aware of and implement newer and safer work practices and get trained in the necessary skills. The tools used to control or eliminate risks include work practice controls (see relevant chapter), engineering controls (see relevant chapter), SOPs (standard operating procedures) (see relevant chapter), quality management, (see relevant chapter), process monitoring and tests of validation (see relevant chapter), audit and surveillance (see relevant chapter), hospital waste management (see relevant chapter), antibiotic policy (see relevant chapter), education and counselling of personnel at all levels.[9]

4. Risk Monitoring

When monitoring risks, always ensure that:

- Safety procedures are workable and effective
- Some of the indicators of risks are recorded. E.g. length of hospital stay, bacteremia, deaths from infectious causes
- Employees understand the need for the procedures and find them acceptable.[13]
- A reporting culture of critical incidents is present to understand the errors in the system

SOME COMMON HAI-RELATED RISKS AND RISK REDUCTION[7, 12, 15]

a. Reducing Risks in Making a Diagnosis/Investigation

Among the various factors involved in this, it is essential that a senior staff member is involved in all diagnostic and investigative procedures of the patient. For example, in the performance of critical procedures such as a lumbar puncture, it is imperative that a senior staff member be present. History-taking, failure to assess and make a differential diagnosis, inappropriate use of tests (overuse or underuse), inappropriate discharge, or leaving a problem unexplained, can all lead to increased risks in making a diagnosis. These can largely be overcome by instituting algorithms, adhering to protocols, following guidelines and preparing and using SOPs.

Reducing risks during invasive procedures

- These can be reduced by carefully considering risk–benefit ratio, discussing with patients, allotting adequate time for performing procedures, ensuring good working equipment with back-up, asking for help when procedures are not going well and having proper protocols of procedure.

- Sterilization and disinfection procedures, proper theatre attire, cleaning and draping protocols, standard precautions and use of personal protective equipment must all be carried out in a sterile environment.
- During surgeries, the anaesthetic procedures like intubation, insertion of catheters and IV lines must be performed under sterile conditions.
- The duration of surgery must be reduced as and when possible to ensure minimum risk to the patient.

b. Reducing the Risks of Drug Treatment

(Figure 8.4)

External retrospective review of case records and critical incident reporting are useful methods in drug-related adverse events.

Computer physician order entry (POE)[16] systems and team-based interventions directed by pharmacists have shown to reduce errors. The POE provides clinicians with a menu of medications and ranges of potential doses, reminders to check drug levels, consider allergies and to note potential drug interactions when appropriate. For some drugs, laboratory results are displayed automatically. It has been shown to decrease serious medication errors from 10.7 to 4.9 events per 1000 patient days.

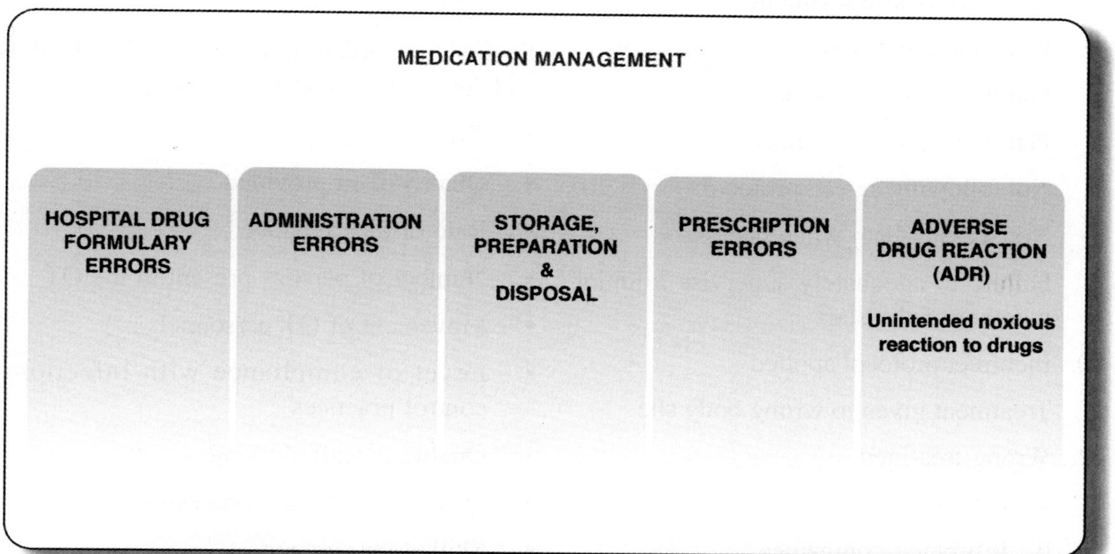

Figure 8.4: Risks due to drugs and drug delivery can be reduced by medication management.

Common factors associated with drug adverse events involve

- Failure to take into account renal and hepatic function
- Failure to check allergies
- Use of wrong drug name or administration
- Miscalculation of dose
- Wrong dosing frequency
- Wrong labelling of drug

c. Examples of Care Management Problems (Acts of Omission or Commission)

1. Failure to monitor, observe or act
2. Delay in diagnosis
3. Incorrect risk assessment
4. Inadequate handover
5. Failure to note faulty equipment
6. Failure to carry out check
7. Not following agreed protocol
8. Not seeking help when necessary
9. Failure to adequately supervise a junior member of the staff
10. Incorrect protocol applied
11. Treatment given to wrong body site
12. Wrong treatment
    a. Patients
    b. Insurance companies
    c. Funding organizations and healthcare providers in a managed healthcare system.

d. Some Common Risks—HAI-Related Process of Risk Management in Clinical Practice

The costs incurred by a payer, a professional, or provider in providing healthcare services varies according to the risks associated with treatment or management and can arise from the doctors' choice between alternative treatments or because different patients respond in different ways to the same treatment. Risk management may not be very well considered by a system where the patient pays for the services, but it is important in a managed care situation where risk managers control clinical operating risks by standardizing clinical protocols and choice of treatment (clinical operating risk).

e. Risks During Surgery

Several factors determine the risks involved in and during surgery, depending on:

- Type of surgery
- Quality of air provided
- Rate of air exchange
- Number of persons present in the OT
- Movement of OT personnel
- Level of compliance with infection-control practices
- Quality of staff clothing
- Quality of cleaning processes
- Skill of the surgeon
- Preparedness for emergency situations and mishaps

f. Handling Risks in the Emergency Room

Careful planning and preparedness is required in the emergency room. Emergency situations are always fraught with dangers of errors on the part of the staff or inappropriate action due to ill-equipped conditions. These can be countered by providing adequate training, reasonable infrastructure and personnel management.

g. Risks and Architectural Segregation

(See Chapter 13)

h. Risks during Outbreaks (Epidemiology)

Outbreaks of infections pose a great risk to healthcare workers, visitors and other hospital staff and thus require samples to be handled meticulously and methodically (see chapter on epidemiology).

i. Risks due to Drug Administration

(Figure 8.4)

Drug administration errors:[16] In the course of managing HAI, various drugs are used, such as antimicrobials, vaccines, sera and other non-drug agents such as interferon.

Hence, there is an ever-present risk of allergies and complications.

Risk assessment can also be carried out in the prescription of antimicrobials. Several factors are taken into consideration here:

a. Age of the patient (nephrotoxicity in the elderly, avoiding fluoroquinolones in children, etc.)
b. Race
c. Weight
d. Concomitant illness
e. Immunocompromised host
f. Concomitant medication
g. Previous antimicrobial therapy
h. Medical and surgical history
i. Expiry dates of medicines

Device-related risks:[3] Their description and handling is dealt with in the chapter on occupational hazards.

j. Risk Groups of Microorganisms

(See Chapter 13)

k. Risks in the Laboratory (Laboratory-Acquired Infections)

History provides us with a rich stock of instances wherein infections have broken out in the laboratory.[17]

- 1957—Reid's report on the incidence of tuberculosis among laboratory workers
- 1973—The famous 'escape' of small pox virus from a London laboratory in which two people died
- 1974—Submission of the Cox report followed by the Godber report after the small-pox incident, which included other dangerous pathogens/threats like the Marburg and Lassa fever viruses. The last mentioned was also believed to be transmitted by the postal route ('Lassa by letter!')

- 1975—Under the chairmanship of Sir James Howie, a report was prepared on a code of practice for the prevention of infections in clinical laboratories and post-mortem rooms (The Howie Code of practice).

  This report includes notes on the need for consultations between designers and users when laboratories are constructed, training of safety officers, assessment of safety and suitability of new equipment and the need to notify laboratory infections.
- 1978—The Birmingham incident of death of a photographer at a small pox research laboratory.

It is reasonable to expect that a person working in a laboratory and working with micro-organisms stands a greater risk of contracting diseases caused by those organisms in comparison to a person outside the laboratory. Microorganisms can enter the body through various routes like mouth, nasal passages, intact or breached skin and conjunctiva.[10] Also, one must remember that the route of infection in the laboratory can be different from the usual or natural route by which the disease is acquired.

Every type of laboratory is capable of predisposing the worker to infections, including research laboratory, diagnostic laboratory, teaching laboratory and biological products laboratory.

The infectious doses for various organisms differ widely, from 1–3 organisms (as in West Nile fever, scrub typhus, measles) to > 10^9 organisms (as in typhoid, cholera, *Escherichia coli* infections).

There are several predisposing activities that may lead to a laboratory acquired infection[12, 13]. These include:

- Spillage/splashes
- Needle and syringe pricks
- Sharps and broken glass
- Opening of culture bottles and ampoules
- Bites/scratches
- Aspiration through a pipette/mouth pipetting and blowing out of the last drop
- Use of blenders/vortex mixers/homo-genizsers/centrifuges/shakers.
- Aerosol production and dispersal in laboratories due to activities such as opening of containers, opening lyophilized cultures, harvesting of infected eggs, pouring, etc.
- Others/unknown

Note: Aerosols include larger droplets that are > 0.1 mm, which settle down and contaminate surfaces, smaller droplets that are < 0.1 mm, which evaporate and the bacteria in them remain in a dried state, are called droplet nuclei, e.g. *Mycobacterium tuberculosis*. The optimum size for alveolar penetration is 0.2 to 0.4 μm .

I. Occupational Exposure Management

It is the practice of identifying and analysing risks or losses and taking those measures necessary to minimize the real or potential losses to levels acceptable to the organization.

Workers dealing with hazardous chemicals must be trained and educated on the use of such chemicals and the hazards explained to them clearly. As far as possible, the use of such hazardous chemicals must be kept to the minimum and managed as follows:

a. Substitute the hazardous substance with a harmless alternative.

b. If substitution is not possible, restrict its use and keep it to the minimum.

c. Store the hazardous substance in an appropriate manner, with clear-cut labels.

d. Encourage the user-staff to adopt protective measures in the form of protective clothing, gloves, goggles, etc. (Photos 8.4, 8.5, 8.6)

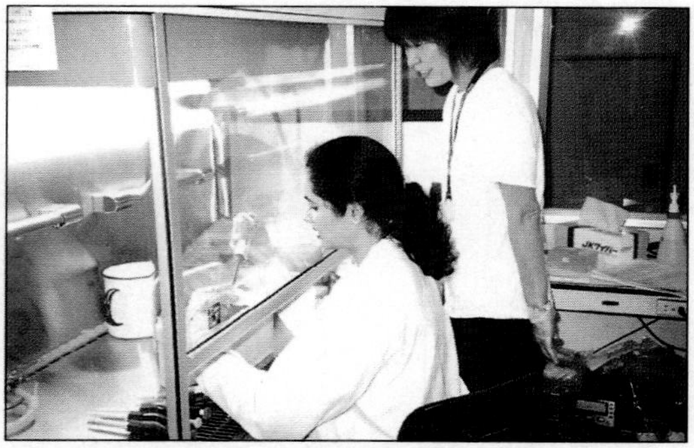

Photo 8.4: A biological safety cabinet for sterile procedures and for laboratory worker protection

Occupational risks due to commonly used disinfectants

Phenols and Phenol derivatives

Classified as a hazardous chemical
Rapid skin absorption to act systemically
Side effects: sinus congestion, phenol burns, skin ulceration, gangrene, dermatitis

Formaldehyde

Highly irritating to eyes and respiratory tract; (<3–4 ppm)

Chronic effects: pneumonitis, pulmonary oedema, residual cardiac impairment, ocular damage, recorded as potentially carcinogenic

Another form of formaldehyde (1,6 dioxhexane, which is chemically bound formaldehyde), gluteraldehyde, benzalkonium + chloride and alkyl urea derivatives are not cleared by the EPA (Employee Protection Agency), USA because of stringent standards but is accepted by the CEN (Committee European Nationalité) and is used in European hospitals as Bacillocid.

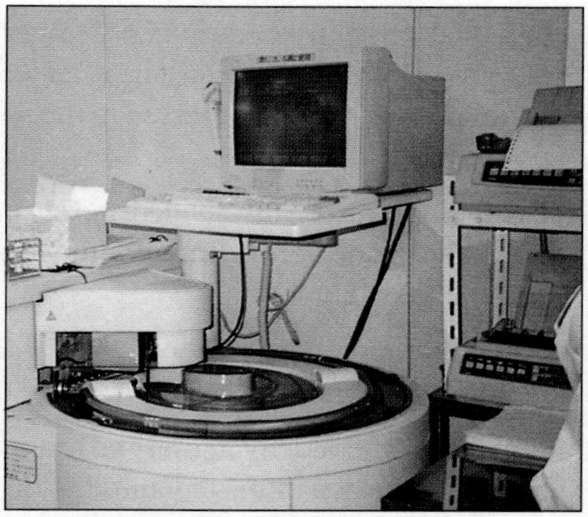

Photo 8.5: Engineering controls have helped design better equipment. Shown here is an automated ELISA processor

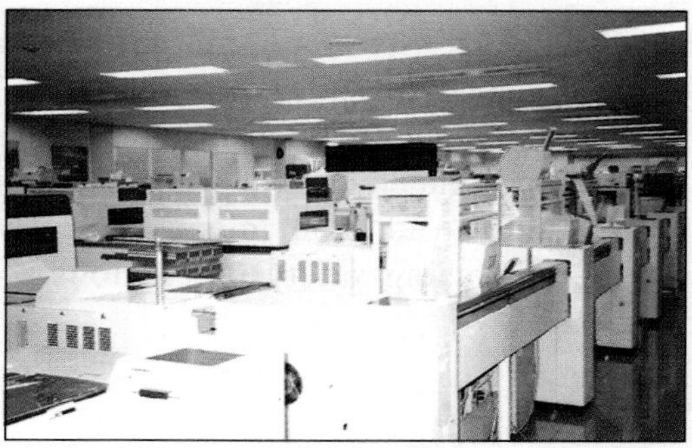

Photo 8.6: A fully automated laboratory in Japan. This considerably reduces risks to workers

Gluteraldehyde

Occupational Safety and Health Organization (OSHA) has adopted 0.2 ppm of gluteraldehyde air vapour as the permissible exposure limit (PEL) in the workplace (1989). Routine monitoring is not recommended.

1. The gluteraldehyde containing trays must be covered at all times except when instruments are being taken out or put in. The trays must be kept in areas which are well ventilated.
2. Personal protective equipment (impervious gloves and aprons) must be used when handling equipment immersed in the solution.
3. Equipment must be dismantled and cleaned with detergent before immersing in the gluteraldehyde solution.
4. Adequate time must be allowed for disinfecting/sterilizing.
5. Residual gluteraldehyde must be removed by adequate washing—manually or by using an automatic washer. The residuals have a number of effects on the body depending on the region they come in contact with (allergic contact eczema, proctitis, etc.).
6. For spills: Use ammonia solution to neutralize small spills and for large spills use ammonium carbonate (500gms per gallon of gluteraldehyde estimated to be spilled). And then, clean after five minutes using safety precautions and PPE.

m. Biosafety or Containment Levels

(See Chapter 13) (Tables 8.3, 8.4)

It is obvious that work with organisms in different risk groups requires different conditions for containment, i.e. ensuring that the organisms do not escape from their specimens, culture vessels or the laboratory. Containment addresses various issues of access, equipment and safety precautions for each group of organisms. The entrance to the laboratory must bear the biohazard symbol to warn the staff and others to take adequate precautions. Entry must be restricted to relevant personnel (Photo 8.7).

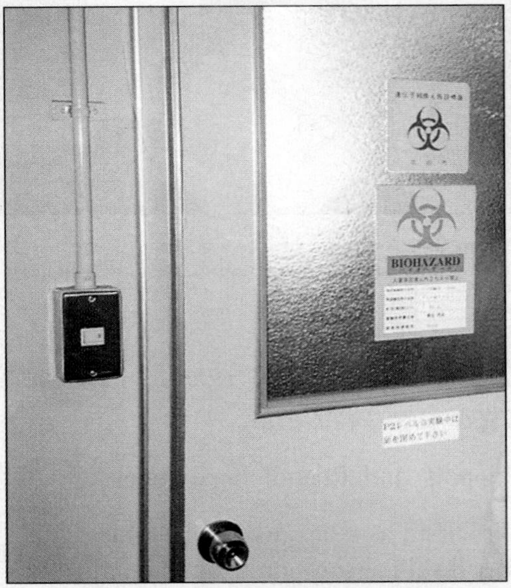

Photo 8.7: A P3 lab has maximum precautions for preventing risks and handling highly infectious organisms Note: the biohazard symbol

Table 8.3: Classification of organisms according to risk

WHO (1979)	Risk Group 1—low risk to individual and community	Risk Group 2—moderate risk to individual, limited risk to community	Risk Group 3—high risk to individual, low risk to community	Risk Group 4—high risk to both individual and community
ACDP (1984)	Hazard group 1—unlikely to cause human disease	Hazard group 2—possible infection to laboratory workers, unlikely to spread to community	Hazard group 3—some hazard to laboratory workers. May spread to community	Hazard group4—Serious hazard to laboratory workers. High risk to community

Table 8.4: Containment by laboratory design and practices

Level	Laboratory practice
1. Basic	Good Microbiological Practice (GMP)
2. Basic	GMP + protective clothing + biohazard signs
3. Containment	Level 2 + special clothing + controlled access
4. Maximum Containment	Level 3 + air lock + shower exit + special waste disposal methods

REFERENCES

1) Kitahara M. Nosocomial infections and risk management.Nippon Geka Gakkai Zasshi. 2003; 104(1): 32-4.

2) John Gosbee and Laura Lin. The role of human factors and engineering in medical device and medical system errors. In: Charles Vincent, ed. Clinical risk management. Enhancing patient safety. 2nd edn. BMJ books. 2001; 301-317.

3) Secker-Walker J and Sally Taylor-Adams. Clinical incident reporting. In: Vincent C, ed. Clinical risk management. Enhancing patient safety. 2nd edition BMJ books. 2001; 419-438.

4) Millar J. System performance is the real problem. Healthc Pap. 2001; 2(1): 79-84.

5) Kuehne RW. Personal hygiene and protection. In: Liberman DF, ed. Biohazards Management Handbook. 2nd edition. Marcel Dekker Inc. 1995; 221-239.

6) Juran JM and Gryna FM. Manufacture In: Quality Planning and Analysis. 3rd edn, New Delhi: Tata McGraw-Hill Pubishing Company Limited. 1995; 393-99.

7) Yamagishi M, Kanda K and Takemura Y. Methods developed to elucidate nursing related adverse events in Japan. J Nurs Manag. 2003; 11(3): 168-76.

8) Carson P, Carson K and Roe C. Management of Health Care Organizations. Cincinnati: South-Western College Publishing. 1995; 351-353

9) Neale G. Reducing risks in the practice of hospital general medicine. In: Vincent C, ed. Critical risk management – enhancing patient safety. 2nd edn. London, BMJ books.2001; 175-191.

10) Unruh L. Licensed nurse staffing and adverse events in hospitals. Med Care. 2003; 41 (1): 142-52.

11) Rogues AM et al. Is length of stay in the recovery room a risk factor for cross infections? Ann Fr Anesth Reanim.2002 21(8):643-7.

12) Farrington M and Pascoe G. Risk management and infection control – time to get our priorities right in the United Kingdom. J of Hosp. Infect. 2001; 47(1): 19-24.

13) Collins C H. Laboratory Acquired Infections. 3rd edn.Butterworth & Heinmann. 1993; 202-213.

14) Collins CH. Laboratory Acquired Infections. 3rd edn. Butterworth & Heinmann. 1993; 184-200.

15) Houston S, Gentry LO, Pruitt V et al. Reducing the incidence of nosocomial pneumonia in cardiovascular surgery patients. Qual Manag Health Care. 2003; 12(1): 28-41.

16) Bates DW, Leape LL, Cullen DJ et al. Effect of computerized physician order entry and a team intervention on prevention of serious medication errors. J Am Med Assoc. 1998; 280(15): 1311-16.

17) Levitt MA. Hazardous chemical management. In: Liberman DF, ed. Biohazards Management Handbook. 2nd edn. Marcel Dekker Inc. 1995; 97-111.

Chapter 9

Epidemiological Concerns in HAI

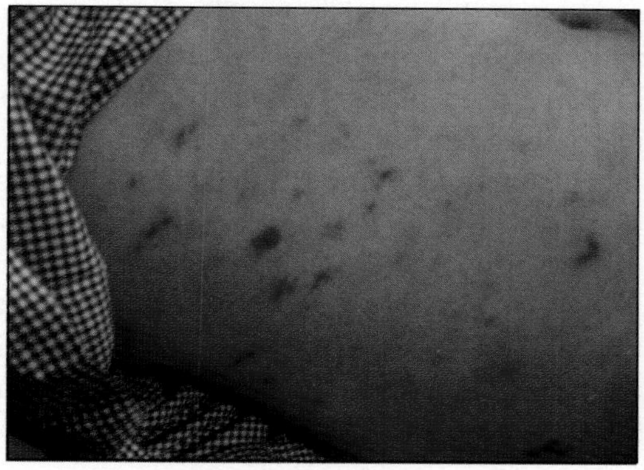

Strategy without tactics is the slowest route to victory. Tactics without strategy is the noise before defeat.

—Sun Tzu

Highlights

The Epidemiological Triad of Disease
The Agent
The Host
The Environment
Community Acquired Infections as HAI
Global Dimensions of HAI
Modes of Transmission

INTRODUCTION

The hospital (or any other healthcare institution) is similar to a small community that is densely populated. It provides a unique environment for the transmission of HAI. The reasons for this are multiple: It provides an interface for transmission of microorganisms between patients, doctors, other healthcare workers and even visitors. This is due to the activities occurring in a healthcare facility—invasive procedures, (mis)use of antibiotics, use of immunosuppressants, blood transfusion, transplantation of organs and laboratory investigations, all of which contribute to an increase in HAI (Photo 9.1). Thus, HAI can occur in primary, secondary or tertiary healthcare settings, as well as in laboratories, animal facilities, dental clinics, blood banks and pain clinics.

Epidemiology

According to Bennett and Brachman,[1] 'epidemiology is the dynamic study of the determinants, occurrence and distribution of health and disease in a population, which, for nosocomial infections, is the hospital population.'

So, like the community acquired infections (CAI), HAI also follow basic epidemiological patterns and are hence amenable to carefully applied control measures. Thus, the epidemiological aspects and measures applicable to a community acquired infection are applicable also to a hospital acquired one. The broad area of patient care is strengthened by the application of epidemiological methods to the many activities encompassed in quality assurance programmes. Yet, there are some differences between a hospital and a community outbreak, thus warranting a few differences in the approach to its control.

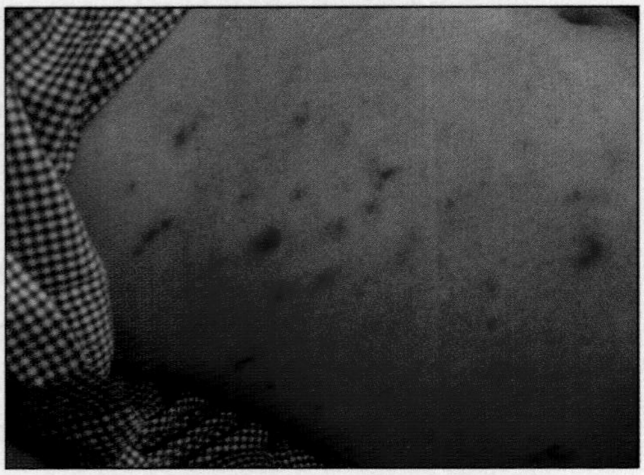

Photo 9.1: A patient of meningococcal meningitis with haemorrhagic spots can spread the disease to other patients, practitioners and visitors.

How Is HAI Different from CAI?

In the hospital set-up, there is

- a continual presence of virulent microorganisms
- selection of resistant strains of microorganisms
- a close association between carriers and susceptible hosts
- low level of host defences in hospitalized patients
- an altered microbial flora in patients on antibiotics, thereby allowing resistant organisms to gain a foothold
- an impairment of inflammatory and immune responses due to certain medications, making the host more susceptible

The good news is that HAI are more amenable to control measures because these infections have certain characteristics that can be controlled: they usually have known reservoirs and are transmitted by predictable routes. They require susceptible hosts for their transmission, and if these are unavailable, due to adequate control measures, the transmission chain is broken. Reservoir hosts exist both in animate (like healthcare workers) as well as inanimate (like food supplies or equipment) environment. All of these are manageable with a well planned-out infection-control programme.[1]

THE EPIDEMIOLOGICAL TRIAD OF DISEASE

(FIGURE 9.1)

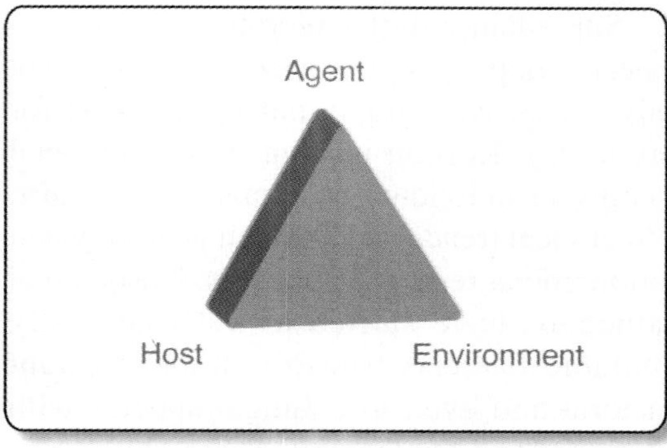

Figure 9.1: The epidemiological triad of disease

It is customary to consider the occurrence of infectious diseases as the end-result of a triad of interlinked factors viz. the Agent, the Host and the Environment. So also, hospital acquired infections occur as a result of complex interactions between the same three factors, which have to be understood in order to plan out control measures.[2]

Source is a site where pathogenic organisms grow and from which they are transmitted and colonize or cause an infection in another site on the same or in another person. A source is usually an infected or colonized patient or staff, or less frequently, inanimate environment.

Nosocomial infections may be classified according to source as endogenous infections or exogenous infections.The majority of nosocomial infections are endogenous in origin, that is, they originate from the patient's own microbial flora. E.g. translocation from gut flora (commensals).

Commensals

Commensals are organisms which exist on the host (skin, oral cavity, gut, etc.) serving a mutually beneficial symbiotic relationship. This is in contrast to colonization, which is the first step to a pathological state. The choice of a prophylactic antibiotic depends on the commensals in that region of the body.

Reservoir

These are sites in the environment where organisms grow or contaminate, but do no necessarily transmit infection. Removing or destroying a reservoir will not prevent transmission of infection, unless it is also a potential source.[3-4]

RESERVOIRS

Source → → Sharps
→ IV fluids and cannulae
→ Surgical instruments (contaminated)

AGENT FACTORS

These include properties or qualities of the

nosocomial pathogens which favour their spread or lodgement in the host, thus leading to the occurrence of HAI. A knowledge of agent factors is required in order to identify them correctly, institute appropriate treatment and to eliminate the microorganism effectively from the host and thus prevent its spread. Properties of the agent:

- Pathogenicity (ability to cause disease)
- Virulence (quantitative ability of an organism to cause disease)
- Toxigenicity (ability of an organism to produce toxin)
- Invasivenes (ability to enter host cells or tissues and spread in the body)
- Load (its numbers)
- Resistance (its ability to resist antimicrobial action). Processes like conjugation, transduction (phage mediated) and transformation confer resistance to antimicrobials agents
- Special appendages to counter the host defence mechanisms: Bacteria may have flagella, fimbria, capsule, slime layer and sometimes highly resistant forms like spores
- Ubiquitous presence and independent existence
- Biofilm formation
- Choice of body sites as targets of invasion

Colonization

Colonization is the persistent survival of microorganisms on the surface of the human body.[1] There is a difference between colonization and infection, and it is often difficult to differentiate between the two, although it is important to do so, because the former does not require treatment while the latter does. Medical equipment and devices are prone to colonization, depending on the type of material, which may progress to full-fledged infection if not contained adequately.

Infection

It is the lodgement and multiplication of an infectious agent in the body. Multiplication of organisms which are a part of the normal flora is not considered infection, while multplication of pathogenic agents in the body even if the body is asymptomatic is an infection.

Surveillance of the microbial aetiology in special groups over prolonged time periods not only can provide important information for day-to-day decision making in antimicrobial therapy in individual hospitals, but can also reflect local trends and shifts in aetiology and antimicrobial resistance patterns. Nosocomial pathogens have shifted away from easily treatable bacteria towards more resistant bacteria and even to a fungal species with fewer options for therapy. These shifts continue to present challenges for nosocomial infection control and prevention.[5, 6]

HOST FACTORS

A number of host factors have been implicated as increasing the risk for HAI. Host factors include:

- General state of health
- Integrity of surface defences
- Special risk groups (COAD, diabetes)
- Capacity for inflammatory and immune response

- Level of immunity
- Impact of medical intervention
- Relevant clinical details
- Date and time of onset
- Clinical symptoms/signs
- Information about treatment
- History of travel abroad
- Details of allergies to drugs
- Certain groups of patients have a vulnerability to certain infections. Patients with transplants, neonatal group, patients with neoplasms or burns, ventilated patients, etc. stand a high risk of acquiring infections.

The hosts involved in HAI may be patients or hospital staff. Among the latter, there are certain groups at high risk, although every HCW needs to be protected. The high risk group includes the laboratory personnel, blood bank workers, surgeons, anaesthetists and nurses. The predisposing factors identified are diabetes mellitus, use of steroids, obesity, extreme age, poor nutrition, distant infection, malignancy, systemic humoral or cellular immune defects and local abnormalities of host defences. These factors can be controlled to some extent by procedures like following aseptic precautions at all times, controlling diabetes, immunization against possible diseases, etc.

Risk factors for acquisition of MRSA

- Prolonged hospital stay (often >14 days)
- Preceding antimicrobial therapy
- Surgical procedure(s)
- Presence in intensive care or burn unit
- Proximity to a known MRSA case

Infections Relating to an Underlying Disease or Immunocompromised Status

1. Humoral immunity impairment (hypogammaglobulinemia IgA, IgM, IgG): Patients with chronic lymphocytic leukemia and multiple myeloma have hypogammaglobulinemia due to impaired number and function of polyclonal B cells. Common infections in such patients are due to Gram-positive bacteria *(Staphylococcus,Streptococcus)* and Gram-negative bacteria *(E.coli, Klebsiella).* Viral and fungal infections are uncommon. These conditions, however, may have associated cell mediated, complement activity or opsonizing antibody defects also. They have an impaired response to vaccination.
2. Cell-mediated immunity defect: Patients with Hodgkin's disease have a cell mediated defect, but have normal granulocyte and humoral function. These patients are prone to infection by the following microbes: *Listeria monocytogenes,* Candida spp, Herpes simplex virus, *Pneumocystis carinii, Streptococcus pneumoniae* and *Coccidioides immitis.*
3. T-cell dysfunction: Patients with hairy cell leukemia have a T-cell dysfunction. They also have defects in their granulocytes and monocytes and have an impairment of the cell-mediated immunity.
4. Neutropenic patients are prone to bacterial Gram-positive infections around the mucosal sites—skin, perineum, sinuses,

oesophagus, colon, etc. The infections are commonly due to organisms colonizing these areas. Common Gram-positive infections are by: *Staphylococcus, alpha haemolytic Streptococcus*. Gram-negative bacilli including *E.coli, Klebsiella* and *Pseudomonas*. Common fungi include Candida, Aspergillus and Zygomycetes (mucormycosis). A functional defect in the granulocytic function is also seen in diabetes mellitus.

5. Monocytopenia: Such patients are prone to disseminated infections due to Candida, Aspergillus, *Pneumocystis carinii,* CMV, atypical mycobacteria.
6. Drugs for immune suppression such as fludarabine, 2-chloro deoxy adenosine deoxycoformycin can cause T-cell defects which may persist for even a year after stoppage of the drugs. These purine analogs are prone to infections by Listeria, Nocardia and Aspergillus. The other older drugs cause infections by Candida, Aspergillus, VZV, HSV.
7. Steroids cause a qualitative defect in phagocytic function and a decrease in immunity
8. Radiation damages mucosa and makes tissues prone to infection.
9. Iatrogenic procedures also have a detrimental effect at times.
10. Local pressure effects of tumours can lead to obstruction to secretions, which then lead to infection.
11. Splenectomy: Impairs antibody function and also mononuclear-phagocytic cell function necessary for removing opsonized and non-opsonized bacteria.

ENVIRONMENT FACTORS[7]

Areas in a hospital that need special measures for HAI control: HAI can occur in all areas of healthcare settings. Some areas have their own unique problems when it comes to transmission of HAI, e.g. blood banks. Therefore, one needs to address these issues and develop protocols, strategies, laws, regulations and guidelines for the respective areas.

Some Important Areas

1. Individual clinical areas

- Intensive care units: surgical, medical, neonatal, burns, etc.
- Operating rooms
- Haemodialysis units
- Labour rooms
- General wards
- Solid organ transplant units
- Paediatric and neonatal units
- Burns wards
- Pain clinics

2. Clinical investigation/diagnostic areas

Spirometry, endoscopy units, neurosciences and cardiology units as also the general laboratories (biochemistry, microbiology, cytology, histopathology).

3. Other areas

- Physiotherapy, hydrotherapy units
- Blood banks

- Pharmacy
- Laundry
- Housekeeping areas
- Food and catering centres
- Autopsy units/mortuaries
- Biomedical waste management department
- CSSD

COMMUNITY ACQUIRED INFECTIONS AS HAI

Any infectious disease brought into the hospital from the community can result in a hospital acquired infection if transmitted by a patient/carrier to a susceptible host in the hospital set-up. Such infections need to be recognized in order to institute proper control measures. Emerging infectious diseases such as the SARS and anthrax can also be rapidly transmitted to other patients and healthcare workers in healthcare facilities.

According to the occurrence of disease, HAI may be epidemic, endemic or sporadic in nature.

GLOBAL DIMENSIONS OF HAI[8]

Newer infections in this jet age may not be limited to a single country or continent. They have the potential to spread quickly and need equally quick solutions that can limit their global impact. This calls for awareness, utilization of facilities at a global level, network for notification at a state, national and international level and rapid mobilization of resources.

MODES OF TRANSMISSION

(FIGURE 9.2)

There are six steps involved in the transmission of an infectious disease, and this also

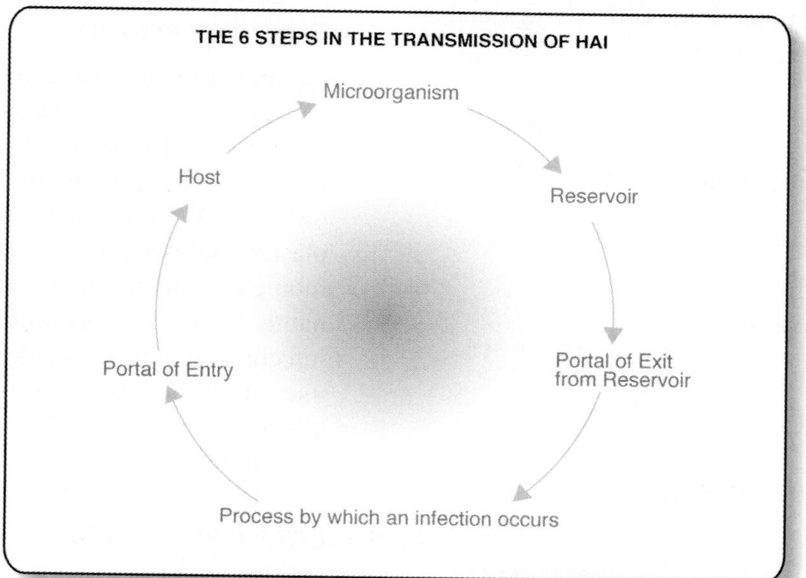

Figure 9.2: Transmission of HAI: There are six steps in the transmission of HAI.

applies to HAI. When any one of these factors is prevented from interacting with the other five, infection or disease does not follow. Therefore, the control measures should aim at breaking the link between these factors.

- Standard precautions are applied to all cases
- Special precautions are applied in addition to standard precautions, wherever necessary
- Special precautions are developed on the basis of the mode of transmission

Portals of exit

All secretions are infectious and should be handled with standard precautions. All secretions should be considered infective: blood, saliva, tears, nasal and tracheal secretions, stools, urine, peritoneal and pleural secretions, bile, CSF, tissues and other patient specimens.

Modes (Process) of Transmission

- Contact (direct, indirect)
- Airborne
- Droplet
- Inoculation (blood-borne)
- Food-borne
- Water-borne

Infections by contact

(Table 9.1)

This is the commonest mode of transmission.

1. Direct contact: Here, the organism is directly transferred by contact, between the host and the infected or colonized person.
2. Indirect contact: Transmission occurs when there is no direct contact but the organism is transmited indirectly on a fomite (needles, dressings, infected hands, etc.)
   a) Staff to patients: With resident and transient flora on skin. Common organisms are *Staphylococcus aureus, Klebsiella, Serratia spp.,VRE, C.difficile, Candida albicans*. Rarely *C. difficile,* RSV, Rhinovirus can be transmitted by fomites. Clothing of staff may transmit *S. aureus* and Gram-negative bacteria. These infections can be prevented by handwashing.
   b) Patient to others: *S. aureus, Enterococcus, C. difficile*. This is prevented by stopping transfer of organisms from one patient to another by decontaminating equipment and hands when moving from patient to patient.
   c) Equipment related: These include tongue depressors, gastric endoscopes (can harbour *H.pylori, Salmonella, Pseudomonas),* Bronchoscopes (can harbour *M.tuberculosis*), adhesive plasters, bed pans, urine cans, rectal thermometers, stethoscopes, telephones to name a few. The prevention of these infections requires consideration of the use of disposables or resorting to adequate and appropriate disinfection procedures.

Airborne transmission

Airborne transmission occurs where the size of the airborne droplets is 5μm or less in

Table 9.1: Modes of transmission of common hospital acquired infections

Portal of Entry in certain HAI				
Percutaneous injury	**Respiratory route**	**Skin infections**	**Gastrointestinal infections**	**Eye splashes**
HIV	Tuberculosis	Warts	Viral diarrhoeas	HIV
HBV	RSV	Fungal infections	HAV	
HCV				HCV
CMV				

diameter. Because of the smaller size of the particles, they remain suspended for a long period and can be carried over longer distances and may even be inhaled by people far away from the source. Normal precautions such as surgical face masks are ineffective in preventing the inhalation. Therefore, special masks and special air-handling techniques must be used to prevent spread. Some of the common air-borne infections include: tuberculosis, pneumococcal pneumonia, meningococcal meningitis, viral infections such as rubella and varicella, fungal infections such as aspergillosis. Bacterial surgical wound infections in the OT are also spread by this mode.

airborne routes → persons
→ aerosolised fluids
→ dust

Infections in the Operating Room: These infections occur in patients usually due to their own flora rather than that spread from the OT staff. Even so, adequate precautions are to be taken to avoid such mishaps. These measures include plenum ventilation for flow of air from OT to the outside and not in the reverse direction, adequate and satisfactory OT clothing of staff and patients, restricting the number of staff members in the OT, reduced movement within the OT and its complex, keeping patient's items like blankets, dressings, etc. at a minimum in the OT.

Droplet-borne infections

Large droplets (more than 5µm in diameter) which are generated due to coughing, sneezing and talking have a tendency to settle down in the conjunctiva or upper airway of the host. These, unlike the airborne transmission, do not travel for long distances and do not require stringent preventive measures. They can easily be prevented by the use of surgical masks and goggles. They do not require special air-handling measures either.

Infection by inoculation

These include various viral infections such as the Hepatitis B and C infections, Human Immunodefeciency Virus infection, and are generally transmitted by injections, blood transfusions, organ transplantations, sharps injury or contaminated infusion fluids (e.g. in total parenteral nutrition patients). Such infections

Table 9.2: Most commonly associated infections in primary immunodeficiency disorders

Immunodeficiency	Infections
T-lymphocyte defects	*Pneumocystis carinii* pneumonia Listeriosis Candidiasis Salmonellosis Aspergillosis Severe, persistent or recurrent viral infections (RSV, parainfluenza, CMV, poliovirus, enterovirus, HSV, EBV) Disseminated or pulmonary mycobacterial infection.
B-lymphocyte disorders	Bacterial sepsis/meningitis *(Streptococcus pneumoniae, Haemophilus influenzae, Pseudomonas aeruginosa)* Recurrent otitis media Recurrent sinopulmonary infections Chronic enteroviral infections Recurrent or chronic gastrointestinal infections *(Giardia lamblia*, rotavirus, *Cryptosporidium spp);* Arthritis due to *Ureaplasma urealyticum*
Complement disorders	Severe or recurrent infections with encapsulated bacteria *(Neisseria meningitidis, Neisseria gonorrhoeae, Haemophilus influenzae, Streptococcus pneumoniae)*
Phagocytic/chemotactic disorders	Pyogenic infections due to *Staphylococcus aureus*, opportunistic Gram-negative bacteria, *Nocardia spp.*, fungi (Aspergillus, Candida spp.)

are also transmitted during various procedures carried out such as: cardiac catheterization, using in-dwelling catheters, using transducers/pressure monitoring devices, blood transfusions, anaesthetic techniques, endotracheal intubation, CNS shunts, gastrointestinal procedures, e.g. colostomies, bronchoscopy/cystoscopy, etc., gynaecological instrumentation, urological instrumentation, interventional radiology, barium enema, peritoneal manipulation and major surgeries. Surgical site infections emphasize the importance of close surveillance of early wound complications and surgical decision-making. This is substantiated by a study on prospective audit of the management and outcome of prosthetic patch infection after carotid endarterectomy (CEA) at Leicester Royal Infirmary, UK. These require protocols for sterilization and disinfection of equipment, blood banking protocols and donor screening for transmission of diseases.

Water-borne infections [9, 10]

Water is a vehicle for transmission of many HAI. Water is not only used for drinking but, also for baths, sauna, hydrotherapy, etc. Water is also used for cleaning and surgical scrub. Therefore, water that is infected can lead to a number of infections. Commonly, Gram-negative bacteria can contaminate water supply. In addition, certain diseases, such as the Legionnaire's disease, are caused by infected water supply. Water contaminated by sewage can lead to a number of diseases too. Intermittent water supply is also a potential source of infection in healthcare institutions as the fall in pressure leads to contamination.

Food-borne infections [9]

Infected food is a potent source of HAI. Improper precautions during preparation, storage, transport and handling can lead to a variety of infections such as diarrhoeas and amoebiasis. Other infections may be due to Salmonella in hospital eggs, and *Clostridium welchii* in meat. Food handlers who are carriers spread organisms like Salmonella and other resistant organisms harboured in their gut.

This forms the basis of development of aseptic techniques and transmission-based precautions.

Important preventive measures based on the modes of transmission are given below:

- Handwashing
- Patient placement strategies (isolation, cohorting, ventilation)
- Attire (masks, eye protection, face shields, respiratory protection)
- Special handling of patient-care articles
- Handling linen and laundry
- Standard precautions
- Transmission-based precautions

The disease: identification, prevention of spread

(Table 9.2, 9.3, 9.4)

Any infection occurring in a patient who has been in hospital for longer than the incubation period suggests a source in the hospital. But, it is also important to have protocols to prevent infection from entering a hospital, to know the kind of host and infection we are dealing with so that adequate precautions can be taken to prevent and treat. It should be noted that each nosocomial infection prolongs the patient's stay in the hospital by five to ten days.

Microorganism (source)

↓

+ Process of infection
+ Risk of infection → Disease
+ Susceptible host

Table 9.3: Common modes of transmission of HAI and prevention

Mode of transmission	Transmission-based precautions
Cross transmission	Patient isolation and barrier precautions determined by infective agents
Hand transmission	Improvements in hand-washing
Droplet transmission	Attire, masks, face shields, goggles
Airborne transmission	Placement strategies, cohorting, patient isolation with appropriate ventilation
Infected equipment	Disposable devices, disinfection, sterilization
Water-borne	Checking of water supply and all liquid containers
Food-borne	Elimination of the food at risk Environmental cleaning (routine and terminal)

Table 9.4: Prevention strategies in primary immunodeficiencies

General measures for prevention of infection in primary immunodeficiencies
• Avoid contact with individuals with infections
• Avoid live viral and bacterial vaccines (oral poliovirus vaccine should not be given to close contacts or household members)
• Immunize normal close contacts against vaccine-preventable disease (i.e. chickenpox, measles, influenza)
• Irradiate all blood products (3000-5000 rad) before administration to avoid graft-versus-host disease
• Use red blood cells for transfusion from cytomegalovirus-seronegative donors or leukocyte-filtered red blood cells
• Avoid splenectomy if possible
• Treat all minor infections with appropriate antimicrobial therapy to avoid severe infections and complications

Risk of infection = dose + time of exposure + virulence of organism + host susceptibility

SOURCE AND PREVENTION

1. Endogenous infection: To prevent or neutralize the translocation of commensal flora

Preventive methods:

- Antibiotic prophylaxis in surgery
- Skin antisepsis before surgery
- Antiseptic bound IV catheter
- Intestinal decontamination of neutropenic patients
- Pneumococcal immunization before splenectomy

2. Exogenous infection: To prevent cross-infection

Preventive methods:

- Hand hygiene for patient-care procedures
- Isolation and decolonization of carriers of transmissible pathogens
- Sterilization or disinfection of invasive devices
- Cleaning and disinfection of fomites
- Outbreak detection and molecular epidemiologic studies to determine the mode and vehicles of spread

3. To prevent common-source infection

Preventive methods:

- Ultra-clean air for prostheses surgery or bone marrow transplant recipients
- Disinfection of *Legionella spp.* in water systems
- Environmental, water and food hygiene
- Sterile parenteral drugs and implantable material
- Outbreak detection and molecular epidemiological studies to identify the source

4. Antimicrobial resistance: To prevent the emergence and spread of resistant genes

Preventive methods:

- Restricted usage of broad-spectrum antimicrobial agents
- Optimized anti-infectious therapy (agents, dosage and duration)

5. To prevent the spread of resistant strains of microorganisms

Preventive methods:

- Detection, monitoring and timely reporting of antimicrobial resistance
- Isolation precautions and treatment of carriers of transmissible resistant strains
- Molecular epidemiologic studies to distinguish between mutant selection, gene or clone dissemination.

REFERENCES

1) Bennett JV and Brachman PS. Hospital Infections. In: Brachman PS, ed. Epidemiology of nosocomial infections. 4th edn. Lippincott-Raven Publishers 1998; 3-16.

2) Park K. Concepts of health and disease. In: Park's textbook of preventive and Social Medicine. 15th edn. 1997; 11-44.

3) Weinstein RA. Clinical Syndromes: Nosocomial Infections. Harrison's Principles of Internal Medicine Fauci AS, Kasper DL, Hauser SL, Longo DL, Jamesonh JL, eds. Mc Graw Hill Publishers E Braunwald, Vol. 1. 15th edn. 2001; 853-856.

4) Weinstein RA and Welbel SA. In: Brachman PS, ed. Hosptial Infection. Epidemiology of nosocomial infections. 4th edn. Lippincott Raven publishers 1998; 741-759.

5) Public health focus: surveillance, prevention, and control of nosocomial infections. Morb Mortality Wkly Rep 1992; 41: 783-787

6) Haley RW. Surveillance by objective: a new priority-directed approach to the control of nosocomial infections. The National Foundation for infectious Disease Lecture. Am J Infect Control 1985;13(2): 78-89.

7) Simmons BP. In: Chap 2. Hospital epidemiology. Hospital Infections. Lippincott-Raven publishers. 4th edn. 1998; 17-22.

8) Wenzel RP. Towards a global perspective of nosocomial infections. Eur J Clin Microbiol 1987; 6: 341-343.

9) Mathai MD. Environmental Challenges: Food and water supply to hospitals. In: Environment Management for Control of Hospital Infections. VII National Conference. Hospital Infection Society. India. CME Vellore. 2003; 80-83.

10) SlaterFM. Water Management.In: Abrutyn E, Goldmann DA, Scheckler WE, eds. Saunders Infection Control Reference Service. WB Saunders Company. 1998; 753-54.

Chapter 10

The Concept of Barriers and Personal Protective Equipment

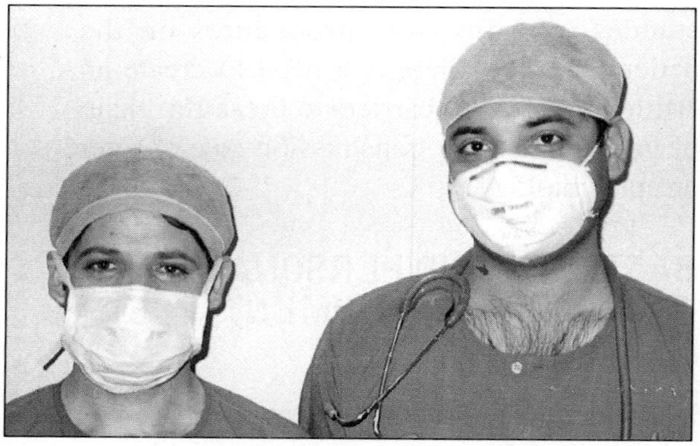

Safety is good technique—a hallmark of technical excellence in which the staff should take pride.

—N. R. Grist

Highlights

Barriers and Personal Protective Equipment (PPE)
Gloves
Masks
Eye protection
Head Covers and Caps
Shoe Covers, Leg covers, Boots
Gowns
Behaviour and Attire Related to Work Area
Importance of Hand-washing
Hand Decontamination
Systems of Precautions
Other Barriers
Role of Institutions

INTRODUCTION

There are certain natural barriers in the body which prevent infection from occurring. These include intact skin, nasal cilia, lung macrophages, white blood cells, acidic environment of the stomach, tears, saliva and the immune system. However, these may be ineffective in preventing infection under certain circumstances (e.g. invasive procedures on the patient). Hence, there is a need to create an artificial system of barriers to break the chain of infection and its transmission (see chapter on epidemiology).

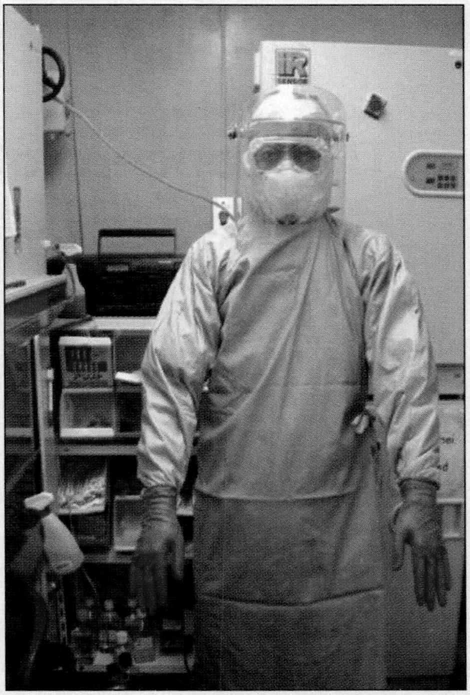

Photo 10.1: Barrier precautions in a P3 laboratory

BARRIERS AND PERSONAL PROTECTIVE EQUIPMENT (PPE)

(PHOTO 10.1)

Historically, the concept of barriers to prevent infection to the patient was introduced long before the concept of personal protective equipment came in. Barrier is anything that separates a person from a hazard (e.g. dressing or drape) and helps in preventing the import of contaminants (CDC, USA). Personal Protective Equipment (PPE) are specialized clothing or equipment (e.g. gloves, gowns, masks, goggles) worn by a healthcare worker (HCW) with the sole purpose of protecting himself/herself against a hazard. The latter is primarily for protection of the healthcare worker. Thus, it means that all PPE serve as barriers but not vice-versa. In other words, PPE is a subset of the group of barriers. Personal protective equipment includes not only barriers for protecting from infection, but which protect from radiation, chemicals, laser, fire, etc. In this section we are referring only to the PPE used for protecting against infection and certain chemicals used for cleaning, disinfection and sterilization.[1-3] The choice of PPE and barriers depends on a reasonably anticipated exposure of the healthcare worker, and on the need for patient protection and the guidelines and level of evidence given by various bodies such as CDC or department of health, UK, which are given below.

Barriers include the following:

- Drapes
- Dressings
- Caps
- Clean linen
- Surgical attire
- Shoes

- PPE (gloves, apron, coat, face mask, eye protection, shoes, clogs, shoe covers, etc.)
- Others

Some Important Guidelines

The references in this chapter are mainly from two important bodies and these concern the use of barriers in clinical practice. They also provide guidelines related to standard precautions, transmission-based precautions, patient placement and systems of barrier precautions.

1. Centre for Disease Control and Prevention (CDC) 'evidence-based recommendations' were developed by Hospital (now Healthcare) Infection Control Practices Advisory Committee (HICPAC) in 1994–95. Systematic reviews and meta-analysis have been conducted by others since the publication of HICPAC guidelines in an attempt to identify reported outcomes clearly linked to evidence.
2. National Health Service, Department of Health, UK[1], evidence-based guidelines and regulations are graded in the following manner:

Category 1: Includes generally consistent findings in a range of evidence derived from a majority of acceptable studies

Category 2: Evidence based on a single acceptable study, or a weak or inconsistent finding in multiple acceptable studies

Category 3: Limited scientific evidence that does not meet all criteria of 'acceptable studies' or an absence of directly applicable studies of good quality

Regulations and controls related to occupation hazards are covered in chapter 21.

GLOVES

Indications

Gloves are recommended for invasive procedures, contact with sterile sites, non-intact skin, mucous membranes and all activities that have been assessed as carrying a risk of exposure to blood, body fluids, secretions and excretions; and when handling sharp or contaminated instruments (NHS, UK, Category 3).[1]

Glove Material

Several varieties of gloves are available to fit all budgets and purposes. Latex, nitrile or vinyl gloves are used for most medical and laboratory procedures. Since gloves can be torn, they should be inspected prior to use.

Latex gloves provide a tighter fit, but contain proteins that can cause allergic reactions in the healthcare worker or patient. Vinyl gloves are less irritating, not assoicated with allergic reactions, but are less pliable and do not fit as tightly. In many countries the use of powdered gloves is prohibited and polythene gloves should not be used in healthcare facilities (NHS, UK, Category 3).[4] Powdered gloves can contribute to dermatitis. Hypoallergenic gloves, glove liners, or powder-less gloves are available to prevent this.

Heavy-duty utility gloves (rubber) are used for housekeeping chores. They must be decontaminated and reused unless they are cracked, peeling, torn or punctured.

Regulations

(Photo 10.2)

Gloves must conform to the regulations of that

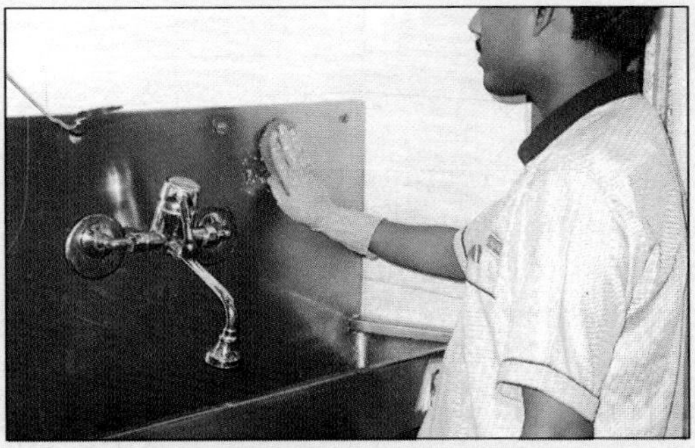

Photo 10.2: Heavy-duty gloves are used for cleaning chores.

state or nation. For example, in the UK, gloves conforming to European Community (CE) standards and of acceptable quality must be available in all clinical areas. (NHS, UK, Category 3). Alternatives to natural rubber latex (NRL) gloves must be available for use by practitioners and patients with NRL sensitivity.

Sterile and Non-Sterile Gloves

Sterile gloves are required to prevent transmission of infection from healthcare worker to patient in surgery and in other procedures associated with a high risk of infection due to interruption of normal host defences. (Examples: insertion of central venous catheters and urinary catheterization).

Non-sterile gloves are used to reduce transmission of infection in situations where sterility is not required (cleaning a spill, emptying suction containers, urine drainage bags, peripheral IV catheter insertion). Disposable single-use gloves must be replaced as soon as possible if contaminated, punctured or damaged during use.

Double gloving or puncture-resistant liners can be used to decrease the risk of percutaneous injury and exposure to blood/body fluids.

Usage, Decontamination and Disposal

Gloves should preferably be worn as single-use items (gloves used for sterile procedures or contaminated nonsterile gloves—preferably disposable), and it is not recommended to re-sterilize or decontaminate them. They must be put on immediately before an episode of patient contact or treatment, and removed as soon as the activity is completed. They must be changed between caring for different patients, or between different care/treatment activities for the same patient (NHS, UK, Category 3). Gloves must be disposed of as clinical waste and hands should be decontaminated following the removal of gloves (NHS,UK,Category 3). They are not to be washed, disinfected, or sterilized for reuse (except utility gloves). Gloves must be changed between patients, and hands must be washed after gloves are removed.[5]

MASKS

Types of Masks

Surgical masks have two functions: first, to protect the patient from a potential source of infection—the wearer (contaminated nasal and oral secretions from the wearer during a procedure); second, to protect the wearer from another potential source of infection—the patient[6-7] (to protect the wearer's eyes, nose and mouth from exposure to splattered or splashed blood or body fluids). Masks with modification for special purposes are also discussed below.

When to Wear

As a barrier: According to the Association of Operating Room Nurses (AORN) and the Operating Room Nurses Association of Canada (ORNAC), 'all persons entering restricted areas of the surgical suite should wear a mask when open sterile items and equipment are present.' This is a controversial area as Skinner et al prescribe that surgical mask is to be worn only by the scrub team and not required by other Operation Theatre (OT) staff.[6] Sound scientifically-based evidence exists that, in the setting of a modern operating theatre with laminar flow/steriflow systems, surgical masks should no longer be considered mandatory for anaesthetists and non-scrub staff during most surgical procedures. (It is assumed here that the theatre air conditioning meets prescribed standards and that standard infection control and transmission-based precautions are in place. Whenever in doubt, it is better to use the masks). However, they recommend that masks must be worn by all OT staff in the following situations: implant surgery, use of power tools and trauma management.

Face masks as PPE: Face masks should be worn where there is risk of blood, body fluids, secretions and excretions splashing into the face (NHS, UK, Category 3). Masks should cover both mouth and nose and should be adjusted for proper fit to primarily act as filters rather than mere barriers. However, masks with eye protection or visor mask protection should be worn by all OT staff during implant insertion surgery, the use of surgical power tools and trauma management.

Filtration Characteristics of Masks

(Photo 10.3)

Another important consideration here is the type of mask worn. The ordinary filter type gauze masks were found to be ineffective in reducing overall airborne contamination, e.g. tubercle bacilli. In such situations, high filtration masks are indicated. There is a common misconception amongst healthcare workers that a surgical mask is quite efficient in the prevention of inhalation of all types of infectious microorganisms. This has been proven wrong because of two important reasons. Firstly, the surgical mask does not provide an airtight fit/seal, and the air moves around the edges, along the path of least resistance and enters the airway of the wearer. Secondly, the mask is not effective against organisms less than 5μm in diameter. In these situations, it is mandatory in some countries to use better devices (high-filtration masks). Therefore, the CDC states that ordinary masks are not adequate in these situations. N-95 mask is also acceptable for protection from small droplet inhalation such as with tubercle bacilli. Positive Air Purifying Respirators (PAPRs) may be worn as an alternative to N-95 type respirator.[7] Other fresh air respirators have been introduced, but they are much more expensive. Particulate respirator is used to filter out,

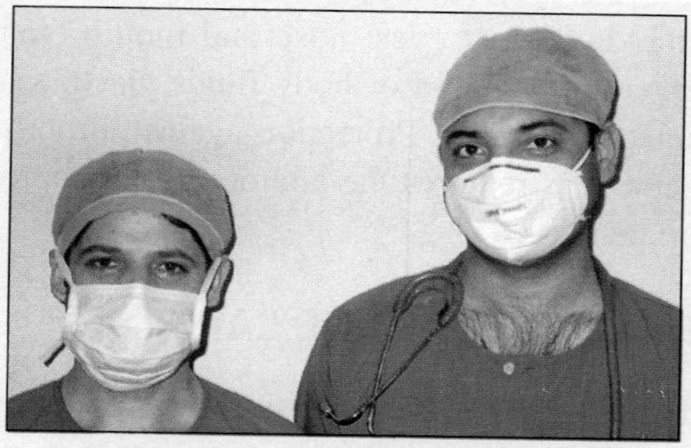

Photo 10.3: A normal surgical mask (left) and a N-95 mask (right)

and protect the wearer from, inhalation of airborne infectious particles of specific sizes. A good face seal around the edges of a particulate respirator is essential for its effectiveness. If it is loose fitting, contaminated air will be drawn in around the edges of the mask, instead of the air being drawn through the filter. Respiratory protective equipment should be selected and used when clinically indicated (Category 3).[1]

EYE PROTECTION

(PHOTO 8.1)

Goggles, safety glasses or face shield should be worn during all major surgical procedures and whenever splashes/sprays of blood or body fluid may be generated.[1, 2, 3] Ordinary glasses are not acceptable unless a solid side shield is added. Protective equipment must be selected on the basis of an assessment of the risk of transmission of microorganisms to the patient and the risk of contamination of healthcare practitioners' clothing and skin by patients' blood, body fluids, secretions and excretions. These are worn when there is a risk of blood, body fluids, secretions or excretions splashing into the eyes (Category 3, NHS, UK). Face shields protect eyes, nose and mouth from exposure to blood or body fluids via splash, splatter or spray. Protection against airborne pathogens requires the addition of an appropriate mask.

HEAD COVERS AND CAPS

These may be plastic disposable or cotton reusable and cover the hair and beards.

SHOE COVERS, LEG COVERS, BOOTS

(PHOTO 10.4)

In some countries shoe covers are used routinely, but they may be used whenever heavy exposure to blood/body fluids is anticipated; e.g. surgery. Shoe/leg covers should be removed or discarded before leaving the Operating Room (OR) suite. Shoes/clogs which protect feet from body fluids are recommended for routine use.

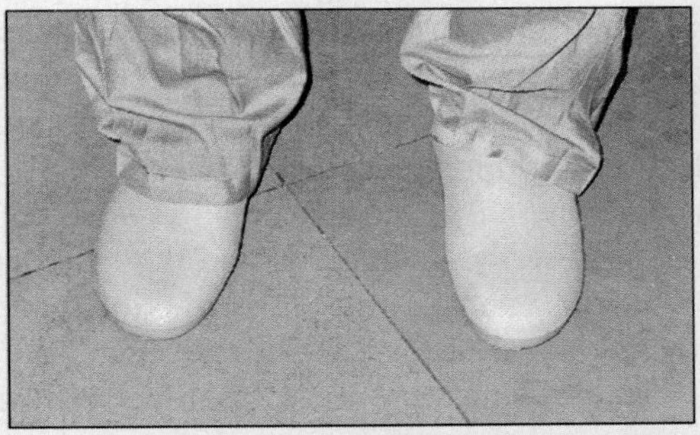

Photo 10.4: Clogs cover the front of the feet preventing exposure

GOWNS

Gowns are used as barriers or PPE. Full-body, fluid-repellant gowns should be worn where there is risk of extensive splashing of blood, body fluids, secretions and excretions, with the exception of sweat, onto the skin of healthcare practitioners, e.g. in labour rooms (Category 3, NHS, UK).[1] Protective clothing should be impervious to fluids, in other words, fluid resistant (i.e., resists penetration of fluids under most but not all circumstances). Protective clothing helps prevent contamination of skin, mucous membranes, work clothes

and undergarments. Regular work clothes, uniforms and surgical gowns are not considered protective attire. Gowns (with sleeves) are used when splashing, spraying, or spattering of blood/body fluids or when blood/body fluid contamination of arms is anticipated. The choice of gown or apron depends on the level of blood or body-fluid exposure anticipated. Fluid-resistant gowns are suitable for most situations, extra fluid-resistant sleeves can be worn over a gown, and/or an impervious apron can be worn under a gown, to improve protection against soak-through during prolonged or high-blood-loss surgical procedures. Aprons (no sleeves) may be worn for lesser degrees of exposure. Plastic aprons should be worn as single-use items for one procedure or episode of patient care and then discarded and disposed of as clinical waste (Category 3, NHS, UK). Other barriers include air curtains, air-conditioning systems and filters, which are discussed in the chapter on environment management and engineering controls.

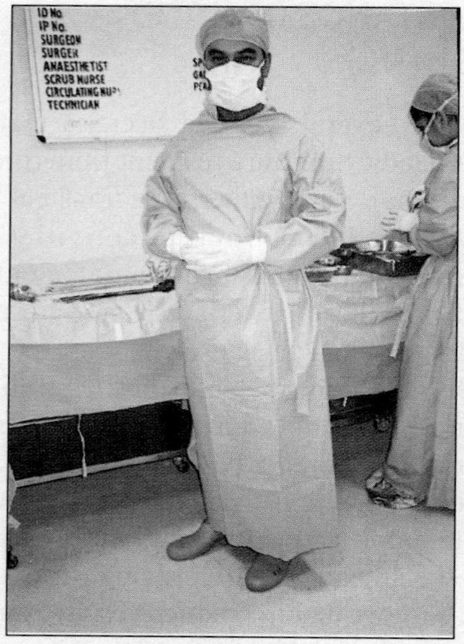

Photo 10.5: The surgical attire

BEHAVIOUR AND ATTIRE RELATED TO WORK AREA

(PHOTO 10.5)

In areas such as operating suites and intensive care units, hospitals follow specialized dressing and behavioural protocols as per the recommendations of their regulatory bodies. In case there are no regulations (as in some countries), guidelines from important organizations are helpful. All persons entering semi-restricted and restricted areas of the operating suite should be in hospital-laundered, surgical attire intended for use only in the surgical suite and wear a surgical mask. As far as possible, facial hair, including sideburns and the neckline should be covered when in the OT. The gown should be loose-fitting and comfortable, with no cords or ends hanging out and interfering with hand movements or work. All items of jewellery and watches should be removed while scrubbing for a case. Nail polish and artificial nails should not be worn while working in the OT complex. Women with long hair should make sure it is covered.[3] Gloves must be worn whenever indicated and in the manner described in this chapter. Feet should be covered with clogs, soft slippers or wrap-around slippers meant for the purpose, as and when indicated. Footwear dedicated for use in the OT complex should not be worn outside the sterile zone. They have to be changed if one has to leave the OT complex, to avoid tracking of blood and debris through to other areas of the hospital. Change of footwear or use of shoe covers is controversial in an ICU setting. Disposable items should not be reused. Reusable items must be properly cleaned and reprocessed before reuse.

IMPORTANCE OF HAND-WASHING[8,9]

There are several types of bacteria that live on our hands. Some are resident flora (present all the time), while others are transient flora (picked up during routine activities like preparing food, domestic cleaning, or outdoor activities). These bacteria can be transmitted to other people, surfaces or parts of the body via physical contact, with the possibility of causing infection, which can be caused by bacteria found on the hands.

Handwashing is the single most effective, and the simplest, of all precautionary measures in the healthcare set-up, although it is often, sadly, sub-optimal in practice. The reasons for this range from lack of appropriate accessible equipment, high staff-to-patient ratios, allergies to handwashing products to insufficient knowledge about the risks, procedures or the time required.[10] When followed meticulously, this simple procedure goes a long way in preventing infections and thereby reducing unnecessary costs of healthcare. It does not require the most expensive disinfectant or cleansing agent as much as it requires common sense and an abundance of it. Although everyone is aware of the 'why' and 'how' of it, a few words spent on hand-washing technique is never a waste, and experience has shown that among every category of healthcare workers, this is a much-required drilling lesson. Hence, at the cost of repetition and ennui we dare to drive home some tenets on hand-washing.

Types of Hand-Washing[8-10]

1. Social hand-washing (ordinary)

This lasts 10 seconds, e.g. personal hygiene, before and after routine contact.

2. Hygienic (procedural or antiseptic) hand-wash (special)

This lasts 30 seconds, e.g. before handling infected patient, material contact with high risk patients, IV lines.

3. Surgical hand-wash (for operative procedures)

Lasts two to five minutes, e.g. for operative procedures, handling burns patients, prior to invasive device insertion.

Several questions arise with regard to hand-washing which need to be addressed and answered

a. Why is hand decontamination crucial to the prevention of HAI?

b. When must you decontaminate your hands in relation to patient care?

c. Is any one hand-cleaning preparation better than another?

d. Choice of decontamination: Is it always necessary to wash hands to achieve decontamination?

e. Is hand decontamination technique important? Does hand decontamination damage skin?

General points to keep in mind about hand-washing

1. The nails must be kept short and clean, because studies have shown that microbial contamination can remain under the fingernails even after scrubbing.
2. Running water should be freely available in the vicinity.

3. Ideally, taps operated with elbow, knee or foot should be used. Some institutions even use sensor-taps which operate on a no-touch technique.
4. Soap or detergent with antiseptic properties should be used.
5. Clean towels should be used for drying.
6. All items of jewellery and ornaments should be removed before washing.
7. A methodical and thorough technique of hand-washing should be followed.
8. Special attention should be paid to the usually neglected parts of the hand.

Hand-Washing and Decontamination

Hands must be decontaminated immediately before each and every episode of direct patient contact/care and after any activity or contact that potentially results in hands becoming contaminated[1] (NHS, UK, Category 3). Hand-washing/decontamination is necessary in the following situations:

- Before handling patients (Photo 10.6)
- After handling patients
- In between patient-handling
- In the same patient—from infected to clean site
- Immediately after contamination with blood, etc.
- After cleaning work
- Before and after eating/drinking
- After handling of infective materials or any exposure incident
- After removal of gloves

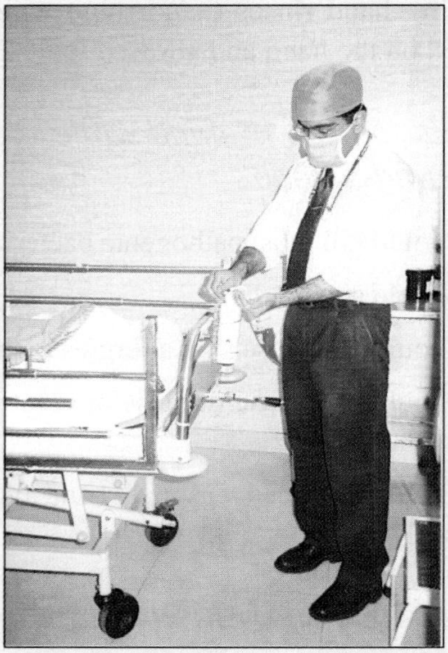

Photo 10.6: Hand decontamination before handling patients

- After using the toilets
- At completion of the day's work
- As and when deemed necessary

Types of Products Available for Hand-Washing[11, 12]

1. Bar soaps
2. Liquid soaps
3. Powder soaps (granules)
4. Paper soaps

Soaps with antimicrobial properties are preferred in OTs, nurseries with newborns, intensive care units and handling of severely immunocompromised patients. Such agents include chlorhexidine, iodine compounds and alcohol. These are also available as foams (sprays), wipes (used to wipe surfaces such

as skin), hand rinses (hand rubs) which are poured on the hand and allowed to dry.

Points to keep in mind while selecting a soap

1. Should kill most pathogenic bacteria
2. Should act rapidly
3. Should not cause skin allergies in the user
4. Should not cause dryness or reactions in the hands
5. Should be priced reasonably and available easily

HAND DECONTAMINATION[13]

(PHOTOS 10.7, 10.8)

As an alternative to hand-washing, hand decontamination (use of hand rubs) can be used, which is equally effective. Compliance to this method is better as it is less cumbersome and does not require running water and wash basins in all areas. It is also less damaging to the skin than repeated hand-washing. Hands that are visibly soiled or grossly contaminated with dirt or organic material must be washed with liquid soap and water first (NHS, UK, Category 3).

When decontaminating hands using an alcoholic hand-rub, the hands should be free of dirt and organic material. The hand-rub solution must come into contact with all the surfaces of the hand. The hands must be rubbed together vigorously, paying particular attention to the tips of the fingers, the thumbs and the areas between the fingers, and until the solution has evaporated and the hands are dry[1] (NHS, UK, Category 3).

Technique of washing or decontamination[14]

All wrist and hand jewellery must ideally be removed at the beginning of each clinical shift before regular hand decontamination begins. Cuts and abrasions must be covered with waterproof dressings. Effective handwashing technique must be practised which involves three stages: preparation, washing and rinsing, and drying. Preparation involves wetting hands

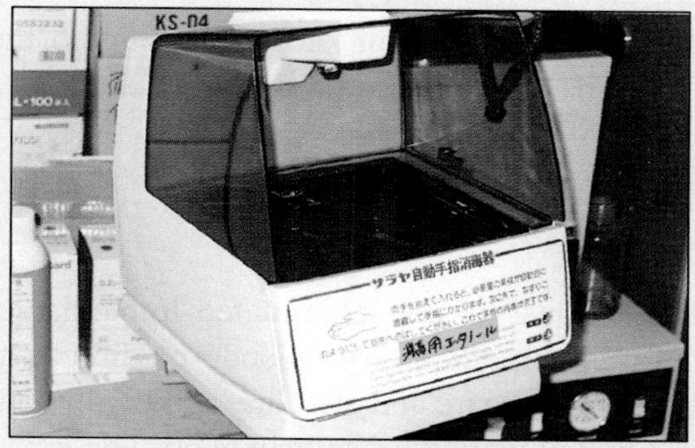

Photo 10.7: Automatic decontaminant dispenser

under running water before applying liquid soap or an antimicrobial preparation. The handwash solution must come into contact with all the surfaces of the hand. The hands must be rubbed together vigorously for a minimum of 10–15 seconds, paying particular attention to the tips of the fingers, the thumbs and the areas between the fingers (the webs). Hands should be rinsed thoroughly prior to drying with good quality paper towels. An emollient hand cream may be applied regularly to protect skin from the drying effects of regular hand decontamination. If a particular soap, antimicrobial handwash or alcohol product causes skin irritation, occupational health advice must be sought (NHS, UK, Category 3).

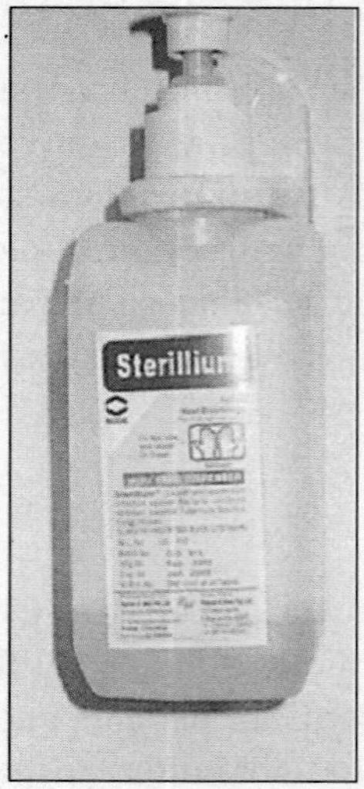

Photo 10.8: Wall-mounted hand decontaminant dispenser

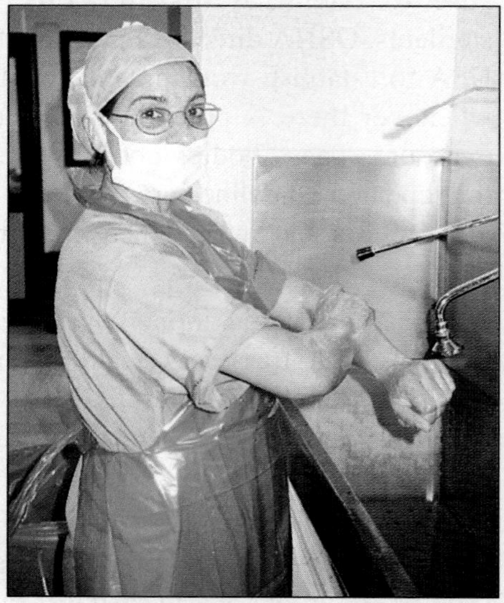

Photo 10.9: The surgical hand scrub

Surgical Hand Scrub

(Photo 10.9)

a. Policies and procedures in surgical hand scrubs should be developed according to the practice in the setting, in association with the Infection Control Committee.[15]

b. A definition of the duration of surgical hand scrub procedures should be made.

c. Approved alternative scrub solutions for personnel with skin sensitivity must be available.

d. A standardized scrub method (standard operating procedure) may be designed and circulated to all staff to standardize the technique. As there is a turnover of staff in the operating room areas, there must be a facility for repeated, regular classes.

e. Gloving technique: There are two standard methods: 1) closed method 2) open method (see photographs in chapter 14).

Regulatory bodies for soaps and disinfectants help in selecting a quality product[16]

E.g. When purchasing or ordering soaps and disinfectants, confirm if it is CEN or EPA cleared, as it ensures quality of the product conforming to European or US standards, respectively.

1. Employee Protection Agency (EPA) of USA is a body that registers disinfectants and sterilants based on microbicidal efficacy data submitted by the manufacturer. EPA is responsible for the regulation of safety and efficacy claims for low and intermediate level disinfectants, and also the toxicity of active ingredients.
2. Occupational Safety and Health Administration (OSHA) gives guidelines for proper usage and minimization of worker expo-

sure to chemical disinfectants and sterilants. OSHA directs employers in the USA to establish work practice controls whenever there is potential for worker exposure. These bodies not only ensure that updated guidelines are available, but also monitor and enforce their implementation.

3. Association for Practitioners in Infection Control (APIC) assesses healthcare professionals in their decisions involving selection and use of specific disinfectants.[14]
4. There are also state and local bodies that are concerned with environmental issues such as hazardous waste disposal methods. The guidelines given by these bodies are now available on their respective websites. The regulatory bodies can be grouped into a) international and b) national bodies. The largest international society for Infection Control Practitioners (ICPs) is probably the Association for Practitioners in Infection Control and Epidemiology (APIC) based in the United States. APIC was founded in 1972, and currently represents some 12,000 members comprising nurses, medical technologists, microbiologists, epidemiologists, physicians and other healthcare personnel whose primary responsibility within their facilities is infection prevention and control.

In the Asia Pacific region, a new organization named Asia Pacific Society of Infection Control (APSIC) was formed in 1998 in an attempt to bring the growing infection control community together. APSIC held its first international conference in Hong Kong in 1999.

SYSTEMS OF PRECAUTIONS

Using the concepts and information we have learnt, it is now time to move on to some special set of recommendations which have evolved to deal with certain clinical situations. These include 1) standard precautions 2) barrier precautions 3) transmission-based precautions.

Standard Precautions

Standard precautions refer to the safety measures and policies adopted by the healthcare workers towards all patients under their care, in order to curtail or minimize the risk of transmitting or acquiring a hospital associated infection. It is called 'standard' because it provides a minimum accepted standard of care in infection-control practice and also is a standard of professional conduct. Earlier these measures were known by the term 'Universal Precautions' and included measures adopted only when handling blood or blood products.[2, 17, 18]

> Essence of Standard Precautions: 'Every conscientious healthcare worker should realize that the spread of infection in the healthcare setting can be prevented very effectively by taking a consistent approach to all patients rather than using precautions only for those with specific diagnosis.'

Thus, by following Standard Precautions, one succeeds in breaking the essential link between the source of infection and the susceptible host, thus disconnecting the mode of transmission.

Who is at risk of acquiring HAI?

The targets include all healthcare workers—physicians, surgeons, nurses, dentists, laboratory and blood bank workers, morticians, etc. Standard precautions for healthcare workers must include an exhaustive list of various tasks as mentioned below:

1. Hand-washing
2. Barrier nursing
3. Handling of sharps
4. Handling of spills
5. Handling of laboratory specimens
6. Patient placement /isolation /transport
7. Housekeeping
8. Waste disposal
9. Handling of disposable/infected items
10. Food and nutrition
11. Patient visitor exposure
12. Linen and laundry services
13. Medical emergencies

Standard precautions apply to

a. Blood
b. All body fluids (CSF, pleural/pericardial/ synovial fluids, vaginal secretions, saliva, breast milk in milk banks)
c. Non-intact skin
d. Mucous membranes

(Usually excludes faeces, tears, sweat, urine, nasal secretions, vomitus)

The present terminology of Standard Precautions (SP) includes the earlier term Universal Precautions (UP) plus a newer term, Body Substance Isolation (BSI). UP includes only blood and body fluids. BSI is designed to reduce the risk of transmission of pathogens from moist body substances.

Thus, SP = UP + BSI

Barrier Precautions

In the early days, the concept of quarantine began as a precautionary measure, wherein patients with infectious diseases were kept in isolation until such time that they ceased to be a threat to other healthy people. Gradually, towards the end of the eighteenth century, with expanding knowledge of diseases, their causative organisms and their modes of spread, the traditional systems of isolation evolved. These, in due course, paved the way for the use of barrier precautions, which includes all measures adopted to create a barrier between the susceptible host and the infective agent. Barrier methods consist of any activity or precaution taken to prevent patient-to-patient transfer of infection.[2, 3] The permutation and combination of these are done according to the type of infection and organism. A barrier precaution may include the following:

1. Prevention of import of contaminants through linen (sheets, drapes, bedsheets, attire, gloves, caps, shoes, gowns, etc.)
2. Prevention of transmission to patients by repeated hand-washing or hand decontamination especially after handling infective areas, excreta, waste, dressings, contaminated equipment
3. Constant monitoring of carrier state and treatment of healthcare workers
4. Isolation of infected or colonized patients

Patient placement

It is sometimes necessary to isolate a patient from others for specific reasons. In such situations, a note must be made in the history sheet as to why the patient required isolation. A private room is usually necessary when:

1. The patient has an infection that transmits by airborne/ droplet route
2. The patient has an infection by microorganisms that can be transmitted by contact
3. Patient has copious amounts of body fluids/discharges from his body or wounds
4. Poor hygiene demands that the patient be isolated
5. Cohorting patients and staff (those detected with same infection are made to stay together)
6. Use of disposable or dedicated equipment (blood pressure instrument, thermometers) for infected patients[17]

OTHER BARRIERS

Other barriers such as wound dressings reduce risk of exposure to blood/body fluids. These are discussed in the chapter on practice guidelines.

There are a number of other barriers, which include air curtains, air-condition systems and filters, which are discussed in the chapter on environment management and engineering controls.

Ultra Violet (UV) Radiation

The efficacy of UV radiation in killing a microorganism will depend on three important factors, namely,

- The type of microorganism—some organisms like airborne fungal and bacterial spores are inherently resistant to UV rays.
- The dose of radiation to which it is exposed—the duration of exposure is also important here.
- The amount of moisture in the air—at typical indoor temperatures, relative humidities above 70% reduce the bactericidal efficiency of UV rays. In general, there are certain points to be kept in mind to maximize the germicidal effects of UV radiation:

  a. Use germicidal lamps that emit short wave UV radiation (254nm).

  b. Install the equivalent of one 30W ceiling or wall fixture for every 200 sq. feet of floor area or for every seven people in the room.

  c. Place labels to warn people to avoid direct eye and skin exposure.

Transmission-Based Precautions (TBP)

These are designed for patients documented or suspected to be infected or colonized with highly transmissible or epidemiologically important pathogens for which additional precautions beyond (in addition to and not instead of) Standard Precautions are needed to interrupt transmission[3]. There are some categories under which these precautions apply:

1. Airborne transmission
2. Droplet transmission
3. Contact transmission

4. Common vehicle transmission: food, water, medications, devices, equipment
5. Vector-borne transmission

Airborne precautions

These are designed to reduce airborne transmission of droplet nuclei which are less than 5μm in suspensions and dust particles containing pathogens. They are spread by air currents or movement of air. A good example of this is tuberculosis. Special precautionary measures for these include negative pressure isolation, special air handling and ventilation techniques. The special type of respirator mentioned earlier may find use in these conditions. It has also been observed that surgical masks are not adequate to break transmission by the airborne route (E.g. *Mycobacterium tuberculosis*). Hence, for preventing these infections one has to use N-95 respirators or HEPA respirators, designed by NIOSH (National Institute of Occupational Safety and Health) and OSHA (Occupational Safety and Health Association). These filter 95% of particles that are 0.3mm in size.[19]

Droplet precautions

These precautions are intended to reduce droplet transmission wherein the droplets are larger particles of more than 5μm. The common sources of these are activities like coughing, sneezing, talking, suction and bronchoscopy. Transmission of these droplets requires close contact (conjunctiva, mucous membrane of nose/mouth). These particles are heavier and hence not suspended. They do not traverse more than three feet and hence, do not merit any special ventilation or air handling procedures.

Contact Precautions

Here, the aim is to reduce risk of transmission of epidemiologically important pathogens by direct or indirect (fomite) contact, which is usually by skin to skin contact. One can be exposed to such risks while performing activities like turning the patient, bathing the patient, etc.

ROLE OF INSTITUTIONS

Protective barriers in providing PPE vary with the laws, regulations and guidelines followed in a country or organization (gloves, masks, goggles and face shields). They should be provided by the hospital and utilized, to reduce the risk of exposure to potentially infective agents. These barrier methods are meant for all those who are at risk of contracting hospital acquired infections, be they the HCWs or patients, or patients' attendants/ visitors. (see earlier on in the chapter). Training programmes must be organized to increase awareness.

Whenever there is a probability of exposure to blood or body substance or when these are likely to be encountered in large amounts or these form a probable route of transmission, barrier precautions are to be followed. (Further details are given in chapter 21.)

It is important to note here that isolation precautions are not required for the following infections: HIV, HBV, HCV and AIDS disease, unless otherwise indicated, but barrier precautions, transmission-based precautions, and standard precautions must be followed at all times.[19]

REFERENCES

1) Standard principles for preventing hospital-acquired infections, Department of Health. Journal of Hospital Infection. 2001;47 (suppl): S21-S37. Available online on http://www.idealibrary.com on IDEAL.

2) Mandated infection control, training course. Available from URL; http://www.laboratoryservices.com/LCSinfectioncontrolcourse.htm (02.06.2006)

3) From Hospitals Infections Programme (HIP) homepage, National Centre for Infectious Diseases, Center for Disease Control Prevention, Atlanta, GA updated 6/2/1999URL; http:/www.cdc.gov/ncidod/hip/iv/jv.htm

4) Korniewicz DM, Laughon B, Cyr W et al. Leakage of virus through used vinyl and latex examination gloves. J Clin Microbiol.1990; 28: 787-788.

5) Olsen RJ, Lynch P and Coyle MB. Examination gloves as barriers to hand contamination in clinical practice. J Am Med Assoc.1993; 270(3): 350-353.

6) Skinner MW and B A Sutton. Do Anaesthetists need to wear surgical masks in the operating theatre? A literature review with evidence-based recommendations. Anaesth Intensive Care 2001; 29: 331-338.

7) Romney MG. Surgical face masks in the operating theatre: re-examining the evidence. J Hosp Infect 2001; 47: 251-56.

8) Simmons B, Bryant J, Neiman K et al. The role of handwashing in prevention of endemic intensive care unit infections. Infection Control and Hospital Epidemiology 1990; 11(11): 589-594.

9) Teare EL, Cookson B, French G et al. UK Handwashing initiative. J Hosp Infect. 1999; 43: 1-3.

10) Ayliffe G, Babb JR, Davies JG et al. Hygienic hand disinfection tests in three laboratories. J Hosp Infect.1990; 16(2): 141-149.

11) Ayliffe GA, Babb JR, Davies JG et al. Hand disinfection: a comparison of various agents in laboratory and ward studies. J Hosp Infect 1988; 11(3): 226-243.

12) Doebbeling BN, Stanley GL, Sheetz CT et al. Comparative efficacy of alternative hand-washing agents in reducing nosocomial infections in intensive care units. New Engl J Med. 1992; 327 (2): 88-93.

13) Ehrenkranz NJ and Alfonso BC. Failure of bland soap handwash to prevent hand transfer of patient bacteria to urethral catheters. Infection Control and Hospital Epidemiology 1991; 12: 654-662.

14) Larson EL. APIC guideline for handwashing and hand antisepsis in healthcare settings Am J Infect Control. 1995; 23: 251-269.

15) Bendig JW. Surgical Hand disinfection; comparison of 4% chlorhexidine detergent solution and 2% triclosan detergnt solution. Journal of Hospital Infection 1990; 15(2): 143-148.

16) Nicoletti G, Boghossian V and Borland R. Hygienic hand disinfection: a comparative study with chlorhexidine detergents and soap. J Hosp Infect. 1990; 15 (4): 323-337.

17) Garner JS. The Hospital Infection Control Practices Advisory Committee: Guidelines for isolation Precautions in Hospitals. Infection Control Hospital Epidemiology 1996; 17(1): 53-80.

18) Curran ET, Riley J and Fletcher AW. Decontamination of reusable instruments in primary care. Br J Nurs. 2002; 12-25; 11(16): 1078,1080-4.

19) Centres for Disease Control Update. Recommendations for Prevention of HIV transmission in healthcare settings. Morbidity and Mortality Weekly Report 1987; 37: 24.

Chapter 11

Environment Management and Engineering Controls

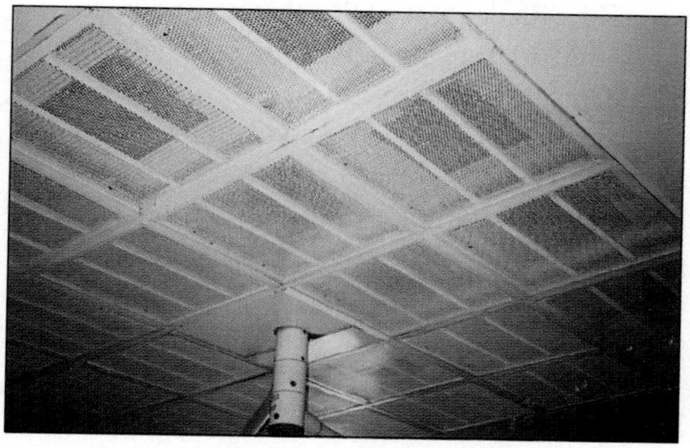

Life is short, and the art long; the occasion fleeting, experience fallacious, and judgment difficult. The physician must not only be prepared to do what is right himself, but also to make the patient, the attendants and externals cooperate.

—Hippocrates

Highlights

Issues in Facility Design
Designing of a Laboratory
Ventilation
Food- and Water-Borne Infections
Water Management in Healthcare Institutions
Pest Management Programme
Containers and Closures for Sterile IV Fluids
Engineering Controls for Laboratory Equipment
Biohazard Material Containers, Bags and Labels
Designing of Bacterial Filters
Designing of Suctioning Equipment/Disposable Suctioning Device
Accessories to Engineering Controls in Environment Management
Environmental Hygiene

INTRODUCTION

The practice of medicine has acquired complex dimensions due to invasive procedures, caring for critically ill patients, implantation of prostheses, organ transplantations and other challenging interventions in various disciplines. In the past, performing such procedures was wrought with dangers of life-threatening infections due to the ever-present reservoir of organisms in the environment.

There are a number of areas in the hospital that pose an increased risk to patient care. Many of the inanimate objects around the patient are a potential reservoir of microorganisms and pose some form of danger to the patient. These include the environmental surfaces, hospital toilets, bathrooms, kitchens, linen, equipment and monitors.These infections have been controlled to a great extent by providing a safer surrounding, be it in the operating room, intensive care or elsewhere in the hospital.

These problems have led to a separate area of management called the environmental management, which includes building design, selection of the right kind of materials used for construction and the use of appropriate technology. It also involves the designing of specific areas in a manner that reduces traffic (people, equipment, trolleys) in certain key areas like the operating suite and intensive care units, and ensures that the spread of infection is eliminated or minimized.

Environment management is a term that encompasses a combination of epidemiology, ergonomics, engineering controls, system operating procedures and other risk management strategies (Table 11.1). This chapter emphasizes the fact that technology and facility design can be used to manipulate and combat risks to patients and healthcare workers. 'Engineering Controls' is the use of technology for reduction or elimination of risks due to various activities in the healthcare set-up, i.e. accidents, fires, laser, radiation and infections. Risk management should be an integral part of the process of strategic quality management process. It demands meticulous planning, careful consideration and an in-depth knowledge of possible hazards. It is a scrupulous study and practice of:

1. Ergonomics, which is the science of fitting the equipment or the task, to the worker
2. Designing of equipment
3. Designing of premises—designing of hospitals/operating rooms and suites/ICUs/ and other areas
4. Containment processes
5. Ventilation processes
6. Management of equipment and use of protective barriers and filtration methods
7. Safety devices, spacing modern devices and materials so as to minimize the hazards of infection in the healthcare setting
8. The effective training of staff in the appropriate use and maintenance of it all

In modern hospitals, environment management and engineering controls go hand in hand. Each complements the functions of the other in every area, e.g. use of air-conditioners, autoclaves, ethylene oxide machines, washing machines, transporting equipment and laboratory equipment.[1] This can be amply seen in the comparative table given below:

Table 11.1: Comparison of environment management and engineering controls

Problem	Environment management	Engineering controls
Air contaminated with dust and microorganisms	Clean air—through restricted entry, ventilation and other measures	Air-conditioning, HEPA filters, etc.
Hospital waste hazard	Minimizing waste generation, segregation, packaging and waste storage	Incineration, autoclaves, washing machines, microwave, etc.
Water contamination	Introduce ideal storage and distribution system	Filters, distillation plants, purifiers, etc.
Hospital catering and kitchen risks	Hygienic food processing, storage and distribution	Use of automated, non-touch techniques
Laboratory hazards	Proper location, designing, training of personnel laminar flow hoods,	Safer equipment like closed centrifuges, biological safety cabinets, etc.

Note: Several topics dealt with here overlap with topics in certain other chapters like work practice controls, SOPs, etc. The reader is hence advised to read these relevant chapters simultaneously for a better understanding.

ISSUES IN FACILITY DESIGN

Some Areas of Concern in the Hospital Premises

- Emergency room where healthcare workers come in contact with highly infectious patients
- Operating suites where invasive procedures are carried out
- Intensive care and other high dependency areas where a combination of use of antibiotics, invasive procedures and immunocompromised patients are present.
- Specific wards—paediatric, burns, wards and rooms with infective patients
- Dirty areas—corridors, toilets, wash areas and disposal areas could lead to transmission of infection
- Storage areas
- Water supply and storage—baths, stagnant water containing areas
- Kitchen
- Others—mortuary, laundry, CSSD, pathology and microbiology laboratories[2]

Before a healthcare facility building is constructed, several design issues must be considered and planned in order to provide for safety and convenience. Issues of special concern include:

- Building design/materials construction
- Space, including spatial separation
- Location
- Traffic—separation of clean and dirty circuits (clean circuits include ICU, OTs, while dirty circuits include all other areas). Proper movement in areas catering to food and laundry, sterile equipment, pharmaceutical distribution, etc.
- Isolation areas
- Floors and walls
- Appropriate access to hand-washing facilities
- Materials (carpets, walls and floors)
- Design of lighting and ventilation
- Prevention of exposure during renovation and cleaning
- Design of laboratories according to biosafety or containment levels

Some Important Guidelines and Standards for Facility Design

A new process called 'infection-control risk assessment', which describes how an organization determines the risk of transmission of various infectious pathogens, is an essential component of any healthcare facility's functional or master programming. It is carried out by the organizational committee, which is a multidisciplinary panel with expertise in areas of infectious disease, facility design and construction, ventilation, epidemiology, etc. The purpose of this committee is to coordinate the individual infection-control needs and create a safer environment for patients, staff and visitors. This highlights the importance of linking environmental management and engineering controls to infection-control activities at the planning stage itself to ensure safer clinical practice and improved outcome.

There are guidelines giving the basic, minimum requirements in relation to infection control, for construction of hospitals. These are known as 'Guidelines and Standards for Environmental Requirements for Construction of Hospitals'. They have been given by the following bodies:

1. 'Basic Requirements of General Hospital Buildings' Indian standards IS 10905 (part 1,2,3). This gives standards for SSD, door and window size, lighting, ventilation, heating, airflow, plumbing and other relevant issues.
2. The American Institute of Architects Committee on Architecture for Health, US department of Health and Human Services, give guidelines for construction and equipment of hospital and medical facilities, Washington DC. In the American guidelines, in addition to the incorporation of changes in design in relation to infection control, conforming to the most current guidelines for prevention of transmission of *Mycobacterium tuberculosis* in healthcare facilities and guidelines for prevention of nosocomial pneumonia are also important prerequisites (1994).[3]
3. Health building note (HBN) 27; first published by the DHSS in 1967, updated in 1992 (main planning document in UK)
4. Recommendations of the European Society of Intensive Care Medicine (ESICM) task force on minimal requirements for intensive care departments were drafted in 1995.

5. Revised US guidelines for ICU design approved by the Council of Society of Critical Care Medicine and published in 1995
6. Biosafety or Containment in laboratories (See outbreaks and epidemics.)

It is obvious that work with organisms in different risk groups requires different conditions for containment, i.e. ensuring that the organisms do not escape from their specimens, culture vessels or the laboratory. Classification of laboratories according to use have caused problems and have hence led to the conclusion that three or four types of laboratories are required according to the class of organisms handled. According to the WHO (1983), there are three levels of laboratory: basic laboratory, for organisms in risk groups 1 and 2; containment laboratory for organisms in risk group 3; and maximum containment laboratory for organisms in risk group 4. The US Public Health Serices (USPHS) (1984) has four biosafety levels, and the Advisory Committee on Dangerous Pathogens (ACDP) (1984), which appears to have been drafted earlier to the draft of the US system, also has four containment levels (explained under Risk Management).

Facility design: general designing principles to prevent HAI

Facility design is a specialized area with a variety of designs and building material to choose from. But whatever may be the complexity of the design, the basic principles remain common. These designing principles take into account the principles of epidemiology and transmission of organisms commonly encountered in a healthcare facility, the general work pattern, the total workforce, traffic, quality of air required, kind of procedures to be carried out, etc. The basic architectural design is then blended with the technological planning. The recommendations given by important bodies are a good reference point. However, modifications may be made according to the economic constraints and the local guidelines.[4,5] In every healthcare facility, there are some departments or areas that carry a greater risk of causing hospital acquired infections than others. A graded example of risk areas would be:

Microbiology > Morbid Anatomy > Mortuaries > Haematology > Clinical biochemistry > Others

ICU

The unit design should take into consideration not only the workload, but also the scope for future adaptability and expansion. A central station must allow visualization of all patients, and one must be able to see patients in cubicles. The resource of space and equipment must be maximized in an affordable way. Specialized units may be modified according to specific requirements, e.g. ICUs of burns, cardiac, surgical, dermatological, neurosurgical, etc. For every eight beds, two may be made isolation rooms.

Segregation or Isolation Room

(Photo 11.1)

Three patient segregation categories have been identified:

a. Airborne infection isolation room: Protective isolation for a hyper-susceptible patient may require a pressure gradient from inside to outside.

b. Protective environment room: If air-conditioning facilities are present, pressure gradients from outside to inside can be maintained.

c. Immunocompromised host in airborne infection isolation

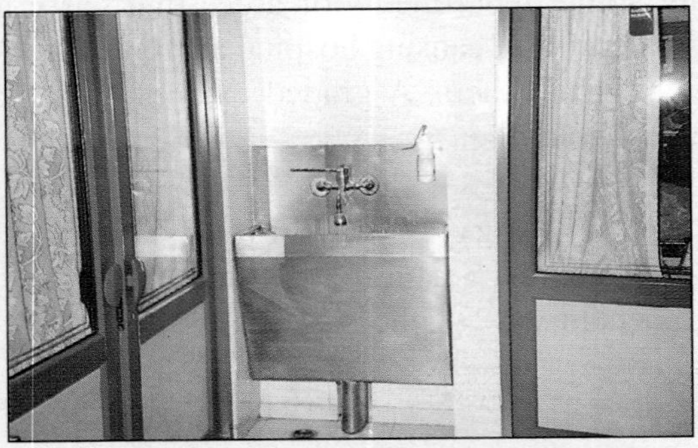

Photo 11.1: Isolation rooms with a sink for two rooms

Isolation in ICU[6]

A facility for isolation of infected or immunocompromised patient must be present. If no air-conditioning facility is available, the isolation may be carried out with barrier precautions.

Standard Requirements Dictate the Following

- 10–12 feet distance between the centres of beds
- Patient area: 150–200 sq ft in a cubicle or per patient
- One washbasin for every two beds
- A utility area, containing a sink and a marked-out area for washing
- Areas for emptying and cleaning bedpans and urine pans, covered bins for soiled linen and contaminated waste
- There must be a well worked-out mechanism for disposal of waste.
- Clean rooms must have separate areas for storage of clean linen.
- The unit should be located near a lift with easy access to the emergency department, operation theatres, laboratory and radiology departments. There should be no unnecessary traffic of people and patients near the ICU. Clean and dirty streams of traffic should be segregated as far as possible. Sorted and sealed waste/dirty linen may be transported through clean corridors although separation is preferable.
- Temperature and humidity are also important considerations in order to contain the generation of contaminants. Humidity levels of 40%–60% are considered optimal for comfortable working.
- Furniture should be minimum and safe with no sharp or jagged edges.

Wall mounting

(Photo 11.2)

Monitoring equipment, suction apparatus and electrical connections should be wall mounted to prevent the clutter and wires on the floor.

Storage area

Storage area should be separate for storage of equipment and should be dust free and clean (wrapped and covered). The equipment must be decontaminated before storage.

Ventilation for ICUs

Plenum ventilation with at least 10 air changes/ hour (99% filtration)

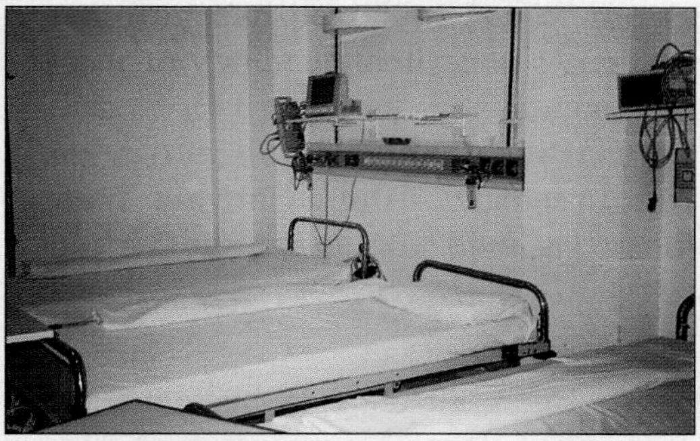

Photo 11.2: Wall-mounted monitors and equipment

OPERATING SUITE[7,8]

Design of Traffic

Clean and dirty streams of traffic should, as far as practicable, be segregated. Although when adequately bagged (sorted and sealed) soiled equipment or waste can be routed via a clean corridor without the risk of bacteriological contamination, the provision of a separate disposal corridor has certain advantages.[7] Such a corridor provides direct access to the point of disposal and reduces traffic congestion in the clean circulation areas.

There should be a transfer or changeover zone section at the entrance of the operating room.

The zonal arrangement is generally followed where each area mentioned forms one zone.

- Sterile area (operating room or sterile storage area)
- Clean area (scrub area [Photo 11.3], anaesthesia room)
- Protective area (entrance, lobby, corridor, changing rooms and recovery rooms)
- Disposal area (sink, disposal corridor)

Interior Finishes

- The walls, flooring and ceilings must be non-dust-shedding with minimum-joint surfaces because dust attracts and carries microorganisms.
- The walls should be non-hygroscopic. The walls could have epoxy resin paint, laminated plastic, vinyl sheets. If epoxy resin is used then the plaster should be of the high-impact type incorporating fibre glass. Tiles are not ideal as crevices are formed. Again the walls should be able to withstand the washing and cleaning. Walls may be tiled or made of stone, but these are not ideal if they contain crevices. Therefore, they must be interlinked in a joint-free manner. Epoxy-painted walls and epoxy-coated floors are good alternatives in OTs and ICUs. They should be

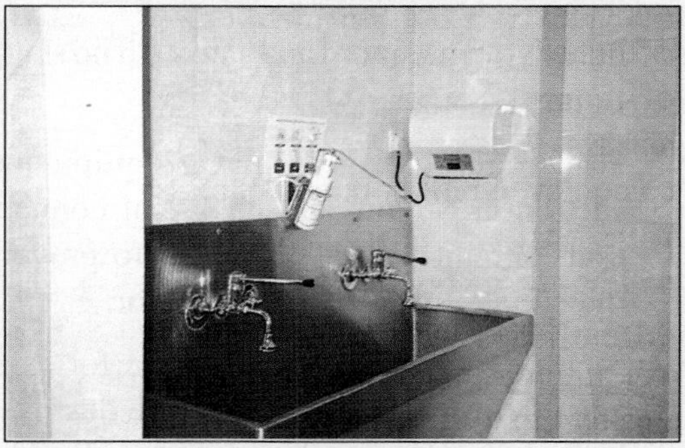

Photo 11.3: Scrub area in an operating room with elbow-operated taps and wall-mounted soap dispenser

washable with detergents and disinfectants. Walls may also be made of laminated plastic, or vinyl sheet, which are easier to maintain, although these are more expensive.

- Floors may be of stone, combination of concrete and stone chips, (terrazo) vinyl or rubber although it must be borne in mind that synthetic floors are difficult to maintain and replace. The flooring materials are also impervious and antistatic. Preferred materials include terrazo (concrete with stone chips), vinyl or stone. Tiles are not ideal as crevices are formed. The material should also bear the effect of detergents and cleaning agents.

Remember: It is not necessary to go for expensive or good-looking materials for floors, walls, etc. It is more important to consider the utility, hygiene and maintenance factors.

- Temperature and humidity are also important considerations in order to contain the generation of contaminants. Humidity levels of 40–60% are considered optimal for comfortable working.
- Furniture: minimum and safe with no sharp or jagged edges
- Wall mounting: monitoring equipment, suction apparatus and electrical connections should be wall mounted to prevent the clutter and wires on the floor.
- Storage area should be separate for storage of equipment and should be dust free and clean (wrapped and covered). The equipment must be decontaminated before storage.

Critical Parameters for Operating Rooms: Recommendations by Hospital Infection Society of India

- Air filtered in series: 1st filter bed > 30%; 2nd filter bed > 90 % filtered
- HEPA filter, which removes particles larger than 0.3µm may be reserved for operating rooms, where high risk surgeries such as orthopaedic implants are carried out.[8-9]
- Temperature of 20–22°C inhibits bacterial growth.
- Minimum air changes per hour recommended: 15 with a minimum of three air changes of fresh air (20%)
- Relative humidity 30–60% to slow down bacterial growth
- Should not be shut down
- Do not use fans
- Regular inspection of filters
- Check pressure differentials between areas and across filters: by smoke test
- Manometer tests for low-efficiency filters
- Dicotylphthalate (DOP) test for HEPA filters
- There is no evidence to suggest that duct cleaning, beyond what is recommended for optimal performance, reduces the risk of infection.
- In hospitals that lack HVAC (heating ventilation, air-conditioning systems) the quality of air cannot be guaranteed.
- When window air-conditioning is used, proper maintenance is required.
- Laminar flow is an optional facility and may or may not be combined with HEPA filters.

DESIGNING OF A LABORATORY[9]

Several aspects have to be taken into consideration in the planning and designing of a laboratory, starting from the siting, access and location (whether the laboratory should be free-standing or contained within an existing facility), to the utilities, security and safety considerations, like safety during fire, electricity and laboratory accidents.

The laboratory and its support spaces demand that every attempt is made to restrict or prevent chances of infection. A typical laboratory must have enough space to accommodate the following:

a. Main workstation space
b. Support spaces including:
   i. Reagent storage areas
   ii. Glassware washing area should have good access from all laboratory spaces. Wide doors for wheeling in carts
   iii. Autoclaving/sterilization area
   iv. Media preparation room
   v. Heavy equipment area
   vi. Cold room/walk-in incubator area
   vii. Photography room
   viii. Distilled water system
   ix. Vacuum and compressed air systems
   x. Storage room
   xi. Refuse room
   xii. Waste treatment area
   xiii. Animal house
c. Laboratory staff chambers and offices
d. Toilet facilities
e. Laboratory administration area
f. Ventilation for microbiological control can be of two types—general ventilation or local exhaust ventilation. These are especially indicated for sterile work environments

VENTILATION[10]

There are a number of surfaces which are associated with known pathogens. This knowledge has led to cleaning and other maintenance protocols specific to those pathogens. The protocols and policies have to be cost effective and also some to specific areas, structures and equipment, taking into consideration the pathogens and probability of their transmission, e.g. high-risk areas like the ICUs and OTs.[11]

Some of the Common Pathogens Associated with Ventilation Systems are:

1. Aspergillus species in air filters
2. Rhizopus species in false ceilings
3. Aspergillus species in some fire proof material

A clean environment refers to an enclosed space where levels of contaminants (having a detrimental effect on people/processes/products) are kept under specified levels. As per US federal standards, 'class of cleanliness' has been defined as the maximum number of airborne particles (size 0.5m) per cubic feet of air. Contaminants could be dust, bacteria, fungi, viruses, fibres or aerosols. Airborne bacteria-carrying particles are of the mean size of 12μm and 99.99% of all bacteria in an environment can be eliminated by effective air filtration. So also, the airborne fungal spores, which are approximately 5μm in size, can be effectively eliminated by air filtration. Airborne viruses, on the other hand, are nanometers in size and filtration is not very successful in removing them.[15]

Clean air systems and impact on outcomes: It is an established fact that the hospital environment requires a particular level of cleanliness or asepsis for the various procedures or activities that are performed, especially in the operating rooms and the intensive care units. This is because pollutants and contaminants have a detrimental effect on the human body and its internal tissues and can thus lead to a greater incidence of infections and other untoward events. Clean rooms and clean air systems came into existence to provide the necessary environment conducive to healthcare. The infection rates, particularly in specialities like orthopaedics, neurosurgery, cardiothoracic surgery and transplant surgery departments, were seen to dip by up to 50% when performed in a clean and aseptic environment. Thus, it is seen that in hospitals, air-conditioning is not merely a comfort requirement, but essential for patient management and even disease treatment. There are several cost-effective ways of preventing or controlling contamination in closed spaces and improving natural ventilation in healthcare institutions. These are essential aspects to be looked into, especially in the operating rooms, ICUs, isolation rooms, nurseries, biosafety cabinets and laboratories.[12]

Ventilation and Temperature Control

In non-air-conditioned areas

1. Design rooms appropriately with adequate windows that are placed scientifically to allow light and cross ventilation (except ICUs and OTs where windows are ideally to be sealed) to permit only natural light.
2. Install appropriate heating/cooling systems.
3. Install and properly place the fans.
4. Use floor-standing fans, table-top fans and exhaust fans correctly.
5. Maintain air-conditioners properly.
6. Pay attention to arrangement of furniture.
7. Educate personnel on the precautions to take while entering/leaving rooms.

In air-conditioned areas[12]

(Table 11.2)

- Adequate ventilation
- Inlets and exhausts
- Filters and their maintenance
- Humidifiers
- Zoning of air
- Positive pressure isolation
- Negative pressure isolation

Operating Rooms

Sources of microorganisms in the operating room are dust, lint, skin squames (epithelial cells), aerosols and respiratory droplets. The microbial level in the operating room is directly proportional to the number of people and turbulence. Swinging doors create more turbulence than sliding doors. The bacterial count can be checked by appropriate ventilation and air-conditioning, i.e. air distribution, air flow and air changes. Air intake should be free from dust particles, for which primary filters are used. Plenum (Photo 11.4) (positive-

Table 11.2: Recommended ventilation rates (air exchanges). Note: There could be variations in recommendation in the various guidelines by different bodies.

Area	Type of pressure	Total air changes/hour
1. Operating room	Positive	15–25
2. Recovery room	Less than operating room	6
3. Intensive care unit	Positive	6
4. Microbiology Laboratory	Negative	6
5. Isolation room	Negative/positive	6

pressure) type of ventilation is recommended for most operating rooms. Here, the air is evenly distributed within the space via ceiling diffusers. Air changes within the room dilute the contaminants. A combination of airflow and pressures create a gradient in flow, which then determines the direction of flow of air. The air flows from a higher-pressure area to a lower-pressure area.[13, 14]

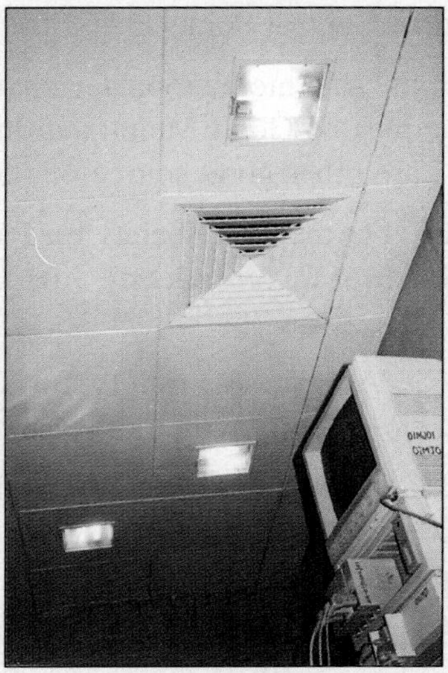

Photo 11.4: Plenum air flow from the ceiling

Pressure gradients in the operating suite

The following pressures determine the gradient:

Sterile zone 25 Pa

Clean zone 14 Pa

Protective 3 Pa

Disposal 0-(-5) Pa

Note: Air-conditioning if switched off overnight, or during the weekend, must be switched on at least one hour before subsequent use of the operating room.

Ultra clean air systems (Photo 11.5) are recommended only for operating rooms where implant, prosthetic valve, or transplant surgeries are carried out. The air exchanges are in the order of 300 changes per hour. The flow is laminar and is re-circulated through HEPA filters. The flow is normally vertical but may be horizontal.[6]

Contaminant exclusion or elimination by filtration/isolation

The most effective filtration of the air can be

6. Testing of chemical disinfectants and sterilants: Dilution Kelsey-Sykes capacity test to check disinfectant when introduced to the hospital. Use process monitoring to check the effectiveness of the disinfectant or sterilant.
7. Testing of carriers amongst staff: Nasal, throat, rectal and stool culture as per protocol of the hospital. Recommended at entry and during outbreaks, but not routinely.

FOOD- AND WATER-BORNE INFECTIONS[17-18]

Factors involved include:

- Source
- Handlers
- Raw food
- Environment
- Purchasing
- Refrigeration
- Cooking
- Personal hygiene
- Clean-up
- Pest control
- Enteral feeding
- Parenteral nutrition

Basic measures to exclude pathogens

1. Consumption of food as soon as it is prepared
2. Storage of prepared food at low (< 10^0C) or high (>70^0C) temperatures as the case may be
3. Protection of food items from rodents, insects and other animals
4. Avoidance of cross contamination during preparation, from other raw food, hands or contaminated equipment
5. Avoidance of cross contamination during storage and transport
6. Re-warming before use
7. Maintaining a good working environment (hygienic equipment, working surfaces and kitchen tools)
8. Maintaining strict personal hygiene by education of food handlers, managers of food establishments, kitchen workers and the consumers
9. Ensuring minimum possible microbial contamination of food obtained from retail

Sources of guidelines and standards

1. Food processing standards or guidelines are given by bodies such as Hazard Analysis Critical Control Point (HACCP).
2. National and international legislations and principles of Good Manufacturing Practices are other good source of standards.
3. ASPEN (American Society for Parenteral and Enteral Nutrition) http://www.clinnutr.org
4. ASCN American Society for Clinical Nutrition) http://www.ama.fasb.og/ajcn
5. ASHP (American Society of Health-System Pharmacists) http://www.ashp.org
6. National bodies providing guidelines on nutrition are IPEN Centre for Research on Nutritional Support Systems (CRNSS),

7. ASHP Technical Assistance Bulletin on Quality Assurance for Pharmacy-Prepared Sterile Products. Am.J.Hosp. Pharm.1993;50:2386-2398.

Enteral nutrition[19]

(Photo 11.6)

There are a number of feeds (benderised, digested and semi-digested) that are available. The feeds can be made in the hospital kitchens or purchased in ready-to-use form. The cost of the hospital-made enteral feeds are far less than the commercially available ones. Feeds should be hygienically and freshly prepared as far as possible, especially in smaller healthcare set-ups where no refrigerators may be available. Storage time must be mimimal with a maximum of eight hours, but stored in refrigerators either at the place of preparation or in the wards. Storage refrigerators for food must be separate from refrigerators meant for other uses.

Feeds are re-warmed to room temperature before feeding. Leftover feeds must be disposed of in a specific manner. Food is transported in sterilized bottles or containers. Intermittent feeding involves handling of food by nursing staff; so they must be educated about food handling.

Diarrhoea is a complication of administering contaminated feeds, but this must be distinguished from other non-infective causes of diarrhoea in the intensive care. Engineering controls provides for this by designing feeding catheters made of non-irritant material with thinner or finer bore catheters, smaller delivery systems and containers for enteral feeding.

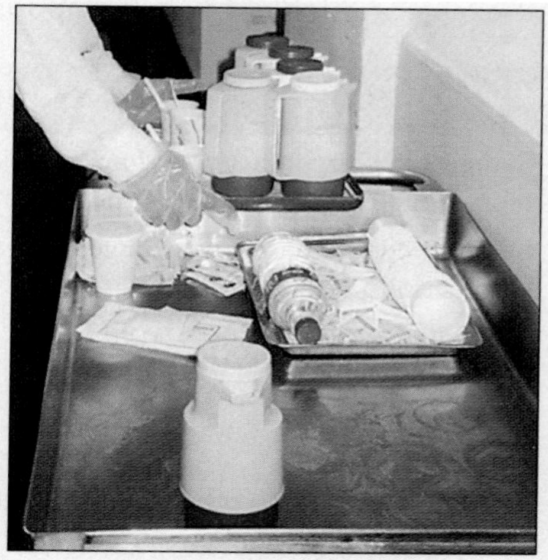

Photo 11.6: Environment management and engineering controls are used for preparation, storage, handling, transport and delivery of enteral nutrition.

Engineering controls and parenteral nutrition[20]

(Photo 11.7)

Providing this form of nutrition constitutes a major source of infection and sepsis, which may be of bacterial or fungal origin, and can be potentially fatal. This is because parenteral nutrition solutions are a good medium for the rapid growth of organisms. The common organisms are *Staphylococcus aureus, Staphylococcus epidermidis, Candida albicans and Malassezia furfur*. Engineering control measures in the prevention of infection by parentral nurtrition are:

1. Dedicated line for infusion of parenteral nutrition solution
2. Decreased handling, aseptic handling and port decontamination techniques
3. Meticulously following recommended hang time for solutions.

Table 11.3: Comparison of air sampling methods

Settle plate	Slit sampler
1. Samples the large, faster-settling particles more efficiently than small particles	1. Samples all particles, irrespective of size
2. Samples continuously over longer time periods	2. Samples over short periods of time and hence, sampling can be repeated
3. Individual events are lost	3. Indicates the occurrence of individual events that may compromise the quality of air in OT. E.g. unnecessary opening of theatre doors or influx of personnel
4. Provides an accurate measure of the rate at which particles land on surface	4. Measures the air in circulation
5. Impossible to sample low numbers of small particles	5. Possible to sample even low numbers of small particles that may pass through a defective HEPA filter*
6. Fungal spores deposit with lower efficiency	6. Can detect fungal spores with high efficiency

*Current guidelines are that there should be no more than 0.5cfu/cubic metre (i.e. 1 cfu in 2 cubic metre; around 3mins. sampling for a high volume slit sampler) in air that has passed through HEPA filters in ultraclean theatres.

early 1990s, CDC developed an extensive set of recommendations for the control of TB in the healthcare settings as 'Guidelines for Preventing the Transmission of *Mycobacterium tuberculosis* in Healthcare Facilities'. The guidelines recommend a TB control plan comprising of hierarchical control measures (See hierarchy of controls in chapter on occupational hazards):

- Administrative: Protocols for identifying, evaluating and treating patients who may have TB
- Engineering: General and local exhaust ventilation, HEPA filtration and Ultraviolet Germicidal Irradiation (UVGI)

Here, the engineering controls are designed to reduce the concentration of infectious droplet nuclei in the air, prevent their dissemination, and render them non-infectious by killing the tubercle bacilli they contain. CDC recommends the following engineering controls to reduce microbial contamination of air:

- Local exhaust ventilation (i.e., source control)
- General ventilation
- Air cleaning

It is very often seen that the airborne pathogens are not adequately diluted in closed rooms and wards. There have been instances wherein a patient with unsuspected tuberculosis has transmitted the infection to no less than 13 of the people who were present or working in the same ward. Usually, the air-conditioning unit merely re-circulates the room's air without filtering out the airborne pathogens.

UVGI radiation has been shown to kill or inactivate *M.tuberculosis* in air. Two types of UVGI are used in TB control: in-duct and upper room irradiation.[16]

In-duct consists of use of UVGI lamps inside an air duct or air cleaner. An appropriately designed, installed and maintained induct UVGI system should effectively disinfect most re-circulated air and therefore, significantly reduce the risk of TB exposure from recirculated air. For TB control purposes, such a system would be almost equivalent to a 100% outside air system (ideal for high-risk settings). But it is expensive to install and operate.

Upper-room consists of use of mounted UVGI lamps in a room where there is a risk of TB spreading. Advantages of UVGI include its use as an upgrade to an existing system and its ability to remove most infectious particles from air without significant reduction to the airflow.

The designing of treatment rooms can be crucial in the treatment of tuberculosis.

- Personal respiratory protection[10, 11,14,16]
- Airborne infections such as tuberculosis need special masks

Microbiological surveillance of the operation theatre

Checklist: Protocol to be established in consultation with the local hospital infection control committee.

1. Airflow and ventilation check: Check the direction of airflow by smoke test. Check air velocity by hot air anemometer. Only used during commissioning and re-furbishing and after repairs of the ventilation system.
2. Check the contamination of the air (Monitor the process of sterilization and disinfection of the environment). Settle plate/slit sampler air sampling.
3. Healthcare workers are often faced with the baffling situation of how, when and with what they should sample air in operating theatres. There is no single consensus on this, although years of experience and toil have clarified some aspects. The microbiological quality of theatre air is one of several significant parameters for controlling surgical wound infection, and sampling is performed to assess both the quality of air entering the theatre, as well as its ability to dilute or exclude contamination. There is a direct relationship between airborne contamination and infection rates in theatres.
4. Surface sampling: Rodac plate method and swab rinse test. Only used during commissioning and refurbishing and during outbreaks.
5. Monitor the sterilization and disinfection processes of equipment: Steam sterilizer and ethyleneoxide sterilizer: Monitor physical characterstics of every cycle. Monitor the effectiveness of chamber daily by Bowie Dick's test. Monitor the effectiveness of the sterilization process by calorimetric change (every load) and by *B. stereothermophilus* spores.

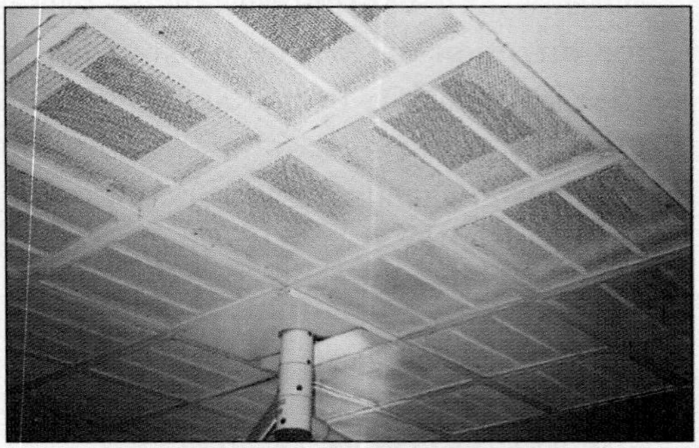

Photo 11.5: Laminar air flow inlet from ceiling

carried out by installation of the laminar-flow clean air systems, which use the HEPA (High Efficiency Particulate Air) filters having an efficiency of 99.97%. These are recommended in critical areas. The other filters used are ASHRAB filters with an efficiency of 90–95%. Both these systems use the principle of multiple-stage filtration. A number of companies specialize in the designing of laminar-flow systems. The filters are to be changed as per manufacturer's instructions. Filter replacement is required periodically (every six months or so) and this may require shutting down of the operating room for a day. While replacing the filter, the process of purging and cleaning may contaminate the operating room. The proper working of the filter at the time of commissioning and change needs to be validated with bacterial tests. Clean room testing and validation also involves testing of air samples, acquisition by checking flow, isokinetic probe or an optical particle counter and bacteriological tests (see process monitoring). It has to be mentioned at this point that HEPA filtration is very expensive and is not a prerequisite for all operations.

HEPA filters, also referred to as ultra-high efficiency air filters or absolute filters, are capable of removing viable and non-viable particulates from air streams, producing ultra-clean, microbiologically sterile air. These filters are composed of continuous sheets of borosilicate glass filter paper. Although glass may provide the best mesh of fibres of circular cross sections and a small diameter, there are other materials that have been used, like-cellulose, asbestos and other mineral fibres. Today, many HEPA filters use fibres of plastic materials. By definition, HEPA filters have an efficiency of 99.97% for particles 0.3 microns in diameter.

HEPA filter units remove essentially all particles in the size range of droplet nuclei. The self-contained units (portable, ceiling or wall mounted) will provide cleaned air to dilute infectious particles and to remove airborne particles. Advantages of HEPA units include improved air quality, ease of installation, maintenance, services and flexibility.

HEPA filtration in other healthcare areas

- No area of the hospital requires more careful control of environmental contaminants than the surgical suite. The Laminar airflow in ORs is defined as ultra-clean (HEPA-filtered) air flow that is predominantly unidirectional, either vertical or horizontal, when not obstructed. In an alternative to laminar airflow in the OR, HEPA-filtered air is delivered from the ceiling, with downward movement to several exhaust inlets located low on opposite walls. This is probably the most effective air movement pattern for maintaining the concentration of contaminants in the OR at acceptable levels.

- HEPA filtered air supply systems have also been recommended for rooms used for clinical treatment of patients with a high susceptibility to infection, such as leukaemia, burns, bone marrow transplants, organ transplants or AIDS.
- Stand-alone bench-type laminar-flow units routinely provide protective sterile environments in hospital pharmacies, tissue banks, blood banks, etc.
- Biological Safety Cabinets (BSC), which combine HEPA filtration and controlled airflow, have found a place in hospital laboratories to protect laboratory workers from exposure to potential pathogens.
- Portable in-room HEPA filtration systems are also available, which can remove particulates and recirculate uncontaminated air into the isolation rooms.

The utility of laminar airflow devices in preventing prosthetic joint infections is controversial. Reports have ranged from no difference to increased infections, depending on the positioning of personnel, to reduced infections. Definitive recommendations on this method of prophylaxis await clinical trials.

History-HEPA filters were developed during the 1940s and 1950s by the US Army Chemical Corps and Naval Research Laboratories and the Atomic Energy Commission to provide respiratory protection from biological warfare agents for military personnel and to contain radioactive dust and other airborne radioactive particles generated in the developing nuclear materials industry. Since then, HEPA filters have found use in medical, research, electronic, pharmaceutical and industrial settings where clean air is essential to work or where emissions of toxic particulates or hazardous biologic agents must be controlled.

Air-sampling in OTs and other clean areas

(Table 11.3)

There are several significant differences between slit samplers and settle plates that are used for sampling of air. These can be summarized as follows:

Although it may seem that slit samplers are superior to settle plates as a method of air sampling, it is important to bear in mind that in the context of artificially ventilated clinical areas, such as isolation rooms or OTs, air sampling should be carried out for a specific reason with a scientifically validated method, the results analysed and then action taken accordingly.

Engineering controls in the prevention of tuberculosis[15]

While engineering controls are applicable to all aspects of healthcare and all pathogenic microorganisms, their relevance holds a special place in the prevention of tuberculosis. This is because *Mycobacterium tuberculosis* is one of the hardiest of organisms and not easy to get rid of. Thus, it is believed that if a control measure or procedure can be applied successfully to control *Mycobacterium tuberculosis*, then it must be good for other pathogenic organisms too. With this in mind, we proceed to describe the application of engineering controls in the prevention of *Mycobacterium tuberculosis*.

In response to the increase in nosocomial outbreaks of tuberculosis in the late 1980s and

4. Collapsible bags rather than bottles
5. Avoiding access of the bottles or bags when additives are added
6. Use of three-in-one bags rather than separate infusions for various constituents[20]
7. Use of microbial filters—although this is still controversial and may not be recommended for routine use

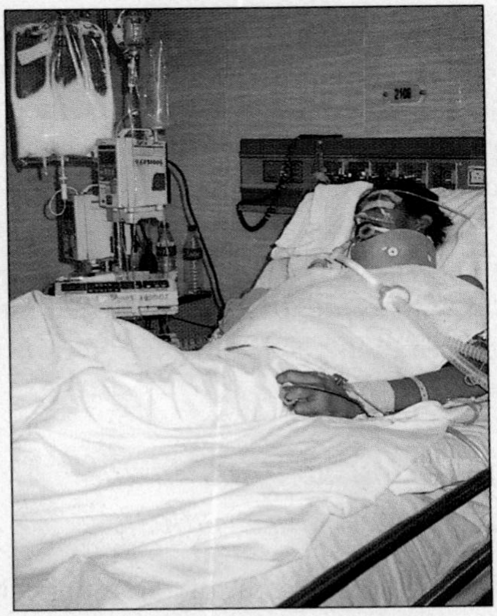

Photo 11.7: Engineering controls for parenteral nutrition. Improved design of bags and delivery systems has reduced HAI.

WATER MANAGEMENT IN HEALTHCARE INSTITUTIONS (DRINKING WATER, BATHS, MEDICAL WATER)[18]

There are a number of pathogens which are commonly associated with water in hospitals. Common pathogens in various water sources include potable water *(Pseudomonas aeruginosa, Serratia, Acinetobacter, Aeromonas, Legionella)*, sinks (*Pseudomonas*), tub immersion (*Pseudomonas*) and water baths (*Pseudomonas, Acinetobacter*).[15-19]

In addition, diarrhoeal epidemics are common in the paediatric wards especially in the developing nations where a large number of patients are treated in smaller areas and there is a storage of the ORS (oral rehydration solution) in the ward. Extreme aseptic precautions must be observed in handling stored water. Patients or their relatives should never be allowed to handle stored water. A plan for managing quality of water, its storage and distribution must be in place for preventing waterborne HAI. One of the important problems of distribution is the intermittent supply of water in many countries where there is a shortage of water. This has been proven to lead to low or negative pressure in the pipeline and subsequent contamination. Staffing patterns and adequate ratio of nurse : patient is important for preventing spread of water-borne diseases. Preventing contamination by sewage and standards for assessment such as the coliform count are given by the local municipalities but those standards need to be strictly enforced.[18]

Preventing legionellosis

One of the important infections transmitted by water is legionellosis. It is responsible for both community acquired infections and HAI.[17] Person-to-person transmission is not reported. It is transmitted by potable water. The highest concentrations are found in storage tanks, cooling towers and condensers. Effective methods of disinfection include chlorination, thermal eradication, UV light, and metal ionization (copper-silver ionization). Routine culturing of water is not recommended.

PEST MANAGEMENT PROGRAMME[21]

Every institution should consider pest management issues at the very beginning, while setting up the healthcare facility, and maintain it as an ongoing activity. The pest management programme should be a 'least chemical means' one, wherein the use of chemicals is avoided or kept to the bare minimum to avoid the cumulative and harmful effects. Wherever research is being carried out with human pathogens, the pest levels must be zero. For tissue culture and media preparation area of the microbiology laboratory, a non-chemical approach is advisable. For a research laboratory doing DNA and genetic work, the NIH pest control guidelines may be followed.[22]

CONTAINERS AND CLOSURES FOR STERILE IV FLUIDS[23, 19]

IV fluids were initially made available in glass bottles and containers. There were several disadvantages in this. They were liable to contamination by foreign particulate matter. Soft glass containers may contain flakes of glass. Fragments of rubber from the closure sometimes get detached during autoclaving. Some insoluble ingredients of rubber like carbon black, zinc oxide, chalk and clay get released into the fluids. Mold spores may get released into the fluid by bursting of blisters in the closure. Bottle closures may be stressed to the limit during sterilization due to pressure changes. Air may escape from some bottles when the closures are a poor fit on the bottlenecks and on cooling such bottles develop a partial internal vacuum. Bottles in this state can take up contamination more readily than those without an internal vacuum.

To overcome all these disadvantages, the plastic containers were designed. There are two types of plastic used widely for intravenous infusion packs: polyvinyl chloride (PVC) and polyethylene.

Advantages of plastics bags (for IV infusion)

- Lighter in weight
- More resistant to breakage during handling and transport
- They are all single-use and disposable and so the problems of washing and decontamination are not there.
- Absence of rubber closures ensures fewer chances of contamination.
- Sterilization, storage and use are fraught with fewer chances of contamination.
- Absence of an airway offers another safeguard against contamination during infusion.

Yet another example of designing for safety can be seen from the improvements in blood collection bags in blood banks. Over time, there has been a gradual but steady improvement in the manufacture of the blood collection systems. Some of the changes that have revolutionized blood banking systems include:

a. Use of frosted tube, free of tackiness, and thus easy to knot
b. Rounded corners of the bag, offering smoother transfer of blood components during separation and transfusion
c. Ultra thin-walled siliconiszed surface, short beak bevel needle, which offers minimum resistance for the needle in penetrating

the skin as also less trauma to the donor by smooth insertion.

d. Blood bags with in-line Leuko-reduction filters.

e. Tamper evident integrated outlet ports, which let one have a 'see and believe' assurance that the seal is intact (complying with ISO 3826 regulations).

Infectious aerosols, droplets and splashing may be produced by some instruments capable of introducing large amounts of energy into liquids being processed, e.g. mixers, centrifuges, dessicators, culture shakers, stirrers and agitators, freeze driers, homogenizers, tissue grinders, sonicators, ultrasonic cleaners, blenders and ultrasonic devices. They create a risk of microbial transmission by airborne and surface contamination. Mixers and blenders and ultrasonic devices should be operated in biological safety cabinets when there is risk of infectious aerosol production.

ENGINEERING CONTROLS FOR LABORATORY EQUIPMENT

Biological safety cabinets are workstations designed to protect laboratory personnel working with microorganisms of varying degrees of virulence and infectiousness. When properly used and maintained, the biosafety cabinet offers three types of protection:[22]

- Personal protection
- Environmental protection
- Product protection

In response to the request of NIH and National Cancer Institute (NCI), the National Sanitation Foundation (NSF) was to prepare a standard for Class II cabinets. So, NSF formed a committee of personnel from NLH, NCI, CDC and manufacturers and potential users of safety cabinets from research laboratories. Thus, the NSF standard#49 resulted. This guideline has been generally accepted as the 'state of the art' for manufacturing, performance, testing and periodic evaluation and certification of Biological Safety Cabinets (BSC).

It is the manufacturer's responsibility to conform to the specifications, while it is the user's responsibility to determine its final location before uncrating. Positioning is critical and can affect the performance. It should be placed in an area where personnel movement is at a minimum. Other factors to be borne in mind are: voltage and amperage, turbulence, electrical supply (whether to include it in an emergency category or not).

There Are Three Classes of Biological Safety Cabinets Available

Class I BSC

This is an open-fronted, ventilated cabinet providing protection to the operator by an inward air flow that is not circulated. It is fitted with a HEPA filter to protect the environment from microorganisms released during manipulations within the working space. Class I cabinets are used for working with organisms of low to moderate risk and although they protect the operator they do not protect the material within the cabinet from contamination.

Class II BSC

This again is an open-fronted, ventilated

cabinet giving personal protection to the operator and to the material within. There is an inward air flow and HEPA filtered supply and exhaust air. Class II has two types of Cabinets:

Class II type A is used in microbiology filters and it re-circulates 70% of the air. This may be used for work with low to moderate risk organisms. These protect not only the worker, but also the material within the cabinet and are hence very useful for work with tissue cultures. Class II type B: These cabinets filter and re-circulate only 30% of the air, and are used while working with radioactive and carcinogenic substances.

Class III BSC

The Class III cabinet is a totally enclosed, gas-tight ventilated cabinet maintained under negative pressure. Both the supply and exhaust air is HEPA filtered. The exhaust air is usually passed through two HEPA filters in series. Work is done with long-sleeved rubber gloves, which are integral with the cabinet carcass. These cabinets are used for working with high-risk organisms and provide a total barrier between the operator and work.

Laminar-flow cabinets

There is often confusion between biological safety cabinets and laminar-flow cabinets or workstations. BSCs are designed to protect the worker (and sometimes the work); laminar-flow cabinets are designed to protect the work only and offer no protection to the worker. These cabinets have no place in laboratories where infectious materials are handled. They are useful, however, in the preparation of culture media and sterile solutions.

BIOHAZARD MATERIAL CONTAINERS, BAGS AND LABELS

Serveral types of equipment are used for transfer and safe disposal of hospital wastes, such as screw-capped bottles, leak-proof vessels for collection and transport of infectious materials, autoclaves for safe disposal of wastes, incinerators. Transport of waste and dirty linen in specialized containers reduces the risk of infection transmission. Disposal of waste by the use of incinerator, autoclave, ethyleneoxide sterilizer are all examples of technology being used for reducing risk of infection to the healthcare worker and the public at large. (For more details see chapter on Hospital Waste Management.)

Designing personal protective equipment such that risk to the HCW is minimized. E.g. respirators, goggles or safety spectacles, face shields.[24]

Designing of laboratory and pipetting aids—several improvements have been introduced in these areas, all of which cannot be enumerated in this book.

DESIGNING OF BACTERIAL FILTERS[23]

In-line IV filters—A number of companies (e.g.Vygon) manufacture 0.22mm in-line filters for the prevention of air embolism, endotoxin, particulate matter and fungal spores into circulation and are useful in immunodeficient, immunocompromised and critically ill patients receiving infusions with many additives.

DESIGNING OF SUCTIONING EQUIPMENT/DISPOSABLE SUCTIONING DEVICE

Traditional suction systems use reusable jars which need to be decontaminated before reuse and pose a risk to the handlers. In some places this has been replaced by disposable suction systems. These systems need modification in protocols for incineration of these systems.

Closed Sheathing Suction Catheters

These are catheters that are used for repeated suctioning of the endotracheal tube and are left in place in a plastic sheath, which prevents any contact with the person performing the suctioning. Though the advantage of this system has not been proven by controlled double-blind studies, this offers an option in terms of newer devices although it is expensive and needs to be changed every day.[23]

ACCESSORIES TO ENGINEERING CONTROLS IN ENVIRONMENT MANAGEMENT

General Cleanliness Measures and Special Precautions (Especially in Areas like OTs and ICUs)

- Restriction of entry: Entry only to authorized persons in these areas. It is interesting to note that the greatest amount of bacteria found in the operating room come from the humans
- Prohibition of smoking/drinking/application of cosmetics/lighting of matchsticks/cluttering of unnecessary papers/sharpening pencils, etc.
- Walls, ceilings and furniture must be cleaned according to specified protocol and at specified intervals.
- Operating Rooms: After known infected cases, the operating room must be cleaned thoroughly according to accepted protocols. Most operating theatres prefer to post an infected case at the end of the list just to save the time of cleaning rather than to prevent the transmission of infection.[25]

Garments should be lint free and fine weave in case of textiles, with a low level of particulate shedding, easily washable, durable or disposable. They should be washed as per frequency specified. Special attire defined for the area with change of footwear or foot covers should be strictly adhered to.

Laundry Hygiene

- Usually, hospital linen is contaminated with GNB from intestine or *Staphylococcus epidermidis* from skin. These are unlikely causes of infection.
- *Staph.aureus* is present in <1% and does not present a hazard if regular precautions are taken.
- *Bacillus cereus* has been isolated from clean laundry and can cause rare outbreaks of infection in neurosurgery patients or umbilical infections in newborns.
- Used linen of patients with specific infections (e.g. *Salmonella and Shigella*) is a potential hazard.
- Linen from patients of HBV and HIV are not hazardous unless blood stained.

UK recommendations for laundry

Laundry can be categorized as:

1. Used
2. Infected
3. Heat-labile (thorough washing and rinsing at low temperatures of 40–50°C will remove most of the organisms and should be sufficient.

There is evidence that levels of contamination are similar in linen from isolation rooms to those in linen from other areas of the hospital, and hence double bagging is not necessary.[24] Standard Precautions are followed in the sorting and handling of all used linen. There is no evidence of acquired infections in laundry workers. Hence, in UK the existing guidelines are followed unless evidence-based alternatives are available.

All hospital linen should be heat-disinfected at 65°C for 10 minutes or 71°C for three minutes.

Staff handling linen should be offered immunization against poliomyelitis, tetanus, HBV and BCG if tuberculin-negative. Those with unhealed lesions, rashes or exfoliative lesions should not handle clean linen unless the wound is covered with impermeable dressing.

ENVIRONMENTAL HYGIENE

Standard Principles for Preventing HAI

There is growing evidence linking poor environmental hygiene and transmission of microorganisms causing hospital acquired infections.[1] This has been addressed by the Infection Control Nurses Association and the Association of Domestic Managers, resulting in the adoption and publication by the department of health, of standards concerning hospital cleanliness. In addition to existing statutory regulations, specialists advise the controls Assurance Standards and clinical Governances, which provides a framework within which hospital environmental hygiene can be improved and monitored. More recently, the NHS Plan included action to be taken to improve hospital cleaning.

Standard Principles provide guidance on infection-control precautions that should be applied by all healthcare practitioners, in the care of all hospital in-patients, all the time. These recommendations are detailed procedural protocols and need to be incorporated into local guidelines.

These Recommendations Are Divided into Four Distinct Interventions

1. Hospital environmental hygiene. Good hospital hygiene is an integral and important component of a strategy for preventing HAI. The routine activities that are generally considered to be central to the prevention of HAI include: cleaning and decontamination, laundry and housekeeping; safe collection and disposal of general and clinical waste; kitchen and food hygiene.
2. Hand hygiene (described earlier)
3. Use of personal protective equipment (described earlier)
4. Use and disposal of sharps (See chapter on hospital waste management.)

These guidelines do not address the additional infection-control requirements of specialist settings, such as the operating department.

Standard Principles of Hospital Environmental Hygiene (Intervention 1)

1. The hospital environment must be visibly clean, free from dust and soilage, and acceptable to patients, their visitors and staff. (Category 3)
2. Where a piece of equipment is used for more than one patient, e.g. commode, it must be cleaned following each and every episode of use. (Category 3)
3. Statutory requirements must be met in relation to the safe disposal of clinical waste, laundry arrangements for used and infected linen, food hygiene and pest control. (Category 3)
4. All staff involved in hospital hygiene activities must be included in education and training related to the prevention of hospital acquired infection. (Category 3)

Kitchen Hygiene

Food hygiene regulations in the UK Food Safety (Temperature Control) Regulations 1995 (Department of Health NHS Executive, 1996) state that 8°C is satisfactory for cold storage, but 5°C is preferable, if possible.

Medical examination of staff—for typhoid, paratyphoid, dysentery, persistent diarrhoea, vomiting, tuberculosis, boils, skin ailments, eye/ear discharges, etc. is mandatory.

Food and Catering

The subject of food handling and catering is very important in a large hospital with these facilities, because infections transmitted from these areas are wholly or mostly preventable with adequate measures.

Important infections that can occur due to inadequacies in any of the catering processes are Salmonella and other food poisoning epidemics. The issues which are important here include: preparation of food, food handlers, standards of hygiene, storage of food and its delivery. In addition to maintaining standards of hygiene and guidelines for environmental management in the hospital kitchen, enteral and parenteral nutrition are issues where a lot of research and innovation have gone in to make the catheters and delivery systems safer.

Important guidelines and standards for water management are given by the following bodies.

- Association for the Advancements of Medical Instrumentation (AAMI): American National Standard for Hemodialysis Systems. Arlington, VA: Association for the Advancements of Medical Instrumentation, 1996. Deals with guidelines for device users, specific emphasis on water purity assurance and monitoring.

REFERENCES

1) Girard R, Perraud M, Pruss A et al. In: Ducel G, Fabry J, Nicolle L, eds. Prevention of hospital-acquired infections – A practical guide. 2nd edn. WHO 2002: 47-54.
2) Planning and organization of central sterile supply department. In: Environment Management for Control of Hospital Infections. VII National Conference. Hospital Infection Society. India. CME. Vellore. 2003; 84-92.

3) The American Institute of Architects Committee on Architecture for Health, US department of Health and Human Services, Guidelines for Construction and Equipment of Hospital and Medical Facilities, Washington DC. The American Institute of Architects Press, 1997; 7, v-viii, 23-26, 88-91.

4) De Franco. Planning the physical structure of the PACU. In: Frost EAM, ed. Post Anaesthesia care unit: Current Practices. 2nd edn. St Louis: The CV Mosby Company. 1990; 187-198.

5) Wolfe MI. Design of the facility. In: Liberman DF, ed. Biohazards Management Handbook. 2nd edn. Marcel Dekker Inc.1995; 1-45.

6) Scoott G. Air Quality and monitoring – Isolation wards and ICUs. In: Environment Management for Control of Hospital Infections. VII National Conference. Hospital Infection Society. India. CME. Vellore. 2003; 63-64

7) Brigden RJ. The theatre or operating department. In: Operating Theatre Technique. 4th edn. Edinburgh. Churchill Livingstone. 1980; 1-32.

8) Karlekar R. Air Quality and Monitoring – Operation Theatres. In: Environment Management for Control of Hospital Infections. VII National Conference. Hospital Infection Society. India. CME. Vellore. 2003; 59-62.

9) Liberman DF and Harding AL. Biosafety: The Research/ Diagnostic Laboratory perspective. In: Liberman DF, ed. Biohazards Management Handbook. 2nd edition. Marcel Dekker Inc. 1995; 151-171

10) Melvin WF. Ventilation for biomedical research, biotechnology and diagnostic facilities. In: Liberman DF, ed. Biohazards Management Handbook. 2nd edn. Marcel Dekker Inc. 1995; 47-77.

11) Liberman DF. Biohazards Management Handbook. 2nd edn. Marcel Dekker Inc. 1995: 1-45.

12) Uduman SA, Farrukh AS, Nath KN et al. An outbreak of *Serratia marcescens* infection in a special-care baby unit of a community hospital in United Arab Emirates: the importance of the air conditioner duct as a nosocomial reservoir. J Hosp Infect. 2002; 52(3): 175-80.

13) Consensus Guidelines for the prevention of infections in the operating room. Newsletter of the Hospital infection Society- Mumbai Forum. 2002:1-9.

14) Nester EW, Roberts CE and Nester M. Epidemiology and public health Microbiology- a human perspective. William C Brown Publishers 1995; 03-19.

15) Sutton PM, Nicas M and Harrison RJ. Implementing a Quality assurance Program for Tuberculosis Control. In: Charney W, ed. Handbook of modern hospital safety. Boca Raton. Lewis Publishers. 1999; 246-252.

16) Riley R and Nardell E: Clearing the air, the theory and application of ultraviolet air disinfection. Am Rev Respir Dis. 1989; 139: 1290.

17) Mathai MD. Environmental Challenges: Food and water supply to hospitals. In: Environment Management for Control of Hospital Infections. VII National Conference. Hospital Infection Society. India. CME Vellore. 2003; 80-83.

18) SlaterFM. Water Management.In: Abrutyn E, Goldmann DA, Scheckler WE, eds. Saunders Infection Control Reference Service. WB Saunders Company. 1998; 753-54.

19) ASPEN. American Society for Parenteral and Enteral Nutrition Board of Directors. Safe Practices for Parenteral nutrition formulations. JPEN. 1998; 22: 49-66

20) Hambleton R and Allwood MC. Containers and closures. In: Phillips I, Meers PD, D'Arcy PF. Microbiological hazards of Infusion therapy. Proceedings of an International Symposium held at the University of Sussex, England, March 1976.

21) Alpert GD. Integrated pest management program. In: Liberman DF, ed. Biohazards Management Handbook. 2nd edition. Marcel Dekker Inc. 1995; 87-96.

22) Collins CH. In: Laboratory Acquired Infections. 2nd edn. Butterworths & Co. 1988;1-28.

23) Cheeseman D. Intravenous care: the benefits of closed-system connectors. Br J Nurs. 2001; 10(5): 287-95

24) Spencer EM, Mills AE, Rorty MV et al. Compliance, Risk management and Quality Improvement Programmes. In: Organization Ethics in Health Care. New York: Oxford University Press. 2000; 171-185.

25) O'Grady NP, Gerberding JL, Weinstein RA et al. Patient safety and the science of prevention: The time for implementing the Guidelines for the Prevention of Intravascular Catheter-related infections is now. Crit Care Med. 2003; 31(1): 291-92.

Chapter 12

Surveillance and Monitoring

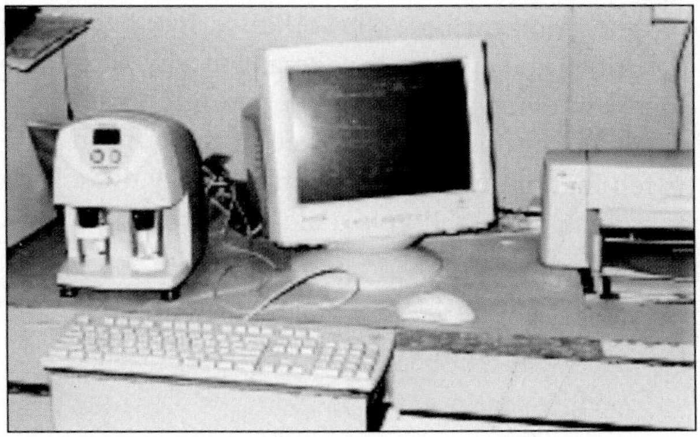

An integrated, organization-wide system for ensuring that standards of quality, of process, and of outcomes are established, communicated and monitored and that performance beyond expectations is effectively remanded.

—Omanchonu and Ross

Highlights

Objectives of Surveillance

Surveillance: How and Why?

Standards for Surveillance

Monitoring

Multicentric Surveillance

Global Initiatives

INTRODUCTION

Many a time it is seen that the words 'monitoring' and 'surveillance' are used synonymously. While this may be justified in a literary sense, it is not so in the healthcare setting, wherein the two terms have taken on rather specific meanings. In a nutshell, it may be stated that 'surveillance' is a broad term that encompasses 'monitoring'. Surveillance has been described and defined in several ways by various workers. Since no single definition succeeds in clarifying the essence of the term, it is felt that more than one definition may drive home the point and give a clearer picture.

- A simple, layman's definition of surveillance would be 'to watch over with great attention, authority and often with suspicion'.
- According to some, surveillance is the continuous scrutiny of the factors that determine the occurrence and distribution of disease and other conditions of ill health.[1]
- In 1990, Benenson defined surveillance as 'the continuing scrutiny of all aspects of occurrence and spread of a disease that is pertinent to effective control'.
- Still others define surveillance as 'the ongoing, systematic collection, analysis and interpretation of health data essential to planning, implementation, and evaluation of public health practice, closely integrated with the timely dissemination of these data to those who need to know',[2, 3] e.g. collection, calculation, and dissemination of surgeon-specific, surgical site infection (SSI) rates to surgeons were found to reduce SSI rates in all published studies.[4] The scientific value of surveillance as a part of the hospital infection control programme was demonstrated by the SENIC study (Study of the Efficacy of Nosocomial Infection Control), which indicated that a highly efficient surveillance and infection-control system could reduce the infection rates by one-third. There should be five criteria for microbiological surveillance—it should be planned, purposeful, scientifically accurate, properly analysed and effectively communicated.[5,6]

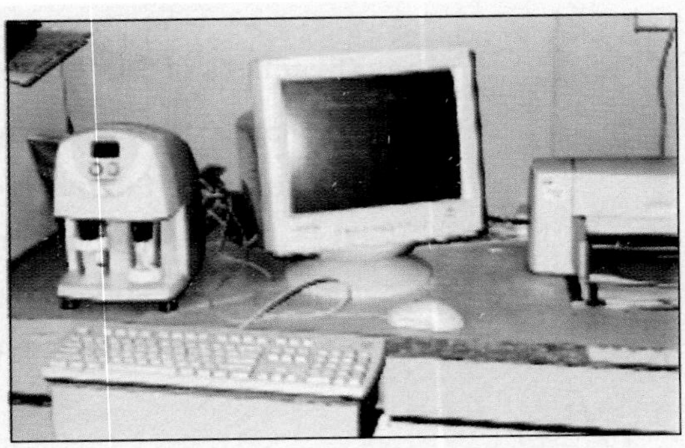

Photo 12.1: Database software and technological advances have revolutionised monitoring and surveillance

Surveillance: Predictive (forecasting, warning), continuous, creates benchmarks

Monitoring: Supervisory (processes), constant, continuous

Surveillance is a process that is applicable to several aspects in the medical field. Thus, it can be epidemiological surveillance, demographic surveillance, nutritional surveillance, equipment surveillance, serological surveillance, environmental surveillance, staff surveillance and so on. It could also be at any level—local, national or international. A unique and useful form of surveillance is the 'sentinel surveillance'. This is a method for identifying cases occurring in a community that have escaped the notification system and are hence not 'caught' by the system. This type of surveillance would prove valuable in minimizing reporting biases. While sentinel surveillance mostly refers to the community at large, it can be utilized in the hospital set-up as well.

It is not possible to restrict the surveillance to hospitals alone, because more often than not, the patients' stay in the hospital is short, which requires that the surveillance system must extend to the community too in order to obtain accurate data. It is important to note that passive reporting of cases is not surveillance. It is a systematic collection of accurate morbidity and mortality data, the meticulous consolidation of these data accompanied by special field investigations if and when necessary, and rapid dissemination of the final information to those responsible for disease control or prevention.[7]

A surveillance system cannot be termed useful if it fails to 'warn' the healthcare personnel about impending disease outbreaks or problem areas, for which the system can arm itself adequately to combat at the earliest.

Surveillance of nosocomial infections is important for the following reasons (Fig. 12.1):

1. To develop internal benchmarks (incidence rates of important infections like, surgical wound infections, nosocomial pneumonia, catheter-related infections, etc.)

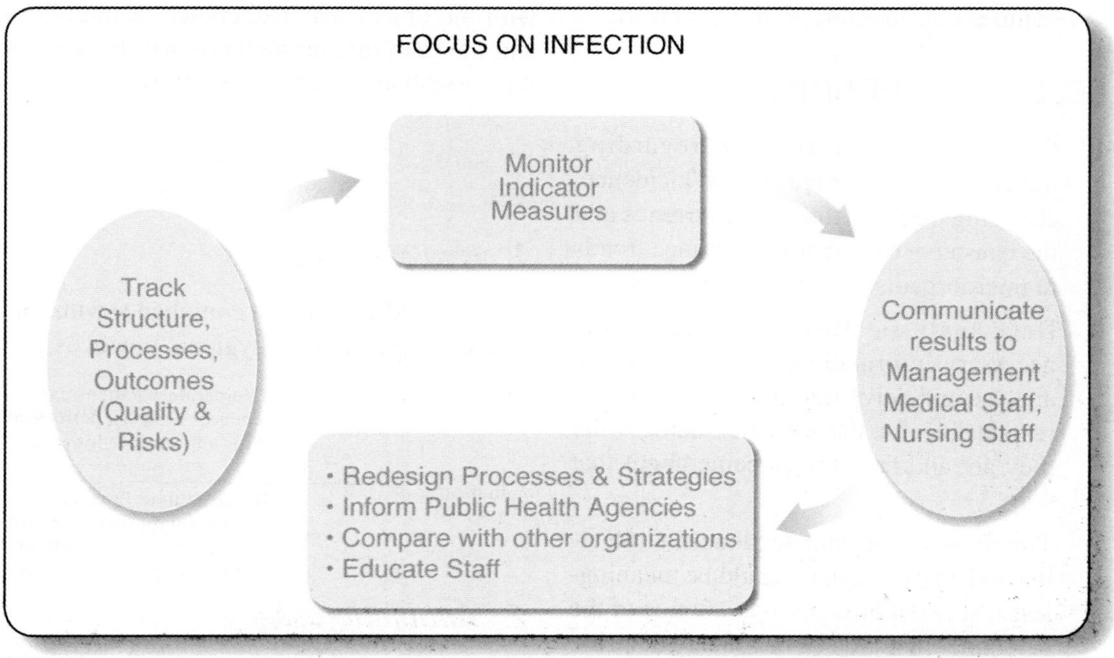

Figure 12.1: Surveillance has a number of objectives

2. To monitor changes in disease pattern of the above-mentioned infections
3. To assess the outcome of nosocomial infections
4. Early recognition and prompt action against impending outbreaks
5. To reduce spread of infection by identifying high-risk patients and to introduce specific control measures in such cases[8]
6. To assess preventive measures followed in the hospital
7. To provide information for planning of preventive measures and resources required
8. Monitoring, with benchmarks external to those of a single hospital's surveillance system, has also been suggested. Developing a system with external benchmarks requires considerable additional effort.

OBJECTIVES OF SURVEILLANCE

1. Collection of information regarding infection rates, their prevalence/incidence, changing trends in disease occurrence and the causative organisms, resistance trends in microorganisms and the like
2. Data analysis: Having collected the necessary information, it is important to analyse and delve into the various factors responsible for the statistics being what they are and how things came about that way.
3. Timely warning and feedback: Collecting and analysing data would be meaningless if it is not brought to the notice of the personnel involved in healthcare decision making. The decision makers need to be made aware of priorities regarding epidemics, outbreaks and situations demanding immediate action.
4. Implement corrective measures: An indirect, yet useful, objective achieved by surveillance is that it helps in the rectification of past mistakes and neglected areas of healthcare. When surveillance reveals poor implementation of policies and healthcare measures, in the form of discouraging statistics, one can take cue from it and incorporate the necessary changes in the existing system in order to reverse the negative trends.
5. Disease prevention: This should be the final and ultimate objective of an efficient surveillance system.

SCOPE

The scope of the surveillance methods vary with the objectives. The choice of indicators and the case finding methods will depend on the surveillance strategy selected.

Examples of Surveillance Carried Out in the Following Areas

1. Hygiene practices

Objective: Monitoring of compliance with, and quality assessment of, hygienic practices

$$\text{Indicators} = \frac{\text{Numerator: Patient care procedures actually performed with appropriate hygiene precautions}}{\text{Denominator: Procedures requiring appropriate standard hygiene precautions/patient census/density of care index}}$$

2. Antibiotic usage

Objective: Continuous monitoring and quality assessment of antibiotic utilization patterns

$$\text{Indicators} = \frac{\text{Numerator: Types of antimicrobial cures/doses and duration used for prophylaxis and treatment}}{\text{Denominator: Surgical interventions/documented infections (e.g. Bacteremia)/ patient admissions}}$$

Source of Data: Pharmacy records, operating room records, medical and nursing records, chart review, computerized patient record

3. *Incidence of hospital infection*

Objective: Continuous monitoring of incidence of infection, hospital-wide or selective areas

$$\text{Indicators} = \frac{\text{Numerator: Infection by site/ ward/procedure or device}}{\text{Denominator: Patient admissions/hospital days/ procedures/device-days}}$$

Source of Data: Laboratory and/ward liaison, chart review, computerized record

4. *Prevalence of hospital infection*

Objective: Periodic assessment of prevalence of infection hospital-wide or selected areas.

$$\text{Indicators} = \frac{\text{Numerator: Infection by site/ ward/procedure or device}}{\text{Denominator: Patient census on the day of survey/procedures/ device-days}}$$

Source of Data: Laboratory and ward liaison, chart review, computerized record

5. *Outbreak warning*

Objective: Detection and cluster analysis of transmissible organisms

$$\text{Indicators} = \frac{\text{Numerator: Colonization or infection by specific microorganism}}{\text{Denominator: Patient admissions/hospital days/ procedures/device-days}}$$

Source of Data: Laboratory-based

Prevalence

Period Prevalence: Refers to the number of cases of infection present in a ward or hospital over a defined period of time, e.g. one week.

Point prevalence: The same as above, but done at a specified point, e.g. one day. These are useful for seeing changes in infection in the hospital over a number of years, e.g. to get information on antibiotic-resistant organisms (e.g. nasal swabs of staff or swabs from lesions of patients).

SURVEILLANCE: HOW AND WHY?[9]

This can be carried out by various methods:

a. Scrutiny of investigative procedures: This is not a laborious process and can be done easily, especially if aided by computerized records. This is a useful method to detect potential outbreaks and to zero in on 'alert' organisms.

b. Ward visits: This can be accomplished by the infection-control nurse who can be assisted by the ward sister, who can provide her with the day-to-day events of infections in the wards.

c. Liaison between the laboratory and the ward through 'link' sisters: These are nurses who form a communicating link between the laboratory and the ward.

Key to Successful Surveillance

There must be a consensus with the patient-care providers on what will be the objectives, indicators and methods of case-finding and validation. There must be an involvement of clinical staff in the collection of data and its interpretation. As surveillance is costly, each hospital must tailor it to its priorities and resources. There are several methods of surveillance of infection in patients, which every hospital would do well to follow.[10, 11]

Aims of Hospital Infection Surveillance[12]

1. To identify high-risk patients and procedures and assign infection control programmes
2. To monitor trends over time of incidence patterns of infections
3. To detect outbreaks of hospital infection
4. To evaluate the efficacy of prevention and control interventions
5. To evaluate quality assurance programmes
6. To educate and motivate healthcare providers and decision-makers

Hospital-Wide Surveillance versus Specific or Selective Surveillance

Select surveillance objectives carefully to avoid unneccessary costs and morbidity. Depending on the scope and objectives, different indicators and data collection methods can be used for surveillance, which may be selective and restricted to specific problems or wards.[13, 14]

Inter-hospital comparisons can be only by standardization of definitions, codes and risk factors. Efficiency of surveillance can be enhanced by computerized records,[15] integrated hospital information that links clinical information with laboratory, radiology and pharmacy records into a single database.

National and international surveillance networks help in comparing data and coordinating control policies (Photo 12.1).

STANDARDS FOR SURVEILLANCE

Two main bodies provide the standards for surveillance of important nosocomial infections:

1. European Prevalence of Infection in Intensive Care (EPIIC)
2. National Nosocomial Infection Surveillance (NNIS)[9]

SENIC study showed that hospitals with surveillance had the lowest infection rates.

Principles used in the surveillance of hospital acquired infections are strikingly similar to those used for CQI (Continuous Quality Improvement) processes in manufacturing. Both emphasize changes at the system rather than individual level.

Voluntary, hospital-based reporting systems were established in the US to monitor HAI and guide prevention efforts of infection-control practitioners. These bodies establish a national risk adjusted benchmark for nosocomial infection rates and device-use ratios by using uniform case definitions and data collection methods and computerized data entry and analysis. Since 1987, ICU infections have been monitored by NNIS by site-specific, risk-adjusted infection rates according to ICU type. The risk-adjusted benchmarks infection rates and device ratios have been published annually for use by the NNIS and non-NNIS hospitals.[1]

The list of important diseases to be notified and the methodology of notification are given by the respective national bodies. Individual practitioners and hospitals have the responsibility of notifying important communicable infections.

MONITORING

Park defines monitoring as 'the performance and analysis of routine measurements aimed at detecting changes in the environment or health status of populations'.[16] This definition may be extended to infection-control measures too, since it is an ongoing measurement of performance of a health service or a health professional, or of the extent to which patients comply with or adhere to advice from health professionals (see chapter on SOPs and process monitoring). Monitoring can thus be thought of as a supervisory process to ensure that procedures are being executed as per plan. It keeps track of achievements, staff movements and utilization, supplies and equipment, and the money spent in relation to the resources available, so that if anything should go wrong, immediate corrective measures can be taken. It is a 'consistent and quantitative monitoring of practices that directly or indirectly contribute to a health outcome and the use of those data to improve outcomes'. Processes to be monitored are to be prioritized. A number of processes may affect the outcome of a particular problem. The outcome of the process to be targetted must be clearly defined. In the case of preventive efforts, it is important to examine the relative importance of risk factors to determine the processes where most effort must be directed.

In India, the National Institute of Communicable Diseases (NICD) is the principal laboratory division that is technically and administratively responsible for the entire nation's health service laboratories for communicable disease surveillance.

MULTICENTRIC SURVEILLANCE

To be successful, a multicentric surveillance system must satisfy three requirements:

a. Use standard definitions, data fields and protocols
b. Identify an aggregating institution to standardize definitions and protocols and to receive the data
c. Assess them for quality, standardize the risk, the benchmarks and interpret and disseminate the data

The National Surveillance Centres also have an epidemiological unit which is responsible for early investigation of reported cases in the community. It is also responsible for contact tracing, laboratory investigations to confirm outbreaks and institute containment measures to control outbreaks of communicable diseases. It is important to carry out microbial monitoring for the control and prevention of outbreaks of infections in highly sterile areas like the bone marrow transplant units. This approach allows significant reduction in the level of contamination not only by improving cleaning procedures, but also by motivating the cleaning staff through making them aware of their responsibilities. Finally, it is also required to notify and report cases to higher levels.

Duties and Responsibilities of Institutions in Disease Surveillance: at Primary, Secondary and Tertiary Levels

I At the hospital/district health centres

1. Early detection of cases/ tracing the index case
2. Making a clinical diagnosis
3. Accurate laboratory diagnosis and confirmation
4. Protocols of management and treatment given
5. Reporting and notifying the cases to relevant authorities

II At the state/regional reference centres for surveillance

1. Receiving data from centres under them
2. Confirmation, collection and compilation of data to confirm the accuracy of the reporting centres
3. Suggesting and carrying out containment measures in the event of an outbreak
4. Analysis and interpretation of surveillance data from other centres
5. Identifying the risk factors and initiating preventive action.
6. Notification to the national surveillance unit, as also the other states for cross-matching of data

III At the national surveillance centre

1. Receiving data and maintaining data inputs from state centres
2. Coordination and dissemination of information and instructions for the containment and handling of the outbreaks
3. Analysis and interpretation of surveillance data from the states and computing national statistics
4. Notification of national data and incidence of communicable diseases to the international surveillance programmes
5. Seeking international intervention and help in the containment/control of communicable diseases

GLOBAL INITIATIVES

International Organization for Surveillance of Communicable Diseases

Every nation, state and district is responsible for the investigation, notification and reporting of communicable diseases including important HAI occurring within its domain. This is done through its hospitals and health centres, which are required to perform surveillance for diseases. At every level, the centres owe a responsibility of appraising the centre at a higher level, of any such occurrences that may be within the purview of public health problems, more often than not, these include communicable diseases. Different strategies need to be employed depending on the existing structure. It is being increasingly recognized by the health authorities that infectious and communicable diseases are capable of posing a major threat to lives and health services if not detected or reported at the earliest. The increase in highly infectious diseases such as severe acute respiratory syndrome (SARS) needs heightened international coordination. The evolution of terrorist threats has also increased the need for international cooperation, information sharing and need for common diagnostic facilities. Without these, highly infectious diseases could spread rapidly within hospitals and also spread to other countries due to increased travel. Thus, a vigilant epidemiology unit strengthened by efficient laboratories is very essential at all levels, be it the international, national, state or district levels.[17]

The WHO has taken up this responsibility by developing an international collaboration network with its member states for the surveillance and reporting of communicable diseases. There is also a network of laboratories to support the public health services. The aim is to ensure early detection of epidemics and facilitate a rapid response before the epidemic becomes a major threat to the population.

> In 1996 the WHO established a global network of epidemiological surveillance units and infectious disease laboratories in an effort to step up the efficacy of recognition and reporting of communicable diseases.

CDC Coding of Nosocomial Infections for Surveillance and Epidemiological Purposes

The Centre for Disease Control and Prevention (CDC) has established the National Nosocomial Infections Surveillance (NNIS) programme to monitor the incidence of nosocomial infections in the US. A companion CDC programme called the Study of the Efficacy of Nosocomial Infection Control (SENIC), keeps statistics on morbidity and mortality of hospital acquired infections.

A list of major and specific-site codes given by CDC includes:

UTI—Urinary Tract Infection

- SUTI: Symptomatic Urinary Tract Infection
- ASB: Asymptomatic Bacteriuria
- OUTI: Other infections of the Urinary Tract

SSI—Surgical Site Infection

- SKIN: Superficial incisional site, except after CBGB
- SKNC: After CBGB, report SKNC for superficial incisional infection at chest incision site
- SKNL: After CBGB, report SKNL for superficial incisional infection at leg (donor) site
- ST: Deep incisional surgical site infection, except after CBGB
- STC: After CBGB, report STC for deep incisional surgical site infection at chest incision site
- STL: After CBGB, report STC for deep incisional surgical site infection at leg (donor) site

For Organ/Space surgical site infection indicate specific site:

BSI—Blood Stream Infection

- LCBI: Laboratory Confirmed Bloodstream Infection
- CSEP: Clinical Sepsis
- BONE: Osteomyelitis

- JNT: Joint or bursa
- DISC: Disc space

CNS—Central Nervous System Infection

- IC: Intra Cranial
- MEN: Meningitis or ventriculitis
- SA: Spinal Abscess without meningitis

CVS—Cardiovascular System

- VASC: Arterial or venous infection
- ENDO: Endocarditis
- CARD: Myocarditis or pericarditis
- MED: Mediastinitis

EENT—Eye, Ear, Nose, Throat or Mouth Infection

- CONJ: Conjunctivitis
- EYE: Other than conjunctivitis
- EAR: Mastoid
- ORAL: Cavity (mouth, tongue or gums)
- SINU: Sinusitis
- UR: Upper respiratory tract, pharyngitis, laryngitis, epiglottitis

GI—Gastrointestinal System Infection

- GE: Gastroenteritis
- GIT: GI Tract
- HEP: Hepatitis
- IAB: Intra abdominal, not specified elsewhere.
- NEC: Necrotizing enterocolitis

LRI—Lower Respiratory Tract Infection Other Than Pneumonia

- BRON: Bronchitis, tracheobronchitis, tracheitis, without evidence of pneumonia
- LUNG: Other infections of the lower respiratory tract
- PNEU: Pneumonia

REPR—Reproductive Tract Infection

- EMET: Endometritis
- EPIS: Episiotomy
- VCUF: Vaginal cuff
- OREP: Other infections of the male or female reproductive tract

SST—Skin and Soft Tissue Infection

- SKIN: Skin
- ST: Soft tissue
- DECU: Decubitis ulcer
- BURN: Burns infection
- BRST: Breast abscess or mastitis
- UMB: Omphalitis
- PUST: Infant pustulosis
- CIRC: Newborn circumcision

SYS—Systemic Infection

- DI: Disseminated infection

The CDC has laid down elaborate guidelines for the diagnosis of nosocomial infections. Apart from providing the above codes for infections of the various systems, it has very clearly given definitions of infection sites and the various criteria necessary to be fulfilled to arrive at their diagnosis. Further, it has also put forth detailed instructions for diagnostic procedures to be carried out, their interpretations and reporting.

Further, the definitions of the following key infections must be understood and used for surveillance:

1. Surgical site infection (SSI) (See chapter 18.)
2. Blood stream infection (BSI) (See chapter 18.)
3. Urinary tract infections (UTI) (See chapter 18.)
4. Nosocomial pneumonia (See chapter 18.)

REFERENCES

1) CDC NNIS System. National Nosocomial Infections Surveillance (NNIS) system report, data summary from January 1990–May 1999, issued June 1999. Am J Infect Control 1999; 27: 520-32.

2) Public health focus: surveillance, prevention, and control of nosocomial infections. Morb Mortality Wkly Rep 1992; 41: 783-787

3) Haley RW. Surveillance by objective: a new priority-directed approach to the control of nosocomial infections. The National Foundation for infectious Disease Lecture. Am J Infect Control 1985; 13(2): 78-89.

4) Cruse PJ and Foord R.A. A five year prospective study of 23,649 surgical wounds. Arch Surg. 1973: 107(2): 206-210.

5) Gaynes RP and Horan TC: Surveillance of nosocomial infections. Appendix A: CDC definitions of nosocomial infections. In Mayhall GC (ed): Hospital Epidemiology and Infection Control. Baltimore: Williams & Wilkins, 1996; 1-14.

6) Banerjee SN, Emori TG, Culver DH et al. Secular trends in nosocomial primary bloodstream infections in the United States, 1980-1989. National Nosocomial Infections Surveillance System. Am J Med 1991;91 (3)(Suppl 2): S86 -89.

7) Emmerson AM, Enstone JE, Griffin M et al. The second national prevalence survey of infections in hospitals – overview of results. J. Hosp. Infect 1996; 32(3): 175-190.

8) Husni RN, Goldstein LS, Arroliga AC et al. Risk factors for an outbreak of multi-drug-resistant Acinetobacter nosocomial pneumonia among intubated patients. Chest 1999; 115: 1378-82.

9) Emori TG, Culver DH, Horan TC et al. National nosocomial infections surveillance system (NNIS): description of surveillance methods. Am J Infect Control 1991; 19:19-35.

10) Hirschhorn LR, Currier JS and Platt R. Electronic surveillance of antibiotic exposure and coded discharge diagnosis as indicators of postoperative infection and other quality assurance measures. Infect Control Hosp Epidemiol. 1993; 14:21-28.

11) Fraser VJ, Jones M and Dunkel J. Candidemia in a tertiary care hospital: epidemiology, risk factors, and predictors of mortality. Clin Infect Dis. 1999; 29: 259-63.

12) Edmond MB, Wallace SE, McClish DK et al. Nosocomial bloodstream infections in United States hospitals: a three-year analysis. Clin Infect Dis. 1999; 29: 239-44.

13) Ducel G, Fabry J and Nicolle L.Prevention of Hospital-Acquired Infection. A practical guide. 2nd edition. World Health Organization. 2002; 47-54.

14) Valles J, Leon C, Alvarez-Lerma F, and the Spanish Collaborative Group for Infections in Intensive Care Units of Sociedad Espanola de Medicina Intensiva y Unidades Coronarias (SEMIUC). Nosocomial bacteremia in critically ill patients: a multicenter study evaluating epidemiology and prognosis. Clin Infect Dis 1997; 24: 387-95.

15) Pert TM. Surveillnace, reporting and the use of computers, In: Wenzel RP. ed. Prevention and control of nosocomial infections. Baltimore: Williams & Wilkins. 1997; 127-162.

16) Park K. Concepts of health and disease. In: Park's Textbook of Preventive and Social Medicine. 15th edition. 1997; 11-44.

17) Wenzel RP. Towards a global perspective of nosocomial infections. Eur J. Clin Microbiol 1987; 6: 341-343.

Chapter 13

Epidemics and Outbreaks

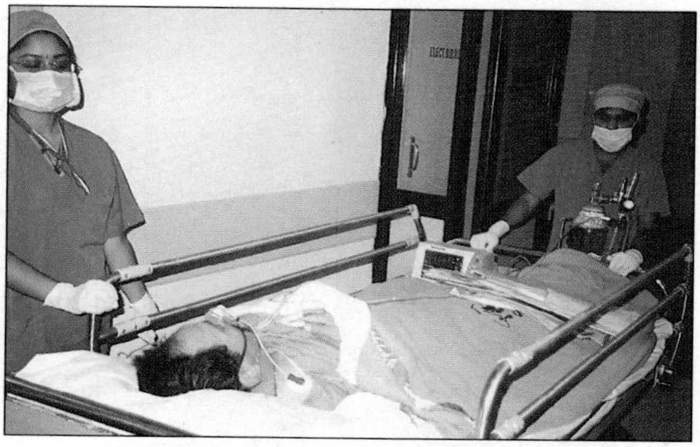

It is easy to sit up and take notice; what is difficult is getting up and taking action.

—Al Batt

Highlights

An Epidemic
The Investigation of an Outbreak
Clinical Situations and HAI Containment
Architectural Segregation
Risk Groups of Microorganisms
Emerging Infections Need Newer Strategies

INTRODUCTION

Outbreaks of infections pose a great risk to healthcare workers, visitors and other hospital staff (Photo 13.1).

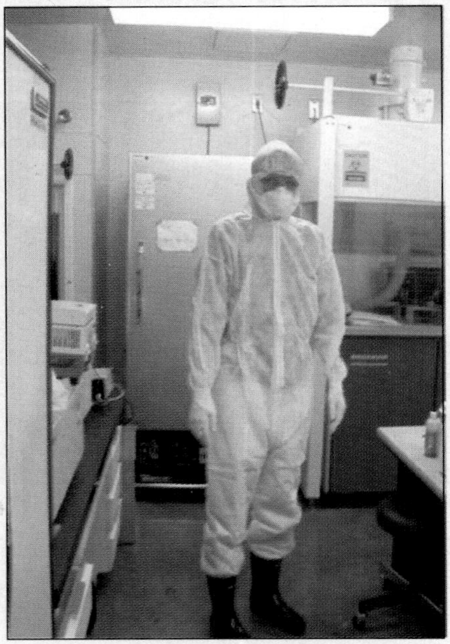

Photo 13.1: Maximum barriers in a P3 laboratory where highly infectious organisms are handled

The WHO recommends that the health authorities of each country should make lists of bacteria, viruses and other organisms in each risk group in the light of the factors affecting the pathogenicity of each organism and according to the local circumstances. There is no international agreement on the composition of such lists and while most states have compiled their own, some have adopted those of other states or organizations. Most lists also specify or make recommendations about mode of transmission and the system of precaution (droplet, airborne, etc.) specific measures for prevention, vaccinations and treatment for handling particular organisms.

CDC: The national Centre for Disease Control and prevention is a part of the US Department of Health and Human Services, and is located in Atlanta, Georgia. It provides support for infectious disease laboratories all over the world, and collects data on diseases of public health importance. An update of all important infectious diseases appears in its weekly report called 'Morbidity and Mortality Weekly Report' (MMWR). The CDC also sends research teams to various parts of the world to assist in controlling epidemics. They also provide refresher courses to update knowledge of laboratory and infection-control personnel.

AN EPIDEMIC

A classic epidemic is an unusual, statistically significant increase in the incidence of a particular disease as compared to the background rate. The other important characteristics are: it occurs in a particular time frame (brief interval), involves a specific patient population with well-defined susceptibility factors, and is caused by a single microbial strain. Any cluster which falls into this category should be identified and controlled rapidly. The clinician, epidemiologist, infection-control practitioner (ICP) and laboratory personnel must work collaboratively to handle the epidemic situation.

AN OUTBREAK

1. Two or more epidemiologically related infections caused by an organism of the

same type: The action to be taken varies with circumstances. Two minor *S. aureus* infections may not warrant any action, but two *S. aureus* infections which are methicillin resistant demand immediate action as also a single case of diphtheria.[1]

2. A single case of rare or serious disease
3. Microbial or chemical contamination of food or water (these are also called infectious incidents)
4. An outbreak can turn into an epidemic

Examples

1. Contamination of infusion products: Outbreaks of infusion-associated septicaemia due to contaminated intravenous fluids were noted (approximately 400 cases reported in 1971). The organisms implicated were Enterobacter groups. 25 hospitals were affected. Organisms were found to gain access to infusion fluids through an elastomer-lined screw cap. When an epidemiological investigation was carried out by CDC (NNIS), the source was traced to a single product (infusion fluid) used across America. The epidemic was reversed after the product was withdrawn.[2]
2. An outbreak of six cases of *Klebsiella* septicaemia in an intensive care unit was attributed to contaminated hand cream used by nurses after hand-washing. Others have found that such lotions may be heavily contaminated with Candida and Klebsiella-Enterobacter.[2]

THE INVESTIGATION OF AN OUTBREAK

This must be done in a sequenced and stepwise manner, taking into consideration several aspects of epidemiological importance.[3] Accordingly, there are several methods of data collection in a hospital set-up, which include:

- Confirming the diagnosis
- Identification of an outbreak

Assessment of the Situation

- Are the infections genuine or are the sites only colonized? Colonization may be an in dication of a spreading organism. E.g. MRSA
- Are the infections hospital acquired?
- Are the infections likely to spread?
- Is there any evidence of existing cross-infection?
- What is the extent of the damage (i.e., the number of cases)?
- Investigate the cause
- Prioritize the plan of action

Outbreaks due to contaminated products reported:[2]

1. Centralized pharmacy-related outbreak in aseptic methods when reconstituting/ preparing fluids (IV) under laminar hood
2. Fungal-related septicaemias (particularly Candida) due to parenteral nutrition
3. Contaminated platelets may lead to outbreaks due to pooling, storage at 25^{0}C
4. Contaminated equipment such as laryngoscopes
5. Contaminated multidose vials. E.g. Propofol
6. Contaminated endoscopes, laparoscopes, bronchoscopes, etc.

7. Infected needles, syringes, surgical instruments.
8. Infected food, water, personnel (colonized or infected)

Steps in the investigation and control of outbreaks

- Establish a case definition and define the population at risk
- Confirm existence of a true outbreak
- Rule out pseudo-outbreaks (contamination of cultures during clinical sample collection or processing)
- Rule out surveillance artefacts (increase in laboratory utilization, or improved laboratory or surveillance methods)
- Determine space-time clustering and/or significant increase of incidence rate versus baseline period in exposed cohort
- Determine clinical severity of infections and number of patients affected to define the degree of emergency, allocate time and resource for further investigation accordingly
- Complete case-finding retrospectively and prospectively; ensure accurate microbiolgic sampling and processing for optimal ascertainment of aetiology; ensure storage and plan the typing of clincial isolates
- Review the literature about risk factors and potential sources and compare with host and exposure factors revealed by reviewing the medical charts of infected patients
- On the basis of descriptive epidemiology of epidemic cases in time, place, patient characteristics, and common exposure to devices, treatments and procedures, formulate tentative hypotheses about host factors, hospital exposure factors, reservoirs, source and mode(s) of transmission revealed by reviewing the medical charts of infected patients
- Reinforce standard hygiene precautions and initiate temporary control measures based on hypotheses defined earlier and follow-up impact on rate of transmission
- If necessary, test hypotheses defined by case-control, cohort and/or intervention studies by epidemiologic typing of representative isolates
- If necessary, initiate targeted culture surveys from potential reservoirs/ sources (patients, personnel, environment, as appropriate); confirm the suspect epidemiologic link by comparative typing of isolates
- Review results of the investigation with all concerned authorities and staff and report to the Infection Control Committee
- Conduct follow-up surveillance to evaluate efficacy of control measures; update control measures if necessary; follow-up evaluation reports for the Infection Control Committee and all staff concerned

Role of the clincial laboratory in the investigation of hospital infection outbreaks

Investigation Steps:

- Outbreak detection
- Outbreak confirmation and descriptive epidemiology

- Identification of reservoirs and modes of transmission
- Follow-up of efficacy of control measures

Laboratory Methods

- Identification and susceptibility testing of clinical isolates
- Epidemiolgic typing of clinical isolates.
- Culture surveys of reservoirs and vehicles
- Typing of environmental isolates
- Typing of clinical isolates, as part of post-outbreak surveillance

Basic Principles for Using Epidemiologic Typing Methods

1. They should be employed with clear epidemiologic objectives and not indiscriminately.
2. All typing procedures must be carried out under the same test conditions in the same test run (preferably).
3. Control isolates from epidemiologically unrelated or environmental sources must be included and must be different from the outbreak strain in order to reach a valid conclusion.

Tracing the Source (Typing)

Bacteria like *Staphylococcus aureus* are present in noses of 20% of healthy people and are usually not a common cause of wound infection. So also, *Pseudomonas aeruginosa* is found in 25% or more of hospital sinks. So, the identification of such bacteria is not relevant unless typing is done. On the other hand, isolation of a specific pathogen or unusual organism like *Salmonella typhii,* from two or more patients in a ward is suggestive of cross- infection and needs no typing. Various typing methods available for bacteria include:

1. Biotyping: Identification using biochemical and other laboratory tests
2. Resistogram: Here the susceptibility is measured to a range of chemicals. E.g. Done for *E.coli, Proteus, Candida*
3. Antibiogram: Various antimicrobials are tested for susceptibility of microorganisms to them
4. Serotyping: Serological testing
5. Phage typing: Susceptibility to bacteriophages is used to type the organisms.
6. Bacteriocin typing: Production of bacteriocin by certain organisms is used for typing.
7. Molecular methods: These newer methods have revolutionized epidemiological studies. They depend on electrophoretic separation of polypeptides, isoenzymes, plasmids or nucleic acids. Comparisons are made of the profiles or 'bands' in a gel or on a membrane.[4, 5]
8. Plasmid (extrachromosomal DNA) typing: This involves extraction of the DNA and comparison of the separated plasmid molecules
9. Restriction Endonuclease Activity (REA): Here enzymes are made to digest plasmid or chromosomal DNA.
10. Pulsed Field Gel Electrophoresis (PFGE): This method separates large molecules of

DNA by the use of alternating electric fields. It is very useful for non-phage typeable MRSA.

11. DNA hybridization or gene probing: Here a known length of DNA is taken and labelled. It is then hybridized with a corresponding DNA from an unknown organism. If hybridization occurs, the organism is identified. This method can be used directly on specimens and is hence useful. Similarly, Ribotyping can be done using rRNA probes
12. Polymerase Chain Reaction (PCR): Is another useful molecular tool in epidemiological studies
13. Restriction Fragment Length Polymorphism (RFLP): Another very useful epidemiological tool used to identify sources of infection as in Tuberculosis

The primary purpose of an outbreak investigation is to:

a. Control the outbreak
b. Limit its spread to other areas
c. Assess how prevention strategies can be further strengthened to prevent such risks in future[6, 7]

CLINICAL SITUATIONS AND HAI CONTAINMENT

Handling Risks in the Emergency Room

Careful planning and preparedness are required in the place of first patient contact, e.g. emergency room. Emergency situations are always fraught with dangers of errors on the part of the staff or inappropriate action due to ill-equipped conditions. These can be countered by providing adequate training, reasonable infrastructure and personnel management.[8, 9]

Proper guidelines must be laid down for infection control in the hospital set-up, taking into consideration the kind of diseases and microorganisms to be handled. One such example is shown in Table 13.1.

Preventing Epidemic and Outbreaks

Step 1: Screening

Identify individuals who show symptoms suggestive of an infectious or communicable disease.

A comprehensive list must be readied, consisting of all communicable diseases with their modes of transmission and the transmission precautions to be adopted. It should also include all diseases that are reportable/notifiable (to the hospital epidemiology department or National Reference Centres). Signs to be looked for:

- Temperature
- Rash
- Cough
- Stiff neck
- Headache
- Draining lesions

Step 2. Deciding the line of action

In case of suspicion of communicable disease, the following line of action help:[9]

a. Inform the physician.
b. Inform the infectious disease control department/epidemiology department, if it

Table 13.1: Preventive measures in high-risk groups: Respiratory syncytial virus (RSV) infection control guidelines

General control measures to prevent nosocomial RSV transmission:
Educate hospital staff about RSV means of prevention Use contact and droplet isolation for RSV-positive patients Maintain good hand-washing procedures Limit visitors with symptoms Restrict staff with upper respiratory symptoms
Control measures during RSV outbreaks:
Avoid elective admissions for high-risk patients Cohort patients (patients with same or similar problems) Cohort staff

could be a cause for outbreaks or epidemics.

c. If then patient is diagnosed to have an infectious disease and is to be followed up at home, discharge instructions should be given.

d. If the disease is reportable, the infection-control department practitioner should be informed.

e. If the patient is to be admitted, procedure for barriers and isolation should be followed.

f. Vaccination and prophylaxis (PEP) treatment (Tables 13.2, 13.3, 13.4) and other preventive measures must be adopted in high-risk groups

g. Initiating isolation precautions in the emergency department must be followed by certain actions:

Admission of the isolation order must be notified, to the nursing unit as this will alert the staff. Nursing unit should inform/notify infection-control committee (for accurate reporting and proper procedure implementation). If the physician disagrees with the isolation order, the infection-control department should be notified (Infection-control team will discuss with the physician and obtain appropriate orders.)[9]

Implemention of Control Measures

- Isolation as and when required
- Meeting of ICT
- Staff movement restriction
- Control new admissions in the same ward
- Send patients home if possible
- Use immune sera if indicated
- Treat contacts of cases
- Inform the administration
- Decide if it is necessary to close the ward
- Sample contacts and the environment
- Carry out active surveillance for cases

Table 13.2: Preventive measures in high risk groups: Vaccination against influenza

Influenza vaccine dosing recommendations			
Age Group	**Dose**	**Number of doses**	**Route**
6–35 months	0.25 cc	1 or 2 (1 month apart)	Intramuscular
3–8 yrs	0.50 cc	1 or 2 (1 month apart)	Intramuscular
9–12 yrs	0.50 cc	1	Intramuscular
> 12 yrs	0.50 cc	1	Intramuscular

Whole virus only beyond 12 years. Below 12 years split virus recommended

Table 13.3: Preventive measures in high-risk groups: Prophylaxis/Ttreatment schedule for influenza

Amantadine and rimantadine dosing recommendations			
Age	**Type of therapy**	**Amantadine**	**Rimantadine**
Age 14 yrs and above	Treatment Prophylaxis	100mg b.i.d. 100mg b.i.d.	100mg b.i.d. 100mg b.i.d.

- Create awareness among HCWs to recognize such incidents
- Carry out special studies to collect information

Architectural Segregation

According to the risk of acquisition of infections, patient care areas can be stratified into four degrees of risk:

- Low risk areas: E.g. administrative areas
- Moderate risk areas: E.g. regular patient units
- High risk areas: E.g. isolation unit, intensive care units, laboratories working with dangerous pathogens
- Very high risk areas: E.g. operating rooms

Compounded Medications

Preventing HAI due to contaminated medications including parenteral medications has elevated concern for safety of compounded medications which include parenteral nutrition, cardioplegia, steroids, analgesics, biologics diagnostics, drugs, baths and soaks for live organs and tissues, implants, inhalations, injections, powder for injection, irrigations, metered sprays and ophthalmic and otic preparations. There are guidelines given by United States Pharmacopoeia (USP) standard (797), 2004. They have also classified compounded mixtures into low risk (made of sterile ingredients,

Table 13.4: Antiviral treatment recommendations

Disease	Valacyclovir	Famciclovir	Acyclovir
Varicella Immunocompetent host			20mg/kg (maximum 800mg) 4 x daily for 5 days
Varicella Immunocompromised host			100mg/kg i.v. every 8 h for 7–10 days
Herpes zoster Immunocompetent host	1g 3 x daily for 7 days	500mg 3 x daily for 7 days	800mg 5 x daily for 7 days
Herpes zoster Immunocompromised host			10mg/kg i.v. every 8 hour for 7 days
Herpes zoster Immunocompromised host resistant virus	Foscarnet 40mg/kg i.v. 3 x daily for 7–14 days		
Immunocompromised host initial episode	500mg p.o. b.i.d. x 10–14 days	125-250mg p.o. b.i.d.x 10–14 d	200–400mg p.o. 5 x d x 10 days 5mg/kg i.v. 8h x 7–10 days

< 24 hrs old) medium risk (more than 24 hours) and high risk (made more than 24 hrs ago). A number of other organizations, JCAHO MM4.20 standard, American Society of Health-System Pharmacists (ASHP), have given specific recommendations on the method of preparation, labelling, training and disposal of these medications to prevent outbreaks.

RISK GROUPS OF MICROORGANISMS

Assessment of the relative risk of handling infectious agents has led to the adoption of a scale consisting of four risk (or hazard) groups, ranging from the least (group 1) to the most (group 4) hazardous to the laboratory workers and the community. Several classifications have been proposed but that formulated and currently used by the WHO is given below:

Classification of Microorganisms on The Basis of Risk

Risk group 1 (no or very low individual and community risk)

A microorganism that is unlikely to cause human or animal disease under ordinary circumstances, e.g. *E.coli*

Risk group 2 (moderate individual risk, low community risk)

A pathogen that can cause human or animal disease but is unlikely to be a serious hazard to laboratory workers, the community, livestock or the environment. Laboratory exposures can cause serious infection, but effective treatment and prevention measures are available and the spread of infection is limited.

Risk group 3 (high individual and low community risk)

A pathogen that usually causes serious human and animal disease but does not easily spread from one infected individual to another. Effective treatment and preventive measures are available.

1. Barriers to be used according to risk anticipated
2. Standard precautions in all cases
3. Transmission-based precautions
4. Prevention, containment, treatment as per guidelines

Risk group 4 (high individual and community risk)

A pathogen that usually causes serious human or animal disease and can be transmitted from one individual to another, directly or indirectly. Effective treatment and preventive measures are usually not available.

The sources of laboratory acquired infections may be any of the following:

- Accident
- Animal/ectoparasites
- Clinical specimen
- Discarded glassware
- Human autopsy
- Working with the agent
- Aerosols
- Intentional infection
- Others/unknown

(Note: 1. Infection with *Mycobacterium tuberculosis* may occur on the fingers of personnel working in the post-mortem room 'Prosector's finger'. Hence, use of protective clothing and appropriate disinfectants are recommended. 2. Creutzfeld-Jacob's disease may result from accidental inoculations/ pricks/ cuts. Hence, working in a safety cabinet is recommended. Also, disinfection with 10,000 ppm of available chlorine for 30 minutes is advised. Instruments must be autoclaved at 121^{0}C for 60–90 mins or 134^{0}C for 18 mins. Alternatively, instruments may be soaked in hypochlorite for 18 hours.[10, 11]

Biosafety or Containment Levels in Laboratories

It is obvious that work with organisms in different Risk Groups requires different conditions for containment, i.e. ensuring that the organisms do not escape from their specimens, culture vessels or the laboratory. Containment addresses various issues including laboratory accomodation, services, access, equipment and safety precautions for each group of organisms.

In USA, there were four physical containment levels for laboratories (P1 to P4). These have now been classified and identified as Biosafety Levels 1 to 4 (USPHS 1984).

There are four biosafety or containment levels (1–4), each designed for work with organisms of the corresponding Risk Groups.

Risk group 1 (basic biosafety level 1)

E.g. Basic teaching laboratory. This does not require any safety equipment and involves open bench work. Good microbiological technique (GMT) is all that is required.

Risk group 2 (basic biosafety level 2)

E.g. primary health services, primary level hospital, diagnostic, teaching and public health laboratories. Here, open bench work along with BSC is used for all potential aerosols. GMT along with protective clothing and biohazard signs are used.

Risk group 3 (containment biosafety level 3)

E.g. special diagnostic laboratory; requires BSC and/or other primary containment for all activities. GMT plus special clothing, controlled access and directional air flow are required.

Risk group 4 (maximum containment biosafety level 4)

E.g. dangerous pathogen units. Here, it is imperative to use a class III BSC or positive pressure double-ended autoclave with filtered air. Laboratory practices include all level-3 ones plus airlock entry, shower exit and special waste disposal methods.

The WHO has classified laboratories according to the kind of organisms they work with.

Basic Laboratories (P1 and P2 laboratories) are those working with Risk Groups 1 and 2 (Biosafety Levels 1 and 2).

Containment Laboratories (P3 laboratories)—those working with Risk Group 3 (Biosafety Level 3).

Maximum Containment Laboratories (P4 laboratories) are those working with Risk Group 4 (Biosafety Level 4).

(* The P stands for Physical Containment.)

Classsification of laboratories according to use have caused problems and have led to the conclusion that three or four types of laboratories are required according to the class of organisms handled. In the WHO (1983) classification, these are: Basic, (for risk groups 1 and 2), Containment (for risk group 3) and Maximum Containment (for risk group 4).

The USPHS (1984), which appears to have four biosafety levels, and that of the ACDP (1984), which was drafted earlier in the US system, have four containment levels.

Special Cases—MRSA

Special solutions for infections of operation theatre origin: Confirm the case, check the staff, sample the nose/hands of staff, sample the floors of the changing room, equipment, etc. 'If the noses and environment are both negative, continue close surveillance and repeat sampling if infections continue, as some healthy carriers only disperse intermittently and for short periods of time.'

For *S.aureus* carriers:

Nose: Mupirocin nasal cream 2% applied to anterior nares 3 times a day for 5–7 days.

Skin: Daily bath with antiseptic detergent (chlorhexidine, triclosan, povidone iodine, hexachlorophane) for one week, then apply antiseptic.

Hair: Antiseptic shampoo with Cetrimide.

Note: No more than two courses of mupirocin should be given either for treatment of nasal carriage or a lesion. If resistant to Mupirocin, use Naseptin (Neomycin+Chlorhexidine) or Bacitracin four times a day for seven days. Also, look for other sites of infection (like rectum/vagina).

Emerging Infections Need Newer Strategies in Specific Clinical Situations

A number of emerging infections around the world have been discussed in the chapter on nosocomial pathogens (Photo 13.2). There are also a number of highly infectious diseases which have emerged in recent years. E.g. SARS. Newer infections need newer strategies of containment and management.

Severe Acute Respiratory Syndrome (SARS)[12-16]

This is a new severe febrile respiratory illness caused by the SARS associated coronavirus (SARS-CoV). It was first recognized in 2003, and quickly spread worldwide involving 8,429 probable cases and 813 deaths in 29 countries. The reservoir of the virus is believed to be the civet cat. The mode of transmission is via direct contact and droplet transmission.

Clinical features

Median period of incubation is 4–6 days with most patients becoming ill within 2–10 days after exposure. Initial symptoms include fever, myalgia and headache, with respiratory symptoms of non-productive cough and dyspnoea appearing 2–7 days later. In 70–90% of cases, pneumonia develops and the overall case-fatality rate is 10% and there are no effective vaccines or treatment for this disease.

Prevention and control

Epidemiological data suggest that transmission does not occur before the onset of symptoms and that most transmission occurs late in illness when the patients are hospitalized.

The early identification of a case is important for immediate single-room isolation to prevent an outbreak. Strict contact and droplet precautions are adequate in preventing further transmission of the virus. The use of proper hand hygiene practices, and careful removal of used gloves and gowns are equally important preventive measures.

For aerosol-generating procedures, it may be advisable to use the N95 mask to prevent inhalation of any droplet nucei created.

Perioperative management of a patient of SARS has been described in great detail by Peng et al.[17-22]

Some important points related to SARS are given below:

1. General [23-30]

- Clear the room of unnecessary or overstocked equipment.
- Post 'SARS Patient' signs on the OR doors to minimize traffic. Keep doors closed.
- Wash hands (before and after patient care)

- Full droplet/contact precaution should be practised, and movement in and out of the room must be kept to a minimum.
- Gown (double gown for high-risk procedure)
- Double glove. Remove and dispose of outer pair after direct patient contact and before touching other areas of the room/ anaesthesia machine. Subsequent interven tion must be performed with double gloves.
- Use N95 mask or equivalent
- Use a full-face disposable plastic shield for eye protection
- Powered air purifying respirator (PAPR) is required for staff member performing laryngoscopy or any other airway interven tion (including extubation).
- Remove gloves/gown and decontaminate hands with alcohol hand wash.
- Remove face shield/N95 mask/hair cover and wash hands again.
- Re-gown, glove, hair cover and mask.
- Transfer directly to the post-anaesthesia-care unit isolation room.
- Remove gown/gloves and mask prior to exiting the isolation room.
- Change surgical scrub suit immediately or as soon as practically possible.

2. Equipment

Intubation kit contains:

- Manual resuscitation bag with viral filter
- In-line suction catheters
- Powered air-purifying respiratory (PAPR) hoods (2 anaesthesiologists and a respiratory technician)

Procedure

- After handwashing, both laryngoscopist and respiratory technician will put on double gloves, gowns, goggles, N95 masks and PAPR hoods in the anteroom, or outside the patient's room
- After intubation, the gowns, hoods, and outer gloves must be removed in the anteroom or inside the patients' room.

3. Circuits

Use disposable circuit with a high-efficiency viral filter placed on the inspiratory and expiratory limbs of the circuit.

Soda lime

- The soda lime does not need to be changed. The end-tidal CO_2 sample line and trap must be changed after the case.

Machine/Surfaces

- Place the anaesthesia machine as far from the patient as practically possible.
- Place contaminated airway equipment in the plastic box for removal from the OR after intubation. Discard needles and syringes immediately after use.

Monitors

- Use axillary temperature probe. Avoid nasal or oesophageal probe.

- The anaesthesiologist, or respiratory technician, is asked to wipe the monitor screen surface with a damp virucidal wipe, if visibly or knowingly contaminated, taking care that the cleaning solution does not drip on the screen.

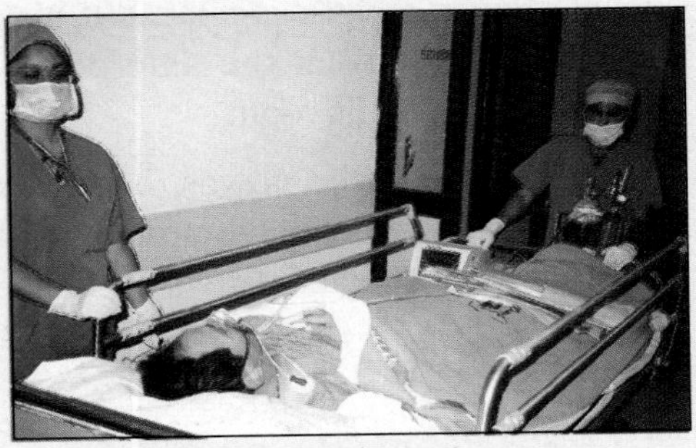

Photo 13.2: Precaution taken while shifting patients can prevent outbreaks of HAI.

REFERENCES

1) Ayliffe GAJ, Babb JR and Taylor LJ. Hosptial Acquired Infections- Principles and Prevention. 3rd edn. Arnold Publishers. 2001; 48-73.
2) Emmerson AM, Enstone JE, Griffin M et al. The second national prevalence survey of infections in hospitals – overview of results J Hosp Infect 1996 ; 32: 175-190.
3) Widdowson MA. An outbreak of diarrhoea in a neonatal medium care unit caused by a novel strain of rotavirus: investigation using both epidemiologic and microbiological methods. Infect Control Hosp Epidemiol. 2002; 23(11): 665-70.
4) Fawley WN and Wilcox MH. Molecular epidemiolgy of endemic *Clostridium difficile* infection. Epidemiol Infect. 2001; 126(3): 343-5.
5) Ayliffe GAJ, Babb JR and Taylor LJ. Hospital Acquired Infections-Principles and Prevention. 3rd edn. Arnold Publishers. 2001; 109-121.
6) Emori TG and Gaynes RP. An overview of nosocomial infections, including the role of the microbiology laboratory. Clin Microbiol Rev. 1993; 6: 428-42.
7) Valles J, Leon C, Alvarez-Lerma F, and the Spanish Collaborative Group for Infections in Intensive Care Units of Sociedad Espanola de Medicina Intensiva y Unidades Coronarias (SEMIUC). Nosocomial bacteremia in critically ill patients: a multicenter study evaluating epidemiology and prognosis. Clin Infect Dis. 1997; 24: 387-95.
8) Kaku M and Kanemitsu K. Outline of the hospital infection control in USA and UK. Nippon Rinsho. 2002; 60(11): 2073-78.
9) West KH. Interdepartmental Infection Control Measures. In: Infection Control in the Emergency Department. Rockville: Aspen Publishers, Inc. 1988; 21-119.
10) Collins CH. Laboratory acquired infections 2nd edn. Butterworths & DO 1988; 66-103.
11) Collins CH. Laboratory acquired infection 2nd edn. Butterworths & Co. 1988: 58-65.
12) Varia M, Wilson S, Sarwal S, et al. Investigation of a nosocomial outbreak of severe acute respiratory syndrome (SARS) in Toronto, Canda. CMAJ 2003; 169: 285-92.
13) World Health Organization. Acute respirtory syndrome, Chine. Wkly Epidemiol Rec 2003; 78:41. Availab le from URL; http://www.who.int/wer/2003/en/wer7807.pdf.
14) World Health Organization. Severe acute respiratory syndrome (SARS). Wkly Epidemiol Rec 2003; 78: 81-3. Available from URS; http://www.who.int/wer/2003/wr7812.pdf.

15) World Health Organization. WHO issues a global alert about cases of atypical pneumonia. Available from URL; http://www.who.it/csr/sarsarchive/2003_03_12/en/.

16) Poutanen SM, Low DE, Henry B, et al. Identification of severe acute respiratory syndrome in Canada. N Engl J Med 2003; 348: 1995-2005.

17) Peng, Philiph WH, Wong et al. Infection control and anesthesia: Lessons learned from the Toronto SARS outbreak. Can J Anaes 2003; 50(10): 989-997.

18) Booth CM, Matukas LM, Tomilinson GA et al. Clinical features and short-term outcomes of 144 patients with SARS in the greater Toronto area. J Am Med Assoc 2003; 289: 2901-9.

19) Ksiazek TG, Erdman D, Goldsmith CS et al. A novel cooronavirus associated with severe acute respiratory syndrome. N Engl J Med 2003; 348: 1953-66

20) Rota PA, Oberste MS, Monroe SS et al. Characterization of a novel cornovirus associated with severe acute respiratory syndrome. Science 2003; 300: 1394-9.

21) Gerberding JL. Faster... but fast enough? Responding to the epidemic of severe acute respiratory synndrome (Editorial). N Engl J Med 2003; 348: 2030; 300:1961-6.

22) Riley S, Fraser C, Donnelly CA et al. Transmission dynamics of the etiological agent of SARS in Hong Kong: impact of public health intervention. Science 2003; 300: 1961-6.

23) Lipsitch M, Cohen T, Cooper B et al. Transmission dynamics and control of severe acute respiratory syndrome. Science 2003; 300: 1966-70.

24) Ferguson NM, Mallett S, Jackson H et al. A population-dynamic model for evaluating the potential spread of drug-resistant influenza virus infections during community-based use of antivirals. J Antimicrob Chemother 2003; 51: 977-90.

25) Centre for Disease Control and Prevention. Severe acute respiratory syndrome – Singapore, 2003. MMWR 2003; 52; 405-11. Available from URL; http//www.cdc.gov /mmwr/preview/mmwrhtml/mm5218a1.htm.

26) Parry J. SARS virus identified, but the disease is still spreading. BMJ 2003; 326: 897.

27) Lee N, Hui D, Wu A et al. A major outbreak of severe acute respiratory sydrome in Hong Kong. N Engl Med 2003; 348:1986-94.

28) World Health Organization. Update 49 – SARS case fatality ration, incubation period. Available from URL; http://www.who.int/csr/sarsarchive/2003_05_07/en/.

29) Health Canada. SARS epidemiologicc summaries: April 26, 2003. SARS among Ontario health care workers. Available from URL; http:/ /www.hc-sc.gc.ca/pphbdgspsp/sars-sras/pef -dep/sars-es20030426_e.html.

30) Kamming D, Chung F, Gardam M. Anaesthesia and SARS (Editorial). Br J Anaesth 2003; 90:715-8.

Chapter 14

Standard Operating Procedures (SOPs)

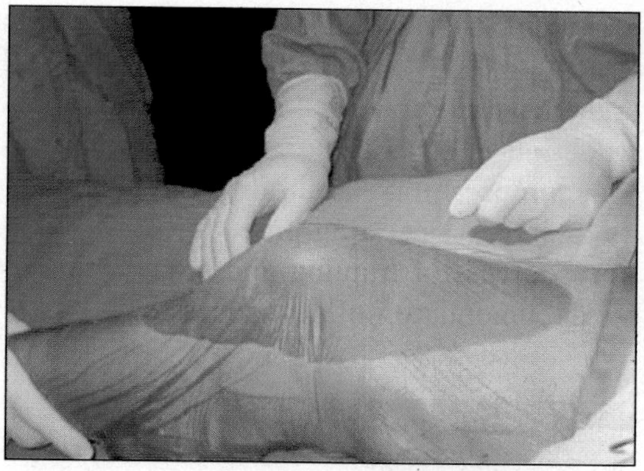

We are what we repeatedly do. Excellence, then, is not an act but a habit.

—Aristotle

Highlights

Design of SOPs

Evidence of Need and Impact of SOPs

Processes, Tasks and Infection Control

Environmental SOPs

INTRODUCTION

The US Environmental Protection Agency (http://www.epa.gov/cgi-bin/printonly.cgi) describes Standard Operating Procedures (SOP) as a quality management tool. SOPs are written documents that describe, in great detail, the routine procedures to be followed for a specific operation, analysis, or action (Photo 14.1, Fig. 14.1). Consistent use of an approved SOP ensures conformance with organizational practices, reduced work effort, reduction in error occurrences and improved data comparability, credibility and defensibility. Standard operating procedures also serve as resources for training and ready reference for documentation of procedures.[1, 2]

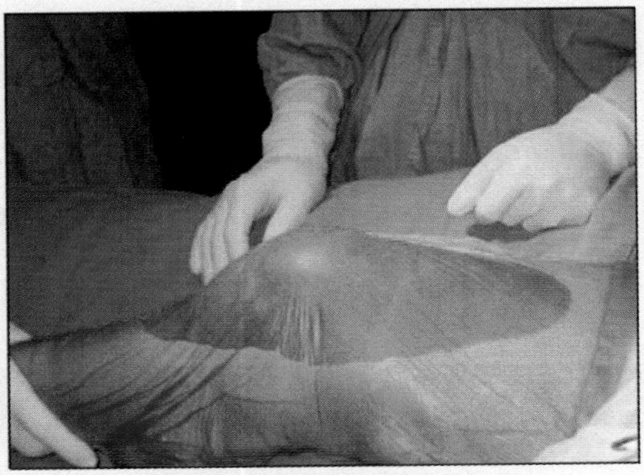

Photo 14.1: Standard operating procedure: Cleaning and draping for a total knee replacement

Maintenance of a written set of SOPs, or a 'procedure manual', serves as a valuable tool in combating HAI. These recommended methodologies are intended to represent what is believed to be an optimal level of practice. Well-written SOPs provide direction, improve communication, reduce training time and also improve work consistency. A very positive sense of teamwork arises when managers, workers and technical advisors cooperate towards common goals.

> SOP + planned training + regular performance feedback ⟶ effective and motivated workforce

DESIGN OF SOPs

Manuals are comprehensive written operating procedure documents covering various aspects of infection control (both analytical and non-analytical). Policies and procedure guidelines reflect variations in practice settings and/or clinical situations, but SOPs determine the degree to which the recommended practices can be uniformly implemented. These could be in clinical or non-clinical areas. Guidance on the development and documentation of standard operating procedures can be found on http://www.cpa.gov/epa/240/B-01/004 March 2001 (guidance for preparing standard operating procedures).

These practices are laid down from guidelines adaptable to various work settings, such as traditional Operating Rooms. SOPs can be formulated for various departments:

- Operating suites
- Intensive care units
- Wards
- Ambulatory surgical units
- Laboratories
- Mortuaries
- Physicians' offices
- Cardiac catheterization suites
- Endoscopy suites

1. Closed Method

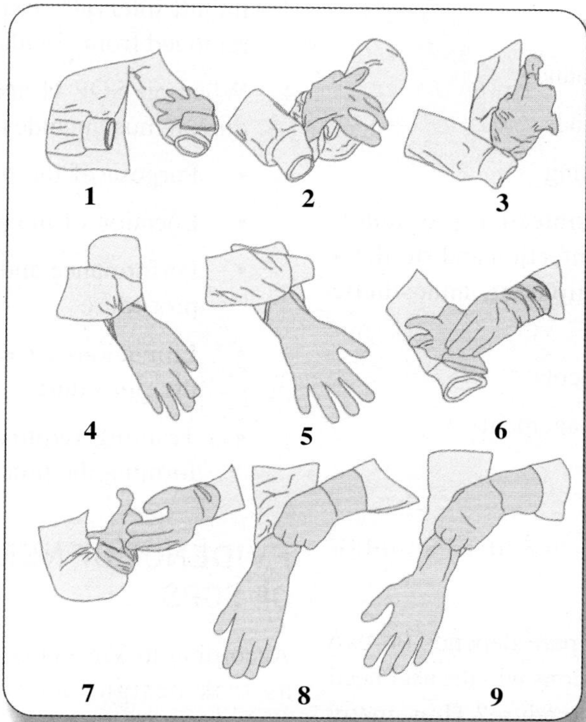

2. Open Method

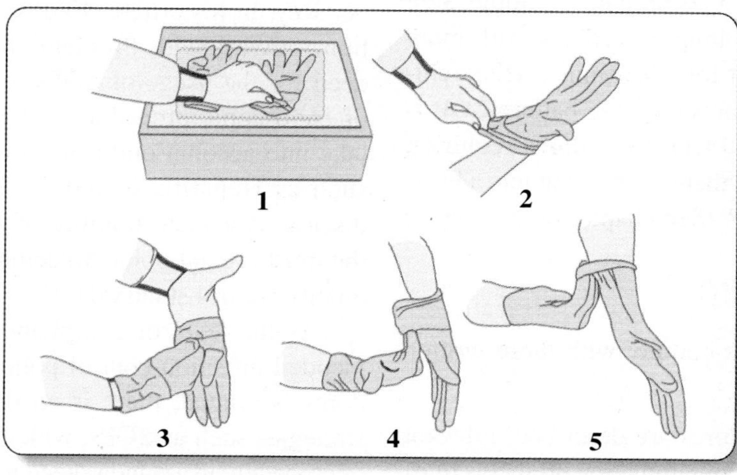

Figure 14.1: Steps of gloving: Standard Operating Procedures ensure conformance with organizational practices, reduced work effort, reduction in errors, credibility, resource for training and ready reference.

- Radiology departments
- Housekeeping
- Engineering maintenance
- Employee health issues
- Environmental cleaning
- Sterilization and disinfection procedures (See chapter on disinfection and sterilization.) Surgical equipment, anaesthetic equipment, etc.
- Intensive care protocols
- Hospital waste management
- CSSD

Points to Keep in Mind in Designing SOPs

The type of SOP to prepare depends on two factors: How many decisions will the user need to make during the procedure? How many steps and sub-steps are there in the procedure? For short procedures with few decisions required, it is best to prepare a simple Step Format SOP. For long procedures with more than 10 steps and few decisions a Hierarchical Step Format or a Graphic pattern SOP is best suited (Fig. 14.1). Procedures requiring many decisions in them are best put into a Flow chart pattern SOP. (See chapter on planning.)

Features of a SOP

1. All staff must comply with these written procedures.
2. When procedures are described, relevant safety and decontamination protocols must also be incorporated.
3. SOPs require regular review at say, 12-month intervals. Expired SOPs must be removed from circulation.
4. When an SOP is applicable to a procedure, it must include the following points:
   - Purpose of the procedure
   - Location of the procedure
   - Performance and methodology of the procedure
   - Limitations and exclusions applying to the procedure
   - Training requirements of staff performing the procedure

EVIDENCE OF NEED AND IMPACT OF SOPS

According to Vincent et al,[3] task factors such as task design and clarity of structure, availability of protocols, and availability and accuracy of test results directly affect clinical practice.

Rey, in his article 'Endoscopic Disinfection—a Worldwide Problem', has stressed the need for the usage of SOPs to ensure safety of endoscopic procedures.[4] This should also take into account outbreak of newer diseases such as Hepatitis C and Creutzfeldt-Jakob disease. Adequate training of staff is one of the most crucial points to achieve the highest quality control standards.[1, 5]

As the level of compliance with recommended infection-control policies and procedures is crucial, there is an urgent need for strategies such as SOPs, which specify a task or procedure in a standardized manner to eliminate ambiguity, control quality, ensure reproducibility and incorporate safety. SOPs assure a correct knowledge of techniques, practices, equipment and agents and are not only for clinicians, but also for a number of ancillary staff who can directly or indirectly prevent HAI.[6]

Infection-control SOPs—who uses them?

a. Doctors
b. Nurses
c. Physiotherapists
d. Dieticians
e. Technicians
f. Radiographers
g. Respiratory technicians
h. Biomedical engineers
i. Cleaning staff (housekeeping)
j. Secretarial staff
k. Social workers

PROCESSES, TASKS AND INFECTION CONTROL

The processes must be responsive to regulatory action in a predictable cause-and-effect relationship in order to minimize variation around a target value. The workers must be trained in the use of the regulating mechanism and procedures. The act must not require undue physical exertion, and the process must be maintained sufficiently to retain its inherent capability.[7]

The SOPs for standard cleaning, disinfection, sterilization and theatre discipline are all important for prevention of infection in the operation theatre and intensive care unit.

Important Monitoring Strategies Must Be Combined with SOPs

- Microbiological surveillance of the operating room
- Air flow and ventilation
- Air microbial sampling
- Monitoring of sterilization (steam; ethyleneoxide; chemical sterilization)
- Testing of sterilants and disinfectants
- Surface sampling
- Testing of microbial carriers amongst the staff

ENVIRONMENTAL SOPs

According to the website for nurses in the US, the earlier phrase 'recommended practice for sanitation in the surgical practice setting' has been renamed as 'recommended practices for environmental cleaning in the surgical practice setting'. The guidelines for environmental cleaning are given by a number of agencies such as Centre for Communicable Disease Control and Prevention (CDC, Atlanta), Environmental Protection Agency (EPA) and Occupational Safety and Health Administration (OSHA).

What Is Environmental Disinfection?

This is primarily the disinfection of all inanimate hospital environment. It includes cleaning and/or fumigation of operation theatres, wards, all ICUs, general hallways, kitchens, toilets, hospital furniture (beds, cupboards, shelves and other work surfaces), hospital linen/laundry and also handling of spills.

The procedures for environmental cleaning in the surgical setting must be written down as Standard Operating Procedure (SOP) for the convenience of healthcare workers involved in the cleaning. This would also help in proper standardization, implementation and enforcement of cleaning protocols. Some of the good examples are seen on AORN website (www.aorn.org).

Environmental Cleaning

1. Operation theatre cleaning
   a. Before the first case of the day
   b. In between cases
   c. Terminal cleaning
2. Cleaning after an infected case
3. Spills handling
4. Fumigation

General Principles of Environmental Cleaning

Use of disinfectants must conform to agreed-upon standards and nationally approved guidelines. They must be used after the recommended dilution. They must be freshly prepared and disposed of after use, since the cleaning solution and equipment could get heavily infected on prolonged storage. Cleaning schedules for each equipment, its frequency, timing, storage and the disinfectant to be used must be specified. In general, the agents used for environmental disinfection have to be employee-friendly, sporicidal and tuberculocidal, apart from being bactericidal and virucidal. The agents used on various metallic surfaces and equipment have to be non-corrosive. The side effects of the various agents used must be made known to the employees so that adequate precautions can be taken against any harmful effects. If a cleaning firm is attached to an organization on a contract basis, the cleaning solutions and equipment should conform to hospital policy.

In the OT—routine cleaning includes

- Floors
- Toilets
- Washrooms
- Washbasins
- Beds
- Locker tops
- Other furniture
- Soap dispensers
- Paper towel cabinets

(Note: It is ideal to make a checklist of all items to be cleaned.)

If there are no national guidelines for choosing a disinfectant or sterilant, then an agent approved by one of the recognized authorities such as Employee Protection Agency (EPA), FDA (Food and Drug Administration, USA) or CEN (Committee' European Normalization) must be selected, as this would take into consideration the safety aspects of the personnel, health workers and environment, in addition to ensuring effectiveness of the agent, with evidence.

Wet cleaning is recommended for floors in which mopping or wet vacuuming is the method of choice (do not use brooms in operating rooms and intensive care units).

Walls and ceilings (which should be of a material amenable to cleaning) of the ICU and

OT are cleaned once in six months, while in the wards they are cleaned once in a year or two; but areas which are contaminated must be immediately cleaned and decontaminated. Use of plaster for walls/ceilings is not advisable.

Managers, doctors, nurses and every other healthcare worker involved in cleaning processes must be fully conversant with all the facts regarding the disinfectant agents they are using, their chemical composition, mode of usage, adverse effects and ways of dealing with them.

Particular staff (nurses, doctors or managers) must be allocated the responsibility of supervising and handling the cleaning procedures, and ensuring employee protection, should there be some untoward incident/accident.

Equipment used for protection of the healthcare personnel are called Personal Protective Equipment (PPE). These must be used in a timely and judicious manner to derive maximum safety and minimize harm to the worker.

Equipment Checklists

The anaesthetic and surgical equipment are classified as per Spaulding's Classification and disinfected accordingly. (See chapter on sterilization and disinfection.) The procedure and agents used must not cause harm to the employees or the patient. Here again, it is important to keep the employees informed of any possible adverse effects of the agents used, and the methods of avoiding such effects.

Operation Theatre Cleaning

(Photo 14.2, 14.3, 14.4)

Before the first case of the day

This is equivalent to 'precurrent (prophylactic) disinfection' and is done before the start of the day's cases.

1. Responsibility for environmental cleaning and supervising must be fixed. For example, the circulation nurse and scrub person should complete preliminary preparation of the operating room before sorting and organizing the supplies needed for the day's cases.
2. Unnecessary tables and equipment should be removed from the room, and the relevant items arranged away from the general traffic.
3. Germicidal solutions should be prepared as per directions.
4. Bags/liners from waste receptacles/buckets/dustbins should be removed and replaced with fresh ones.

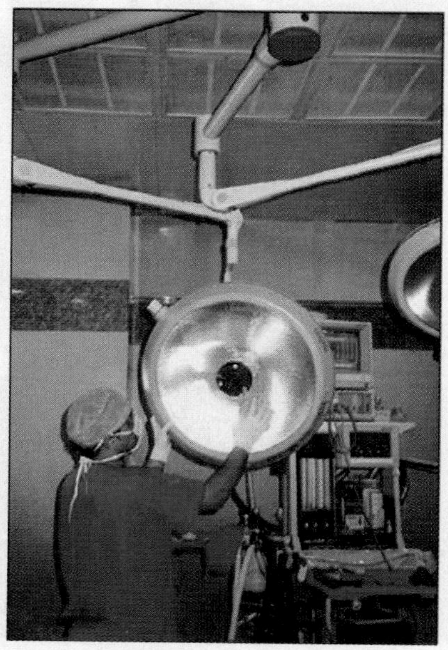

Photo 14.2: Standard operating procedures describe in detail the routine procedures to be followed.

5. Liners (bags) should not be allowed to touch any part of one's body.
6. Damp dusting of the following items should be done with an approved agent:
   - Overhead lights
   - OT table (after dismantling into components and removal of the mattress)
   - Furniture
   - Cabinets
   - Fixtures
   - I-V stands
   - Waste receptacles/buckets/dustbins
   - All flat surfaces (horizontal/vertical) their tops, rims, counter tops

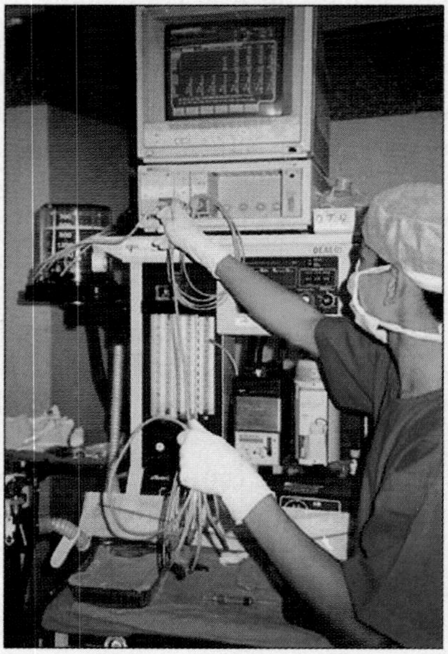

Photo 14.4: Cleaning of anaesthetic equipment

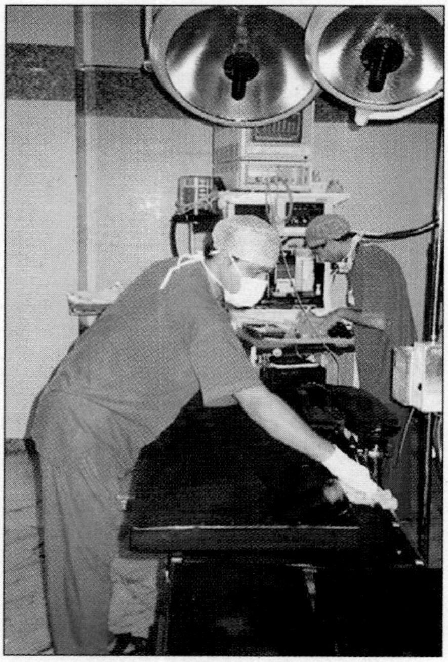

Photo 14.3: SOPs can clearly define environmental cleaning and ensure uniformity and standardization.

   - Walls and wall vents
   - Casters (wheels) of mobile furniture should be pushed through the disinfectant solution
   - Doors and doorknobs
7. The room should be carefully inspected with the naked eye for debris.
8. Floor should be damp-mopped.

Between-cases cleaning

Also called 'concurrent disinfection', this is physically applying disinfecting measures as soon as possible after discharge of infectious material from the body of the infected person, or soiling of the articles with such infectious discharges. After the patient has been wheeled out of the operating room, the following personnel and areas are considered contaminated:

a. Members of the sterile team

b. All furniture

c. All operating room and anaesthetic equipment

d. The floor immediately surrounding the focus area and the patient area

e. The patient transport carts

Decontamination of the above should be done by the following processes (Note: Always check the concentration of the disinfecting solution used for cleaning and follow manufacturer's instructions meticulously):

1. Clean heavy-duty gloves must be worn during the clean-up process
2. OT table and furniture: The horizontal surfaces of all tables and equipment should be washed with a disinfectant solution which is non-corrosive (avoid sprays, as these will aerosolize the particles). They should be damp-wiped with a germicidal solution. The in-between-cases cleaning requires special attention to the OT table. The mattress must be cleaned vigorously, manually or by mechanical friction. Dismantling of the table is essential for removal of all contaminants. Cleaning of the armrests is also mandatory.
3. OT lights: For cleaning of overhead lighting and light reflectors, the disinfectant solution recommended by the manufacturers should be used.
4. If the walls of the OT are splashed with blood or other organic debris, those areas should be washed with a detergent disinfectant and any area where gross debris is evident must be cleaned. The walls, ceilings and floors should be checked for soiled spots. Any spillage of blood must be wiped clean.
5. All liners (bags) from buckets, waste bins and receptacles must be removed, using both hands, but not allowing the bags to touch the body.
6. Equipment such as the electro-surgical units or lasers need special attention while cleaning, to avoid saturation of the internal machine. Manufacturers' instructions for cleaning should be followed wherever applicable.
7. Cleaning of suction bottles: (Photo 14.5)
   a. Suction bottles must be kept dry
   b. 100ml of 1% sodium hypochlorite solution must be added before use.
   c. After use, the sucked material must be drained 30 minutes after completion of the process.
   d. The bottles must be washed and kept dry till next use.
   e. Savlon must not be used for suction bottles.[8]
8. Floor should be mopped. Wet vacuuming may be done instead of wet mopping.
9. If facilities are available, wet vacuuming with a filter-diffuser exhaust cleaner is the equipment of choice for floor care in the operating room.
10. Linen must be sorted out from waste material. The waste must be stored in separate bags as per the protocols, under the supervision of a trained nurse.
11. Sharps should be collected in puncture-proof containers and handled according to waste management rules.

12. Anaesthetic equipment must be disinfected by the technicians as per protocols mentioned elsewhere in this book.
13. All the reusable anaesthetic masks and tubings must be cleaned and sterilized before reuse. This is discussed in greater detail in the chapter on sterilization and disinfection.
14. All disposable masks, tubings and circuits are disposed of according to protocol.
15. Special attention must be paid to cleaning and decontaminating the foot switches.
16. Rubber gloves must be washed in germicidal solution, while they are still on the hands.
17. If the case was known to be an infected one, terminal cleaning protocols must be followed.
18. The operating room must finally be inspected for repairs and deficiencies before the next case is taken up.

Terminal cleaning (at the end of the day)

(Photo 14.6)

1. It is the application of disinfective measures after the patient has been removed, (after completion of surgery), by death or has ceased to be a source of infection. The following must be damp-wiped using an appropriate disinfectant:
   - All walls and wall vents
   - Overhead lights
   - Ceiling and wall-mounted fixtures
   - OT table, after dismantling into its components and removal of the mattress
   - Other furniture, cabinets, fixtures
   - IV stands
   - Waste receptacles/buckets/dustbins
   - All flat surfaces (horizontal and vertical); Tops of surfaces, their rims and counter tops
   - Walls and wall vents (to be spot-washed with germicidal solution)
   - The casters (wheels) of mobile furniture (must be pushed through the disinfectant solution)
   - Cabinets and doors, doorknobs (especially the contact points)
   - Surgical scrub areas and sinks (top to bottom)
   - View charts, blackboards, surgical cabinet glass
   - Air intake grills, ducts and filter covers

Note: For the inaccessible areas germicidal solution must be sprayed

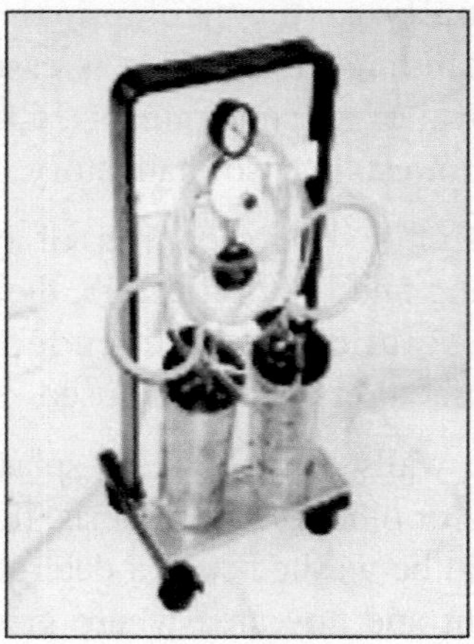

Photo 14.5: Suction apparatus is a major risk for HAI.

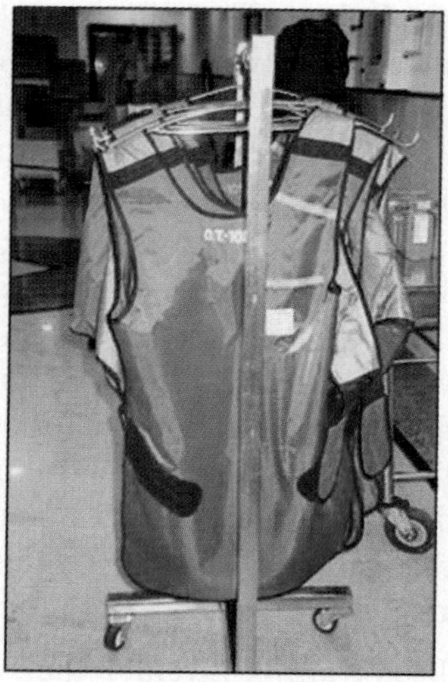

Photo 14.6: Cleaning protocols should include decontamination of lead shields and other ancillary equipment.

2. Floor: All the furniture should be moved to one side of the room. A 'wet floor' sign should be placed at the entrance of the room. The floor should be flooded with germicidal solution, especially if there has been a known infected case in the day's list. Wet mopping should be done to remove the solution. The furniture should be moved to the other side and the floor scrubbing procedure should be repeated.
3. Rubber gloves are washed in germicidal solution while they are still on the hands as mentioned above.
4. The room should be inspected for repairs and deficiencies again at the end of the day.
5. Suction bottles must be cleaned and sterilized as mentioned above.
6. Casters and wheels should be cleared of suture ends, debris, plaster, etc. and washed with disinfectant solution.

Spills

Handling of spills depends on

1. How hazardous the spilt substance is
2. How big the spill is
3. How many aerosols are generated as a result of the spill

It is important to avoid generating aerosols that can be inhaled. If aerosols are generated outside the containment, the room should be deserted for at least 30 minutes for the aerosols to settle.

Procedures for cleaning up of spills of body substances (e.g. blood, faeces, urine, etc.):

- Heavy-duty, puncture-resistant utility gloves such as those used for house cleaning should be worn (and not the latex gloves). This is to avoid tears, which do not occur easily with the heavy duty gloves.
- If the spill contains broken glass or sharp objects, then rigid sheets of cardboard should be used and direct contact with the gloves should be avoided.
- The spill should be absorbed (most disinfectants are ineffective or inactivated in the presence of proteinaceous substances, hence the bulk of the spilled material should be removed before the disinfectant is used). Absorption of the spilled material is done with disposable absorbent material such as paper towels, toilet paper or gauze pads.
- After absorption, all contaminated material should be discarded into a biohazard waste container designated for medical waste.
- The spill-site should be cleaned using any common detergent. Disposable absorbent

materials should be used and discarded into the biohazard waste container.

- The spill-site should then be disinfected. Sodium hypochlorite is widely recommended as the disinfectant of choice for cleaning spills of infectious nature. It is cheap and readily available (3–5 % solution). A 1 in 10 dilution with tap water (100ml of hypochlorite, and 900ml of water) will produce a concentration of 5000 parts per million of free chlorine, which is recommended for dirty spills.
- The disinfectant is left in contact with the spill-site for a period of time recommended by the manufacturer. The spill-site may be flooded with the disinfectant, or sprinkled with a granular absorbent disinfectant, or wiped down with disposable towels soaked in disinfectant. The disinfectant is then absorbed with disposable towels.
- The spill-site is then rinsed with water.
- The spill-site must finally be dried to prevent slipping.
- All the disposable materials used to clean up the spill are placed in a biohazard container and disposed of in the same way as infectious waste.

Spills of blood or body substances

Spill spots should be wiped immediately with a damp cloth, tissue or paper towel. An alcohol wipe may also be used. Discard contaminated materials (tissue, paper toweling, alcohol wipe) in accordance with local procedures.

a. For small spills (up to 10cm in diameter), disposable cleaning gloves, eye wear and a plastic apron should be worn if there is a risk of splashing. The spill should be wiped up immediately with absorbent material, e.g., paper hand towel. Place contaminated material into impervious container or plastic bag for disposal. Clean the area with warm water and detergent, using a disposable cleaning cloth. Where contact with bare skin is likely, disinfect the area by wiping with sodium hypochlorite 1000ppm available chlorine (or other suitable disinfectant solution) and allow to dry. Hands should be washed and reusable eyewear should be cleaned and disinfected before reuse.

b. For larger spills (greater than 10cm in diameter), the area of the spill should be covered with granular chlorine releasing agent (10,000ppm available chlorine) or other equivalent acting granular disinfectant and left for 3 to 10 minutes depending on formulation and labelling instructions. Use disposable (e.g., cardboard) scraper and pan to scoop up granular disinfectant and any unabsorbed blood or body substances. Place all contaminated items into impervious container or plastic bag for disposal. The area should be wiped with absorbent paper towels to remove any remaining blood and placed in a container for disposal. The area must be well ventilated, as small amounts of chlorine are likely to be released. Do not vacuum or sweep the area immediately, as this can disperse contaminants into the air and other surfaces.

Fumigation Protocol

Fumigation has been given up in many countries (including USA) because formalin (both gas and liquid forms) has been found to be carcinogenic. The reports on use of bound formalin (as in Bacillocid), if any, are conflicting, but still are used in many European countries. However, the fumigation protocol with formalin gas is given here for reference:

- All articles likely to be damaged by fumigation are removed.
- The OT should be washed properly.
- Air-conditioners should be turned off.
- 500ml of 40% formalin should be diluted in 1000ml of boiled water per 1000 cubic feet of space.
- The solution should be put in OT care machine.
- The machine should be put on for half an hour.
- The OT should be sealed for 10–12 hours.
- At the end of the procedure, the air conditioner should be turned on and the fumes exhausted. The area should then be washed, cleaned and carbolized before use.

Bacillocid is a new, improved, economical and rapid method of disinfection for OTs, CCUs , ICUs and other high-risk areas.

Advantages over fumigation

1. It is simple and easy to use. Consists of spraying of the prepared solution.
2. Provides asepsis within just 15–30 minutes.
3. No cleaning with detergent or carbolic acid is required.
4. No post-procedure neutralization with ammonia is necessary.
5. No need to shut down the OT for 24 hours.

Mode of use

Bacillocid Special (composition given below) + tap water.

1. 1 bottle=100ml at 0.5% dilution (for non-critical areas, wards, OPDs, etc.)
2. 1 bottle=50ml at 1% dilution for Alternate Day Disinfection of OTs, ICUs, ICCUs, etc. To be mopped or sprayed manually or with OT care machine
3. 1 bottle=25ml at 2% dilution for weekly disinfection of all critical areas including OT, ICCU, ICU, etc. To be mopped or sprayed manually or sprayed with OT care machine.

Important: For emergency disinfection, in between procedures, operations or infected cases, use only 0.5% Bacillocid Special (1 bottle =100ml).

Preparation and usage

(Table 14.1)

Disinfectants must always be used at the correct concentration. Too little is ineffective and too much may be irritant to the skin. The 'use dilution' may be suggested by the manufacturer on the basis of a Kelsey-Sykes capacity test, but the responsibility of ensuring efficacy rests with the user.

The life of a disinfectant varies with its formulation and many deteriorate when diluted with water. Disinfectants also deteriorate during their use due to their inactivation by microbes and other organic materials to which they are applied. Working solution should therefore be renewed each day.

Disinfectants may not kill even susceptible bacteria if these are present in very large

Table 14.1: Commonly used decontaminants

Antimicrobial agent	Gram Positive bacteria	Gram Negative bacteria	*M.tuber-culosis*	Fungi	Viruses	Spores	Initial Action	Residual Action	Remarks
1. Alcohols	Good	Good	Good	Good	Good	Poor			
2. Chlorhexidine gluconate		Good	Good		Fair	Good	Good	Good	Birth defects in pregnant users
3. Hexachlorophene	Good	Poor	Poor		Poor	Poor	Good		
4. Iodine/Iodophors		Good	Good	Good	Good	Good	Poor		Iodine allergy
5. PCMX	Good	Fair	Fair		Fair		Fair	Good	
6. Triclosan	Good	Fair	Fair		Fair		Fair	Good	
7. Phenol and derivatives	Good	Good	Good		Poor				
8. Hypochlorites (Inactivated by bioburden)	Good	Good	Good						
9. Formaldehyde	Good	Good	Good						Irritant, Potential carcinogen
10. Clea-N-Sept tablets (Sodium dichloroiso Cynurate)		Good	Good	Good		Good	Good	Good	
11. Bacillocid		Good	Good	Good		Good	Good	Good	
12. Sterillium hand rub		Good	Good	Good		Good	Good	Poor	

numbers or the disinfectant has been inactivated by excess organic matter or if it is not brought into contact with all the contaminated surfaces. Disinfectant solution must not be overloaded with bacteria or organic materials such as culture media. All articles to be disinfected must be properly immersed in the disinfectant.

Disinfectants take time to act. The time for effective disinfection will vary with the microbial load, the presence of organic material, the temperature, the pH, the nature of exposed surface and the presence of resistant bacteria or spores. Overnight exposure at room temperature, provided fresh contaminated material is not added, is generally considered adequate for most purposes.

Certain disinfectants are easily inactivated by changes in pH, by the presence of soap or detergents of opposite polarity, or by the presence of cork, cellulose, cotton, rubber and other discard materials. Disinfectants therefore should not be mixed with other disinfectants or cleaning solutions, and current procedures should be monitored by regular 'in use' tests.

It is necessary, therefore, to choose a disinfectant that is suitable for the required purpose and each healthcare facility should have a written disinfectant policy specifying the type and concentration of disinfectant for each type of use.

Composition, Contact Time, Toxicological Information of Common Agents

Bacillocid (composition)

1,6 dihydroxy 2,5-Dioxhexane 11.2gms
(chemically bound formaldehyde)

Gluteraldehyde 5.0gms

Benzalkonium chloride 5.0gms

Alkyl urea derivatives 3.0gms

Contact time

For an anti tubercular action

2%—4hrs contact time

2.5%—1hr contact time

1.5%—6hrs contact time

Gluteraldhyde

High level disinfection 2% for 10 hours;
Intermediate level disinfection 2% for 20 minutes

Sterillium (tuberculocidal and virucidal hand rub disinfectant)

Contact time: 30 seconds

Composition

Each 100gms contains

2-propanol	45g
1-propanol	30g
Ethyl-hexadecyl	0.2g

Dimethylammonium-
Ethylsulphate
Skin protecting substances

Hypochlorite (not effective against spores)

Fresh solution to be prepared as it is not stable on storage

SOPs and Categories (level of evidence)

Recommendations for disinfection and sterilization of objects in various categories-Modified and abstracted from CDC Guidelines: http://www.cdc.gov/nciod/dhqp/disinfection.html (18.01.2006)

CATEGORY I

Cleaning: Every object before sterilization/ disinfection should first be thoroughly cleaned to remove organic (Blood/tissue) and other residue

Sterilization/High Level Disinfection:

a. Critical instruments* should be sterilized.

b. All scopes** entering sterile tissue must be sterilized before each use. If this is not feasible, they should at least receive HLD.

c. Equipment that touches mucous membranes† should receive HLD.

Biological Monitoring of sterilizers:

a. If spore tests are positive, use of the sterilizer should be discontinued until it is serviced.

Use of sterile items: An item must not be used if its sterility is questionable. E.g., package torn, wet or punctured.

Reprocessing single-use/disposable items:

a. Items/devices that cannot be cleaned and sterilized or disinfected without altering their physical integrity and function should not be reprocessed.

b. Reprocessing procedures that result in residual toxicity or compromise the overall safety or effectiveness of the items or devices should be avoided.

CATEGORY II

Sterilization methods:

a. Whenever indicated a steam sterilizer should be used, unless the object to be sterilized will be damaged by heat, pressure or moisture. In this case, an alternate appropriate method must be used.

b. Flash sterilization@ is not recommended for implantable items.

Biological Monitoring of sterilizers:

a. All sterilizers must be monitored at least once weekly with appropriate commercial preparations of spores.

b. Every load with implantable objects must be monitored and not used till spore test is negative at 48 hours.

c. If spores are not killed in spore test, the sterilizer should immediately be checked for proper use and function and the spore test repeated. Objects other than implantables do not need to be recalled for a single positive spore test, enless the sterilizer or its process is defective.

Use and preventive maintenance: Manufacturer's instructions must be followed for use and upkeep.

Chemical indicators: These should be visible on the outside of each package sterilized to show that the package has been through a sterilization cycle.

HLD—High Level Disinfection

*Critical instruments are patient care equipment that enter normally sterile tissue or vascular system or through which blood flows.

** Scopes include Laparoscopes, arthroscopes, endoscopes etc.

† Includes- Endoscopes, endotracheal tubes,anaesthesia breathing circuits, respiratory equipment.

@ 270° F (132° C) for 3 minutes in a gravity displacement steam steriliser.

Corrosive on metals

Granular calcium hypochlorite preferred to liquid sodium or ammonium hypochlorite solution

Effective concentrations

1: 100 for HIV

1: 5–1:10 for Hepatitis B virus

1:10 recommended for all blood spills

REFERENCES

1) Palenik CJ. Strategic Planning for infection Control. J Contemp Dent Pract. 2000; 15; 1(4): 103.

2) Otero RB. Healthcare textiles services: infection control. Prof Dev Ser. 1997; 1-13.

3) Vincent C and Adams ST. The investigation and analysis of clinical incidents. In: Clinical risk management. Vincent C ed. 2nd edn. BMJ books 2001; 439-460.

4) Rey F. Endoscopic disinfection: a world wide problem. J Clin Gastroenterol.1999; 28(4): 291-7.

5) Juran JM and Gryna FM. Manufacture. In: Quality Planning & analysis. 3rd edn. New Delhi: Tata Mc Graw-Hill Publishing Co. Ltd. 1995; 343-376.

6) Vignaragah S, Eastmond VH, Ashragh A and Rashad M. An assessment of cross-infection control procedures among English speaking Carribean general dental practitioners. A regional preliminary study. Int Dent J. 1998; 48(2): 67 - 76.

7) Favero MS.Chemical disinfection of medical and surgical materials. In: Block SS, ed. Disinfection, sterilization and preservation. 3rd ed. Philadelphia: Lea and Febiger, 1983; 469-92.

8) Rutala WA, Stiegel MM, Sarubbi FA et al. Susceptibility of antibiotic-susceptible and antibiotic-resistant hospital bacteria to disinfectants. Infect Control Hosp Epidemiol 1997; 18: 417-21.

Chapter 15

Disinfection and Sterilization

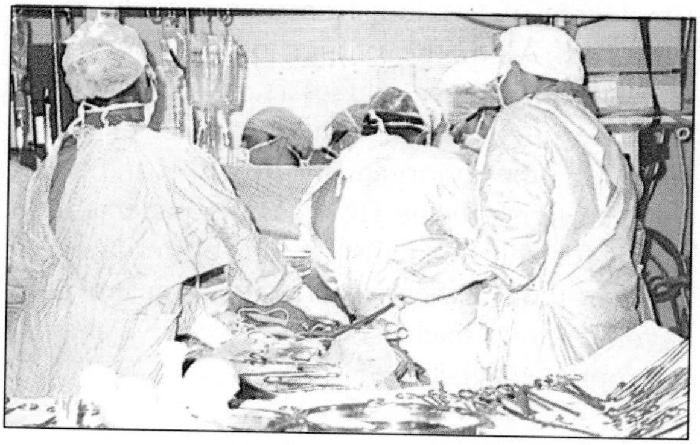

There is no real excellence in all the world which can be separated from right living.

—David Starr Jordon

Highlights

Classification of Instruments and Equipment

Who Sets the Standards for Sterilization?

Monitoring the Sterilization Processes

Anything New in the Offing?

Sterilization Procedures for Special Organisms

Steps for Sterilization and Disinfection

Non-Critical Items and their Disinfection Methods

Environmental Cleaning

INTRODUCTION

The practice of medicine and patient care demands that utmost care be taken in keeping instruments, equipment, surfaces and other materials coming in contact with the patient, as free as possible, from pathogenic microorganisms. This can be achieved by various processes, the selection of which depends on the degree of freedom from microorganisms required. Also, the choice of the method depends on a number of factors, including type of material, level of contamination of the material, types of organisms involved and the degree of risk to the HCW or the patient. In opting for a cleaning, disinfecting or sterilizing process, the healthcare professional must bear in mind several factors, in order to arrive at an appropriate decision.

- What is the material I want cleaned?

  Glass, wood, plastic, enamel, metal, cloth or any other (also, see Spauldings classification of instruments)

- Will the decontaminated material be adversely affected?

  Corroding, loss of elasticity, loss of shape, loss of function

- How clean do I want it?

  Free from every kind of living organism (sterile), free from pathogenic microorganisms (disinfected) or free from soil and dirt (clean)

- What purpose do I want the material for?

  To use on patient's intact skin, for invasive procedures, to grow microorganisms, surfaces to work on, for common patient use like clinical thermometers and so on (see Spaulding's classification).

- Do I want to get rid of a particular microorganism?

  E.g. Prions from instruments (use NaOH), *E.coli* from a drinking water source; (Microorganisms show varying susceptibility to sterilizing/disinfecting agents.)

- What will it cost me/my institution?

  This point is a very relevant one, especially in developing countries. Given the same efficacy of two disinfecting agents, the cheaper one is naturally preferred. (Look at EPA, CEN, national regulations and guidelines and use of planning techniques, quality, risk and performance management.)

- How do I know if the processes and techniques employed are effective?

  Use of process monitoring techniques

- Is there any risk to personnel?

  In the form of skin allergies, hypersensitivity as in iodine. (See chapter on occupational exposure.)

- Which product should I use?
- Which technique should I use?

  (Refer to chapters 14 and 18)

These and several other queries will be answered in the course of this chapter.

Understanding Terminology

Cleaning

A process that removes foreign material from an object. E.g. soil, organic material, microorganisms, etc. Cleaning is carried out before decontamination. It is a must for any process of decontamination to be effective and is carried out by various methods of washing. Enzymatic cleaning is now recommended for removal of soil and organic material.[1] (Figs. 15.1, 15.2, 15.3, 15.4). Personal protective equipment must be worn while carrying out cleaning procedures.[1] A useful method of ensuring high-level cleaning is to use the ultrasonic cleaner as a follow-up to manual cleaning. (Photos 15.1, 15.2, 15.3)

Remember: disinfectants may be inactivated by protein/organic content, hard water, presence of detergents, etc. The organic materials may coagulate or form films or clumps of materials that shield and protect the microorganisms from the disinfectant. Sometimes the disinfectant may combine with the organic materials causing a loss or reduction in germicidal action. E.g. Chlorine.

Decontamination

It is a process that renders an object safe for handling by removing contaminating organisms. It is a broad term and includes cleaning, disinfection and sterilization. The level of decontamination should always be such that there is no risk of infection when using an equipment, neither to the patient nor the healthcare worker.

Disinfection [2]

A process which reduces the number of patho-

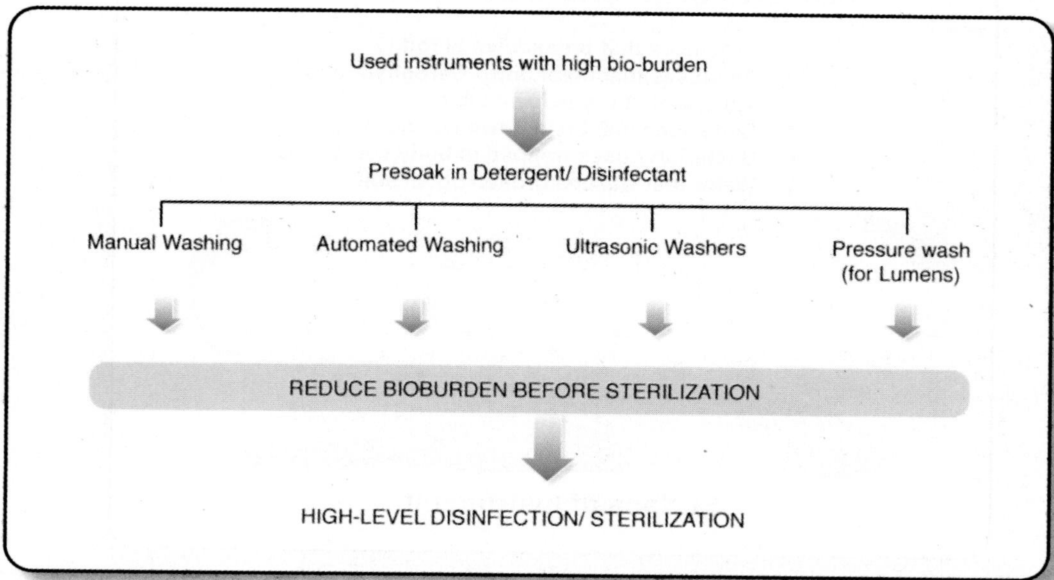

Figure 15.1: Decontamination/sterilization is preceeded by reduction of bioburden (Courtesy 3M India Ltd.)

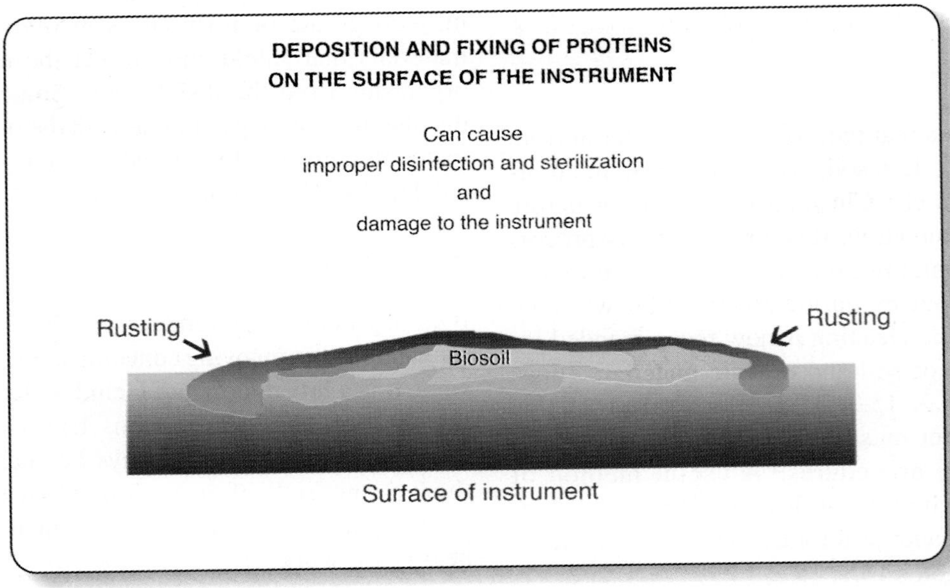

Figure 15.2: Deposition of biosoils leads to rusting of equipment and incomplete sterilization or disinfection (Courtesy 3M India Ltd.)

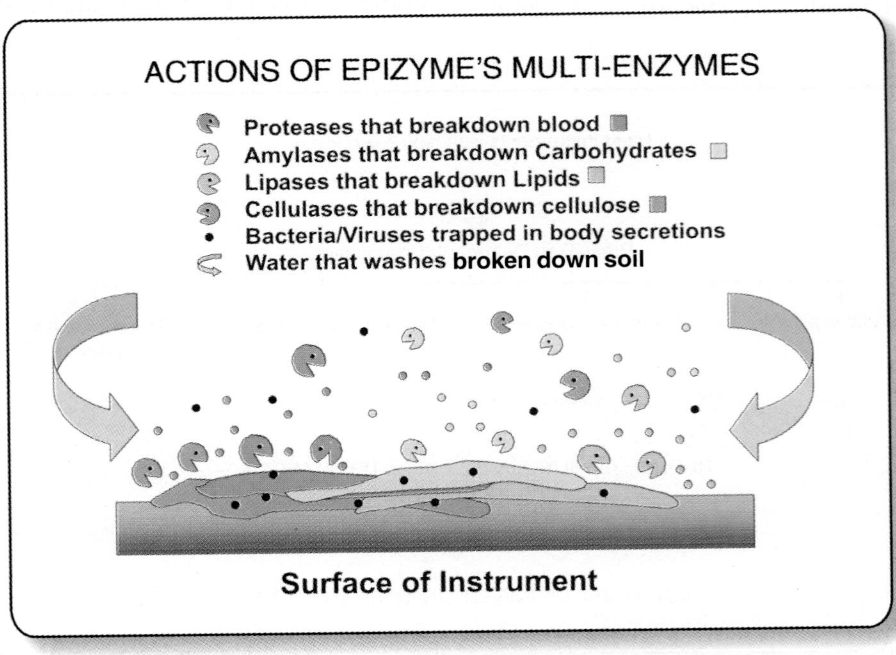

Figure 15.3: A number of enzymatic cleaning agents are avaiable which help break down biosoils (Courtesy 3M India Ltd.)

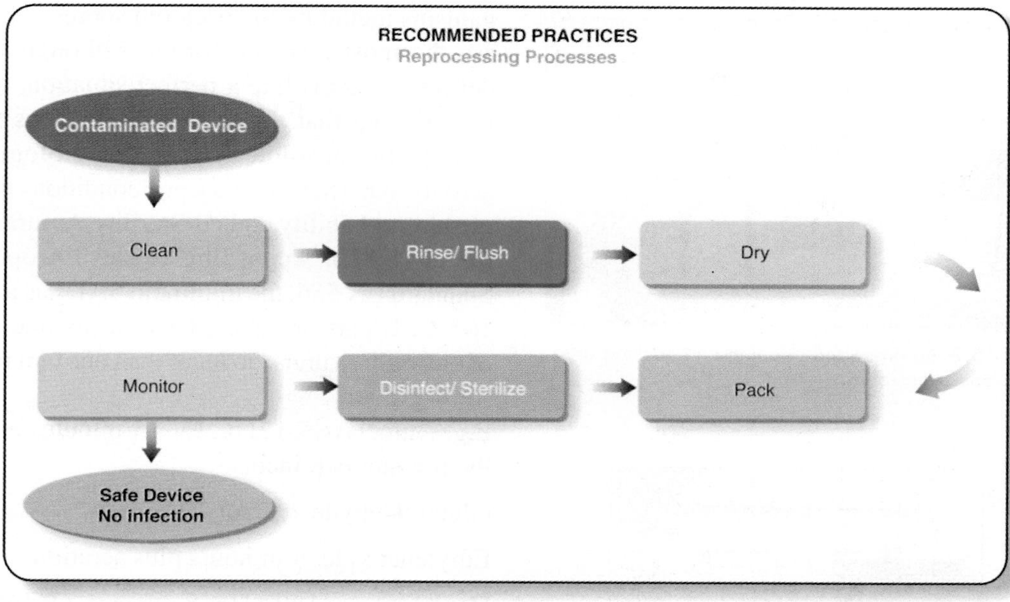

Figure 15.4: Steps of reprocessing a device (Courtesy 3M India Ltd.)

genic microorganisms, but not necessarily bacterial spores, from inanimate objects or skin, to a level that is not harmful to health. The level of disinfection is further graded into low, intermediate and high levels.

Low-level disinfection (LLD)

It can be performed for objects that contact intact skin or mucous membranes, where neither *Mycobacterium tuberculosis* nor spore-forming organisms are a threat. This method is effective for HIV, HBV, HCV, other common viruses, vegetative bacteria, yeasts, other fungi and protozoa. This level of disinfection can be achieved by boiling, microwave, use of chemicals such as alcohol, chlorhexidine, iodophors, cetrimide or sodium hypochlorite.

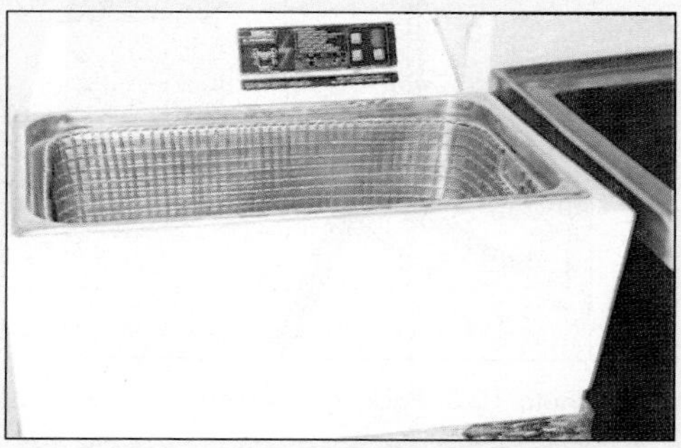

Photo 15.1: An ultrasonic cleaner

Intermediate-level disinfection (ILD)

In addition to organisms mentioned in low-level disinfection, this is effective against *Mycobacterium tuberculosis*. E.g. Glutaraldehyde 2% for 20–30 minutes.

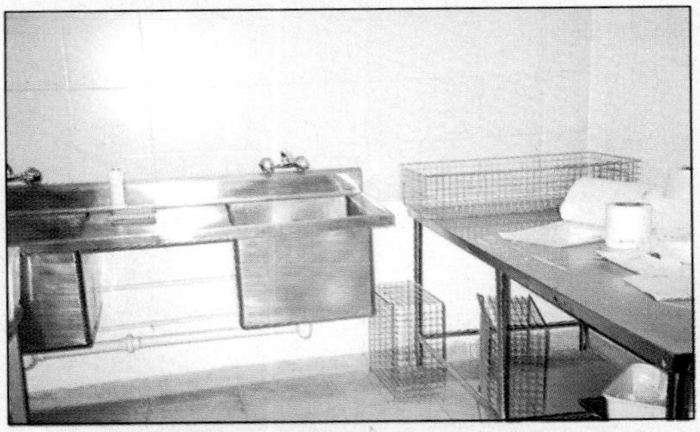

Photo 15.2: An organised cleaning and packing area in the operating room

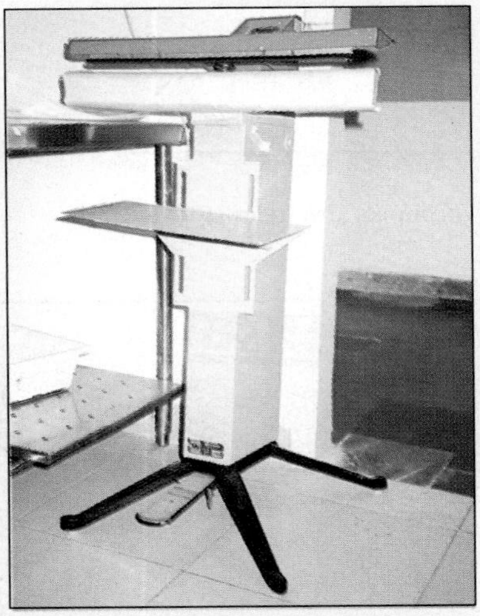

Photo 15.3: Packing machine

High-level disinfection (HLD)

This term is often used for a process which kills *Mycobacterium tuberculosis* and entero-viruses, in addition to other vegetative bacteria, fungi and more sensitive viruses. This again, does not include bacterial spores.

Sterilization [3]

This is a process which destroys all microorganisms including the bacterial spores, which are the most resistant forms. Although this definition seems like a perfect situation, it is now known that the term 'sterile' does not specify the absolute absence of biological activity, but determines aseptic conditions with certain probability, called Sterility Assurance Level (SAL). According to the European Standard EN 556, the minimum SAL has to be 10^{-6} CFU/part or better. This means that out of one million units, no more than one unit may show growth.

E.g. Autoclave—121°C for 15 minutes at 15 lbs pressure/sq. inch.

Glutaraldehyde 2 % for 10 hours

Ethyleneoxide: four hours plus aeration

Hot Air Oven: 180°C for 8 minutes. Or 160°C for 1 hour.

Flash sterilization: 134°C for three minutes

There are a number of other methods of sterilization shown in Fig. 15.5.

Validation (process monitoring)

This is a process of demonstrating that a sterilization process guarantees a certain Sterility Assurance Level (SAL) of the produced sterile goods.

Understanding the processes

Cleaning removes—soil+dust+particulate matter+some microorganisms

Disinfection removes—soil+dust+particulate matter+pathogenic microorganisms

Sterilization removes—soil+dust+particulate matter+ all living forms including bacterial spores

CLASSIFICATION OF INSTRUMENTS AND EQUIPMENT

Spaulding's Classification

According to E. H. Spaulding, there are three categories of surgical instruments based on the risk of infection they pose when used. Accordingly, the level of sterilization or disinfection and subsequent rinsing required can be determined for each category.

I Critical items

Items assigned to this category present a high risk of infection if the item is contaminated with any microorganism, including bacterial spores. These critical items must be sterile, because they come in contact with sterile tissue or the vascular system. Sterile rinse water is required for critical items that have been exposed to a liquid sterilant. E.g. surgical instruments and implants.

II Semi-critical items

These are items that come in contact with mucous membranes or with the skin that is damaged. They must be free of all microorganisms, with the exception of high numbers of bacterial spores. These items require a minimum of high level disinfection. E.g. flexible endoscopes and respiratory therapy equipment. 2% alkaline glutaraldehyde is most commonly used for high-level disinfection of semi-critical items. Although quality tap water has been found to be acceptable, and practical, for the rinsing of these items by many healthcare professionals, it is preferable to use sterile water, especially when dealing with immunocompromised hosts.

III Non-critical items

These items come in contact with the intact skin, but not with mucous membranes. For these items, it is appropriate to use intermediate or low-level disinfection. Such chemicals include quarternary ammonium germicides and isopropyl alcohol. Tap water is sufficient for rinsing of such items. E.g. blood pressure cuffs, bedside tables and bed pans.

STORAGE

A most frequently asked question about sterilization is, 'Once an item is sterilized, how long will it remain so?' This is a difficult question to answer. But, it can be said that the sterility of an item is not so much time-related as it is event-related. This means, instead of setting a time limit to accept its sterility, it is better to consider other factors like whether the packaging has been torn or damaged, or if the sterile item has got wet, etc. Sterility also depends on the manner and number of times a sterile item is handled as also the conditions of its storage.

Shelf-life

(Photo 15.4)

The term 'shelf life' is defined as the period during which sterility can be maintained and is considered valid. In literature, storage times between two days and an indefinite period have been reported, but in most instances wrapping materials and storage conditions were not considered. Thus, it may be said that loss of sterility is considered event-related (e.g. by the frequency and method of handling and storage area condition) and not time related. An optimal sterile storage area is adjacent to the sterilization area and one that protects the sterile

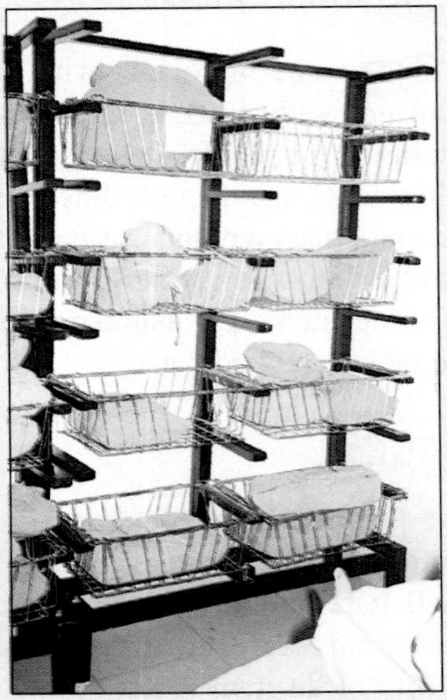

Photo 15.4: Storage of sterilized goods must be organized, clean and dry.

products against dust, moisture, insects, vermin, temperature and humidity extremes. Sterile items should be positioned such that the packaging is not crushed, bent, compressed or punctured.

Transportation

Sterile products transported to the operating rooms and other areas within the hospital should be provided with an additional outer dust-protection cover that can be removed before the items are taken into the clean zone.

Every hospital must specify its policies for the method of cleaning, disinfection, validation and storage (Fig. 15.6). The process must be clinically effective and must implement the recent evidence-based practice. They must utilize proactive concepts of risk management in dealing with problems of disinfection and sterilization:

a. Use standard definitions and protocols.

b. Identify an aggregating institution to standardize definitions and protocols and receive the data.

c. Assess them for quality, standardize the risk, adjust the benchmarks and interpret and disseminate the data.

WHO SETS THE STANDARDS FOR STERILIZATION?

Standards for Chemical Sterilants and Disinfectants

(Table 15.1, 15.2)

For products sold in Europe, sterilants and disinfectants need to have a CE mark. A CEN (Comite European Normalization) standard would have to be met by manufacturers. This deals with various aspects such as:

1. Consumer safety
2. Environmental hygiene
3. Tests of disinfection and sterilization and
4. Toxicity levels

Similarly, in the USA, disinfectants have to be cleared by the EPA (Employee Protection Agency) and sterilants have to get the clearance of FDA.[4]

In countries which do not have an agency that needs to certify the quality of disinfectants and sterilants, it would be prudent to select agents which conform to these standards (CE or EPA cleared).

CDC guidelines focus on strategies for disinfection and sterilization of medical equipment. These guidelines do not recommend specific chemical germicides that are

Table 15.1: Various categories of disinfectants and sterilants, and their action against microorganisms

	Gram Positive	Gram Negative Bacteria	Myco-bacteria Bacteria	Fungi	Enve-loped viruses	Non enve-loped viruses	Bacterial Spores
Phenolic compounds	Good	Good	Fair	Good	Slight	Some	Nil
Hypo-chlorites	Good	Good	Fair	Slight	Slight	Slight	Fair
Alcohols	Good	Good	Good	Nil	Slight	Some viruses	Nil
Formal-dehyde	Good	Good	Good	Good	Slight	Slight	Good
Glutaral-dehyde	Good	Good	Good	Good	Slight	Slight	Good

Table 15.2: Examples of FDA recommended contact time for some of the chemical sterilants and disinfectants. (Note: The same agent from different manufacturers has different recommended contact times. These products are available in the US and may not be available elsewhere.) Source: (http://www.fda.gov/cdrh/ode/germlab.html. Dated. 5/13/05)

Product	Active Ingredient(s)	Sterilant contact conditions	HLD Contact conditions
Sporicidin Solution (Sporicidin International)	1.12% glutaraldehyde 1.93% phenol/phenate	12hrs at 25 °C 14 days maximum reuse	20min at 25°C 14 days maximum reuse
Rapicide (MediVators, Inc.)	2.5% glutaraldehyde	7hrs 40 mins at 35°C 28 days maximum reuse	50min at 35°C 28 days maximum reuse
Cidex OPA solution (Advanced Sterilization Products)	0.55% ortho-phthalaldehyde.	None	12min at 20°C 14 days maximum reuse

Table 15.2: (Contd.)

Cetylcide-G Concentrate and Diluent concentrate (Cetylit Industries Inc.)	3.2% glutaraldehyde	10hrs at 20°C 28 days maximum reuse	40min at 20°C 28 days maximum reuse.
MedSci 3% Glutaraldehyde (MedSci Inc.)	3% glutaraldehyde	10hrs at 25°C 28 days maximum reuse	25min at 25°C 28 days maximum reuse
Endospor Plus solution (Cottrell Ltd)	7.35% hydrogen peroxide	180 min at 20°C 14 days maximum reuse	15min at 20°C 14 days maximum reuse
Sporox Solution (Reckitt & Colman Inc.)	0.23% peracetic acid 7.5% hydrogen peroxide	6hrs at 20°C 21 days maximum reuse	30min at 20°C 21 days maximum reuse
Peract 20 liquid (Minntech Corpn.)	1% hydrogen peroxide 0.08% peracetic acid	8hrs at 20°C 14 days maximum reuse	25min at 20°C 14 days maximum reuse
Procide14N.S. (Cottrell Ltd)	2.4% glutaraldehyde	10hrs at 20°C 14 days maximum reuse	45min at 20°C 14 days maximum reuse
Omnicide Long life Activated Dialdehyde solution (Cottrell Ltd)	2.4% glutaraldehyde	10hrs at 20°C 28 days maximum reuse	45min at 20°C 28 days maximum reuse
Omnicide Plus (Cottrell Ltd)	3.4% glutaraldehyde	10hrs at 20°C 28 days maximum reuse	45min at 20 °C 28 days maximum reuse
Metricide Plus 30 Long Life Activated Dialdehyde solution (Metrex Research Inc.)	3.4% glutaraldehyde	10hrs at 25°C 28 days maximum reuse	90min at 25°C 28 days maximum reuse
Metricide 28 Long-Life Activated Dialdehyde	2.5% glutaraldehyde	10hrs at 25°C 28 days maximum reuse	90min at 25°C 28 days maximum reuse

Table 15.2: (Contd.)

solution (Metrex Research Inc.) Metricide Activiated Dialdehyde solution (Metrex Research Inc.)	2.6% glutaraldehyde	10hrs at 25°C 14 days maximum reuse	45min at 25°C 14 days maximum reuse
Cidex Activated Dialdehyde Solution (J&J Medical Products)	2.4% glutaraldehyde	10hrs at 25°C 14 days maximum reuse	45min at 25°C 14 days maximum reuse
Cidex Formula 7 Long-Life Activated Dialdehyde Solution (J&J Medical Products)	2.5% glutaraldehyde	10hrs at 20–25°C 28 days maximum reuse	90min at 25°C 28 days maximum reuse
Cidex Plus 28 Day solution (J&J Medical Products)	3.4% glutaraldehyde	10hrs at 20–25°C 28 days maximum reuse	20min at 25°C 28 days maximum reuse
Wavicide-01 (Wave energy systems)	2.5% glutaraldehyde	10hrs at 22°C 30 days maximum reuse	45min at 22°C 30 days maximum reuse
STERIS 20 Sterilant (STERIS Corpn.)	0.2% peracetic acid	12 min at 50–56°C Single use only	None

formulated for use on medical equipment or environmental surfaces in the healthcare setting.

Tests for selecting chemical disinfectants and sterilants[5]

The ultimate responsibility for the quality of agent used is the users' (hospital/healthcare institution). A germicidal agent is selected according to some principles. The manufacturer gives certain guidelines regarding the spectrum of activity and the concentration based on the Kelsey-Sykes capacity test, but the responsibility of ensuring efficacy lies with the user. Kelsey-Sykes capacity test and Maurer stability test should be carried out in specialist laboratories. Hospital laboratories should carry out an 'in-house and in-use' test to confirm that the chosen disinfectant is effective under the given conditions. The main disadvantage with Rideal-Walker or Chick-Martin co-efficient tests is that they do not test its activity on organisms present in the hospital. (The test organism in the laboratory is *Salmonella typhii.*) In general, laboratory-cultured organisms are more sensitive to disinfection than primary environmental isolates. Use of phenol co-efficient is restriced only to phenolic disinfectants. Germicidal activity of chemicals is ranked high, medium or low. Germicidal chemicals are regulated in the US and in Europe.

Ranking of pathogens according to susceptibility to germicides [2] (Weakest to strongest)

Enveloped viruses

↓

Vegetative bacteria

↓

Non-enveloped viruses
(RNA →DNA virus)

↓

Fungi (non-pigmented)

↓

Pigmented fungi

↓

Mycobacteria

↓

Amoebic cysts

↓

Bacterial spores and fungal chlamydospores

↓

Prions

STERILIZATION BY HEAT

(PHOTO 15.5, FIGURE 15.5)

Dry heat sterilization requires temperatures of 180°C for 30min. or 160°C for 60min. Activity of techniques using heat are compared by knowing their D-value. Therefore, the same effect can be achieved at different temperatures. What is the D value? It is the Decimal reduction value—the time needed to reduce the population of bacteria to one-tenth of the original population.

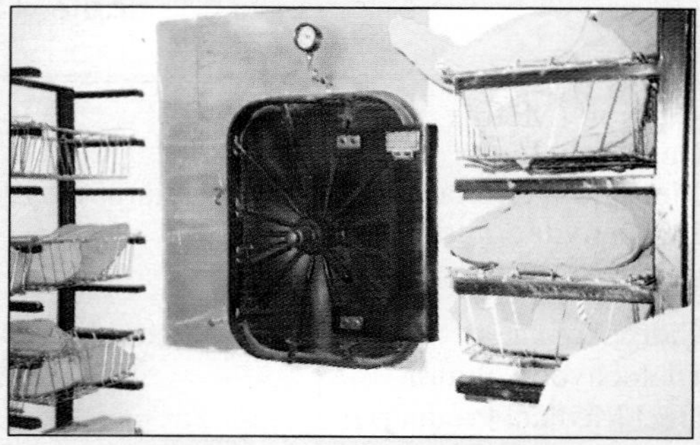

Photo 15.5: An autoclave

Steam sterilization needs lower temperatures. But, steam sterilization process depends on the efficacy of air removal and the kind of air removal process. If the air is not quantitatively removed by an adequate air removal process, dry heat instead of steam is found inside the hollow or porous goods.[6]

Thus, the fractionated vacuum steam sterilization process is suitable for all types of packaged, hollow, solid and porous goods, while the gravity displacement or single vacuum steam sterilization process is suited for non-packaged, solid goods to be used immediately after sterilization or for goods to be sterilized to prevent cross-infections.

The quality of water used as feed water to the steam sterilizers is of special importance for the steam quality and in turn the sterilization process. Water has to be desalted, softened and fed through rust-proof pipes. The transition time to heat up the goods depends heavily on the amount of air, which may insulate the goods to hinder the steam condensation.

Radiation is used to sterilize plastics and drugs (items which should not be damaged by the process or by sterilants).

Variations can be avoided by following standardized practices and validating each

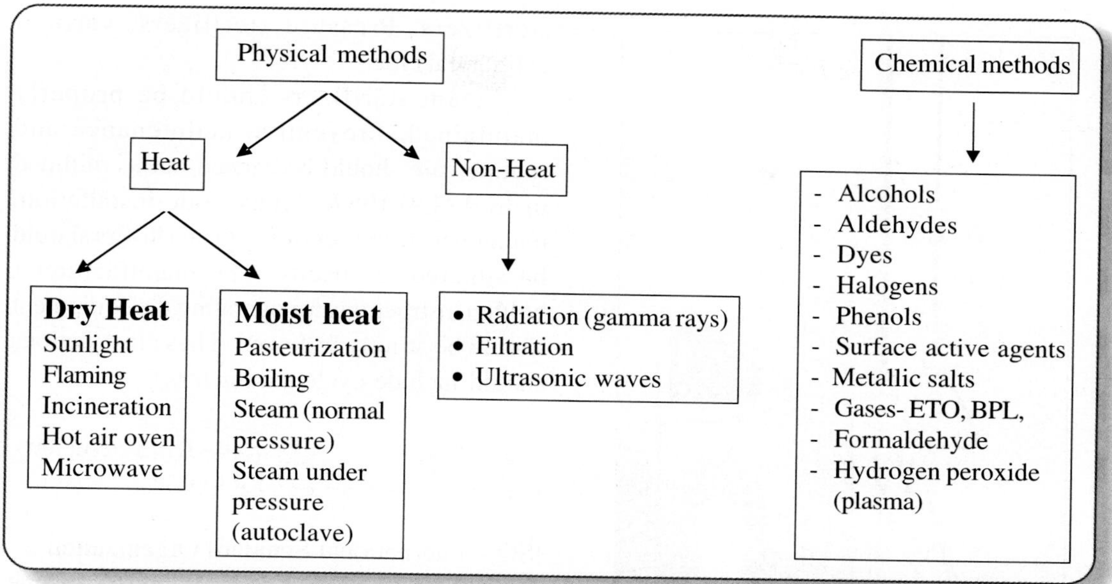

Figure 15.5 : Methods of sterilization

cycle of disinfection and sterilization (Fig . 15.6, Table 15.3).

Every country or a group of countries either formulates its own standards for sterilization, taking into consideration all aspects relevant to their requirements, or adopts the standards set by some of the developed nations with well-documented, satisfactory results.

European Standards (CEN; EN)

These standards are applicable to all member countries of the European union, including the associative countries Norway, Iceland and Switzerland.

CEN—Comite European de Normalisation

EN—European Norm

(In case a European standard is published, national standards with the same content automatically become obsolete within the EC member countries.)

National Standards

These are applicable to individual countries. For example the standards followed in India are given below:

Example

Ethylene oxide sterilization

(Photo 15.6)

Specifications of equipment: The bureau of Indian standards should be consulted: Ethylene oxide sterilizer, DOC MHD 14 (2200)

Written instructions for cycle parameters by the sterilizer manufacturer must be followed.

Dry heat sterilization

Hot air sterilizers should conform to specifications given in the Indian standard IS: 3119-1978.

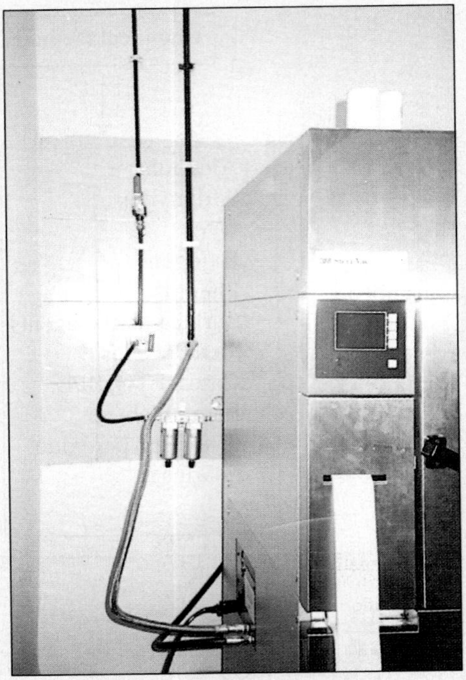

Photo 15.6: Ethyleneoxide (ETO) chamber with exhaust

Process controls are dealt with by Indian standards IS: 12430-1987. Safety code for installation, maintenance and servicing of sterilizers must be adhered to.

Steam sterilization

For purchase of various types of steam sterilizers administrators should insist on specifications laid down by IS 3829 (part 2) – 1978.

Indian Standards specifications for steam sterilizers. Horizontal cylindrical high speed sterilizers, pressure type. IS 3829 (part 3)– 1985.

Indian standard specification for steam sterilizers. Pressure sterilizers, vertical cylindrical type.

Steam sterilizers should be properly maintained. Preventive maintenance and routine care should be carried out as outlined in IS 12430:1987. Safety code installation, maintenance and servicing of sterilizers should be adhered to strictly. The manufacturer's written instructions for operating the equipment should be strictly followed. These instructions should include cycle parameters.[7]

Worldwide Standards—Accepted by Most Countries of the World

ISO—International Standard Organization
Some ISO and EN standards merge to one identical EN-ISO standard.

The member countries of the ISO standards have drafted standard guidelines for every aspect of sterilization and disinfection which fall under the following categories:

1. General requirements
2. Standards for packaging, storing and transport of items
3. Test equipment and methods of use
4. Selection of method of sterilization to be used for different items
5. Standards for validation of various processes
6. Types, indications and methodologies for use of chemical indicators
7. Types, indications and methodologies for use of biological indicators
8. Types, indications and methodologies for use of physical indicators

Table 15.3: Selection of other methods of sterlization/disinfection

Sterilization/ Disinfection method	Advantages	Disadvantages	Remarks
ETO	For heat-intolerant materials	Toxic. Can cause cancer in laboratory animals	
Formaldehyde 10% with 0.5% sodium tetraborate	For heat sensitive items	toxic, carcinogen	Requires ammonia vapour to remove
Ozone		Poor penetration	Used in water works industry to sanitize water
Vapour phase H_2O_2	Less toxic. Leaves no residues Non-inflammable Non-carcinogenic Penetrates fairly well	Capable of degrading incompatible materials	For medical instruments and biosafety cabinets Most viruses are filtrable
Filtration	heal labile items		For sterile pharmaceutical products and vaccines
UV rays	For work surfaces of safety cabinets	Difficult to achieve sterility. Short wave UV rays have poor penetration Photoreactivation is possible if cells are not sufficiently exposed	Avoid exposure to skin and eyes.
Microwave radiation		Sealed bottles may explode due to pressure differentials. Materials wrapped in paper or cloth may ignite	No evident non-thermal lethal effect
Hypochlorite	Good for spills of blood, etc.	Corrosive on metals and textiles	Must be made freshly to be stable
Ultrasound		Extent of decontamination depends on exposure time, intensity and the organism	

Medical-Device-Directive (MDD) of the European Community-Guidelines

- Defines all sterile goods applied to human beings as medical devices
- If hospitals produce sterile goods not only for their own use, but also for a third independent legal party, they require a notified body to validate their sterilization process
- The validation of a sterilization process includes cleaning, disinfection, functional check, sterilization process (including sterilizer/supply media, programme used, goods sterilized, packaging material and procedure), storage, transportation to the end-user and a quality management system
- The objective of validation is to guarantee sterility according to EN 556 (SAL = 10^{-6} CFU/piece)

Sterility Assurance Level (SAL)

Sterilization processes are designed such that all microorganisms are killed after thorough cleaning of the items to be sterilized, leaving minimal bioburden, and that the Sterility Assurance Level (SAL=10^{-6}cfu/device) required by EN556 standards is achieved. A precondition to be observed here is that the sterilant reaches all inner and outer surfaces. This is possible only if the air has been removed before the process or if no non-condensable gases are built up within the hollow instruments during the process.

MONITORING THE STERILIZATION PROCESSES

An essential quality assessment procedure for infection control is the monitoring of the sterilization process. The methods available for this include—physical, chemical and biological indicators (Figs. 15.7, 15.8, 15.9).

Validation or Process Monitoring

What are the various parameters to monitor in a sterilzation process?

1. In steam sterilization—temperature, time, air removal, steam penetration.
2. In ethylene oxide—temperature, time, gas concentration, humidity, gas penetration
3. Dry heat—temperature, time, individual packaging, heat transfer through packaging.

Physical Monitoring

These processes ensure sterilizer functioning (e.g. temperature, pressure, time). They tell us if the sterilization process has been correct. Although sterilization process monitors do not verify sterility, they do indicate procedural errors and equipment malfunctions. Any deviation in these should alert the operator to potential problems.

Chemical Monitoring

(Figure 15.8)

Although biological indicators are ideal to monitor sterilization processes, they are not suitable for daily routine monitoring due to their long response time between two and five days. So, chemical indicators can be used to monitor the processes with the advantage of having the result of the sterilization process available immediately. Chemical indicators include the colour or physical change indicators that monitor exposure to sterilizing agents or conditions. For example, the chemical indicators used to detect the presence of air or steam have a lead-sulphur basis, which are able to produce pronounced colour contrasts between a steam and hot-air atmosphere. Under steam conditions at 134°C, the indicator changes from yellow to black within 1.5 to 2.5min, whereas under hot-air conditions no change to black is effected at 140°C in 30min. Several chemical indicators are available for different sterilization processes.

Functions of indicators

1. Equipment Control: Control of physical parameter—Effective air removal/ steam penetration test (Bowie-Dick Test) (Fig. 15.9). The Bowie-Dick air removal test must be used in every batch.
2. Load Control: Sterility test—with indicators (biological indicator) placed inside the chamber for monitoring the entire load (batch)
3. Batch monitoring with PCD: This consists of a process challenge device (PCD) where the indicator is inserted. The test device replaces a cotton pack or container and simulates the most difficult place to sterilize.The result is available immediately after the sterilization process has ended.

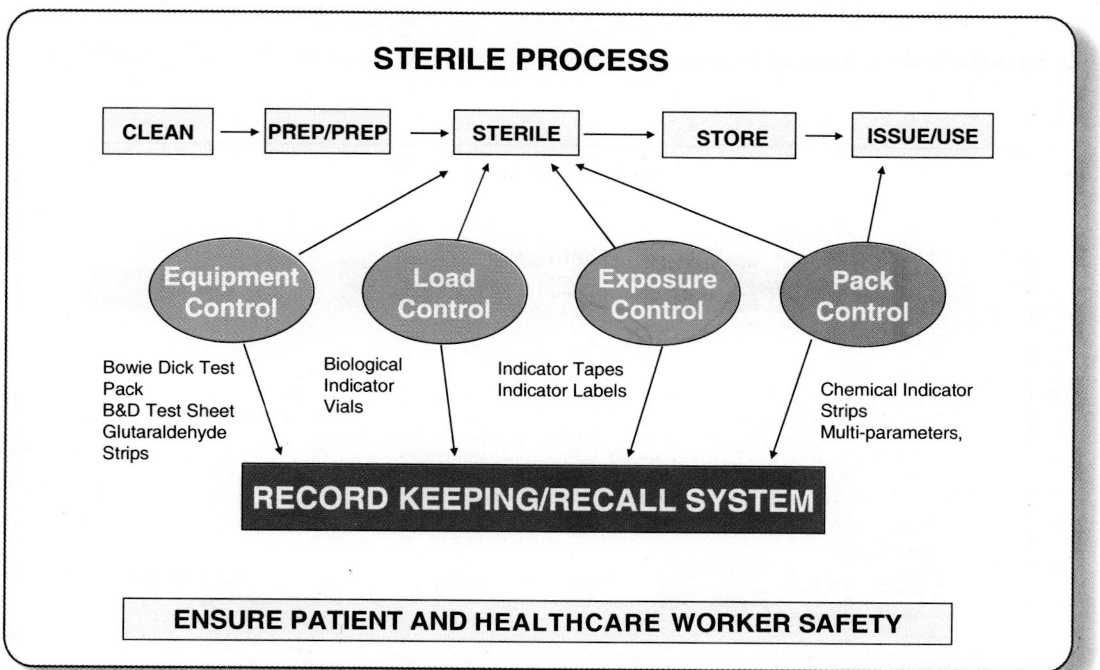

Figure 15.6: The processes which are used must be monitored to ensure sterility. (Courtesy 3M India Ltd.)

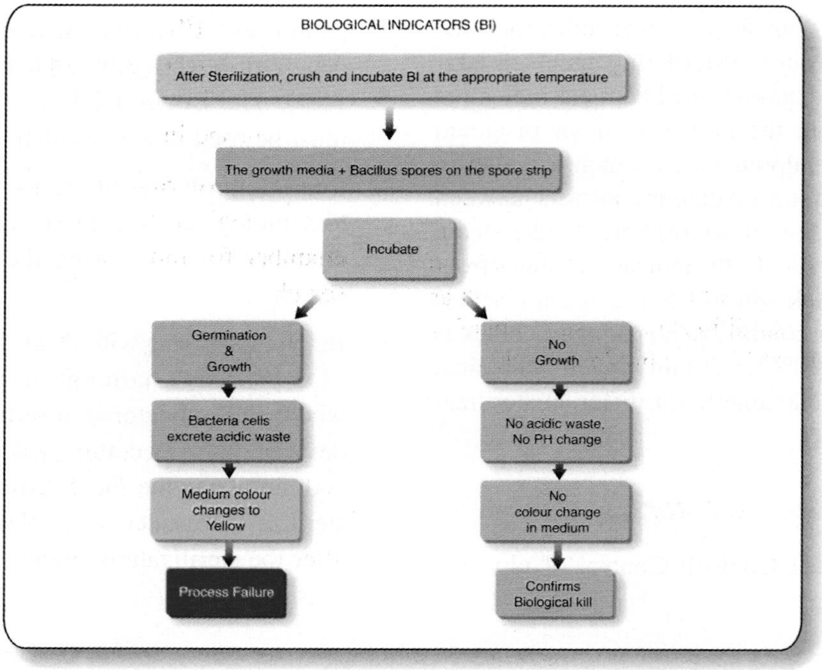

Figure 15.7: Using biological indicator for validating the process of sterilization (Courtesy 3M India Ltd.)

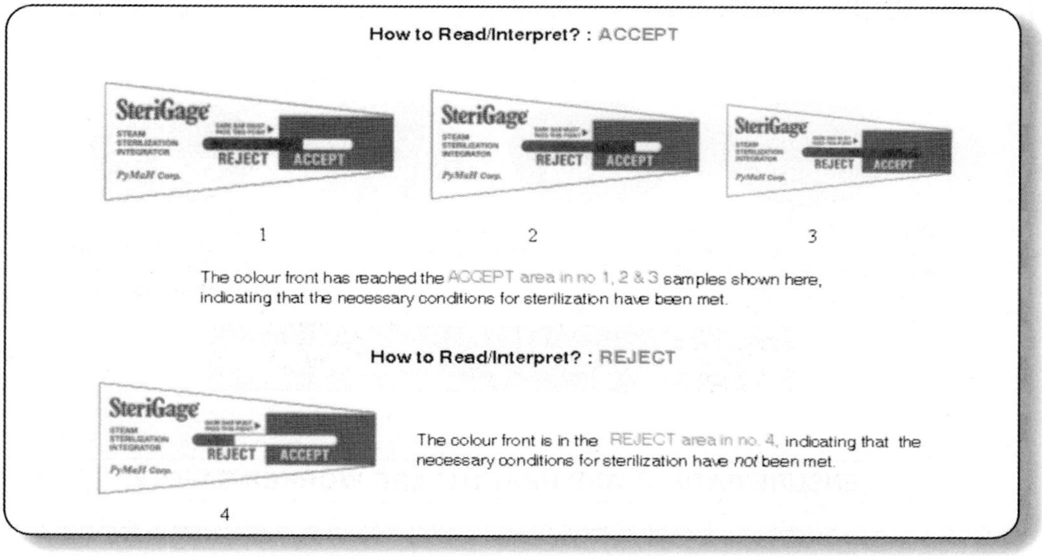

Figure 15.8: Chemical indicators can be used to monitor various sterilization processes (Courtesy 3M India Ltd.)

4. Exposure Control: Logistic information—by placing the indicators on the surface of the package to provide pure handling information (indicator labels)
5. Exposure Control: Here the indicators may be placed on top of packs or containers. They only indicate if the item has been subjected to the process and not the efficacy of the sterilization process.
6. Pack Control: Here the integrated indicators are used to control packs, containers or pouches. They must be placed inside each pack. The result is only available after opening the package or container before use.

   Note: Exposure control indicators placed on the surface of packs, containers or pouches are unable to control the efficiency of a sterilization process.
7. For hospital use, a monitor should
   - be easy to use
   - be inexpensive
   - not be subject to exogenous contamination
   - provide positive results as soon as possible after the cycle so that corrective measures may be taken
   - provide positive results only when the sterilization parameters (e.g. EO concentration, humidity, time, temperature) are adequate to kill microbial contaminants

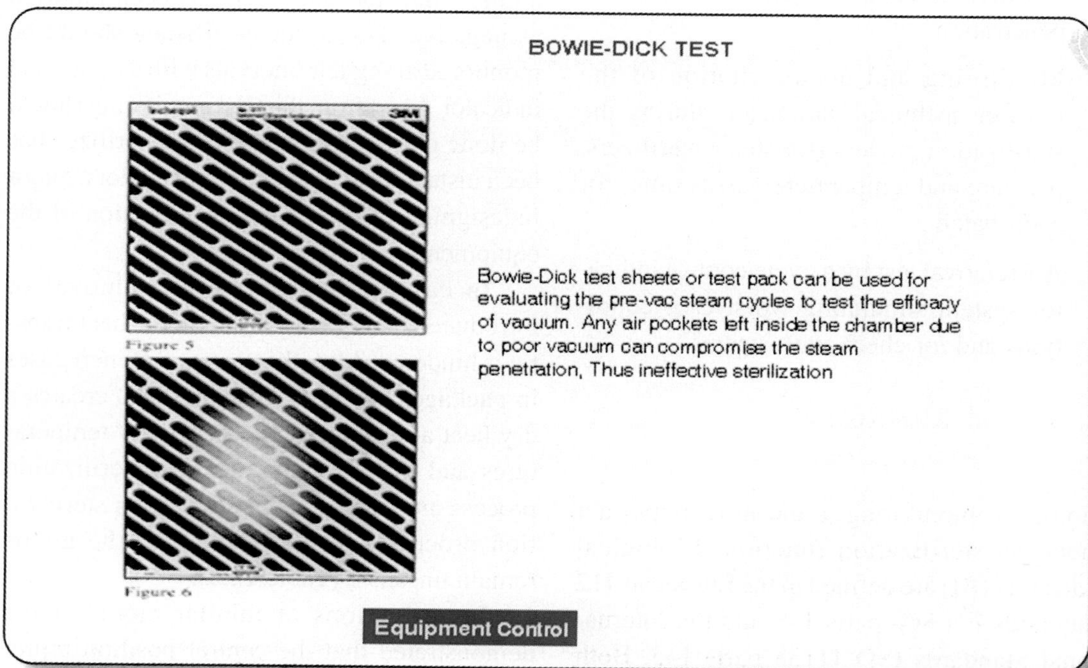

BOWIE-DICK TEST
Figure 5
Figure 6
Bowie-Dick test sheets or test pack can be used for evaluating the pre-vac steam cycles to test the efficacy of vacuum. Any air pockets left inside the chamber due to poor vacuum can compromise the steam penetration, Thus ineffective sterilization
Equipment Control

Figure 15.9: Equipment control by Bowie-Dick test (Courtesy 3M India Ltd.)

Sterilization control of fractionated vacuum steam sterilization

(Table 15.4)

1. Functional control of the sterilizer—after production, after installation and after essential repairs, by means of physical and /or biological tests (commissioning)
2. Validation of the sterilization processes; testing if the machine and programme can sterilize the goods processed
3. Air removal and steam penetration control with Bowie-Dick test (BD) in the BD-Test-Programme (134^{0}C, 3.5min)

   Note: The American test package has approximately half of the weight of the European test package and is therefore less sensitive in testing air removal and steam penetration.
4. Monitoring and documentation of the relevant technical parameters during the sterilization process (for steam sterilizers, pressure and temperature versus time) for each batch
5. Air removal test by a cycle control indicator system simulating worst case conditions and /or check with steam[8]

Biological Monitoring

(Figure 15.6, 15.7) (Table 15.5)

Biological monitoring is the most important check on sterilization function. Biological indicators (BI) are defined in the European 412 Standards EN 866 parts 1–8 and the International Standards ISO 11138 parts 1–3. Both standards are currently merged into one EN-ISO-Standard 11138 parts 1–6. Accordingly, certain reference bacteria have been selected to monitor the sterilization processes. E.g. *Bacillus stearothermophilus* for steam, formaldehyde and hydrogen peroxide sterilization processes, *Bacillus subtilis* for Ethylene dioxide and dry heat sterilization processes and *Bacillus pumilis* for radiation sterilization processes.

The CDC recommends monitoring of steam autoclaves in hospitals at least weekly. *Bacillus stearothermophilus* spores should be used as biological indicators for heat sterilizers and *Bacillus subtilis var niger var globigii* spores for ethylene oxide sterilizers. Every load containing implantable objects should be monitored with a spore test. It is also recommended that sterilizer loads containing implantables or intravascular devices be quarantined until the spore test has been reported as negative. The sterilizer efficacy should be monitored at regular intervals with a biological indicator. Apart from this, the monitoring should be done out-of-turn whenever a sterilizer has been installed, after a major repair, after a major redesigning or after a major relocation of the equipment.

In case of inadequate air removal or introduced inert gases in steam, the heat transfer is hindered. Also, the presence of inert gases in packages and/or hollow products creates a dry heat atmosphere. The necessary temperatures and times for the dry heat sterilization process are not reached in the steam sterilization process with the result that the goods remain unsterile (Table 15.4).

Investigations of tubular models have demonstrated that the central position represents the most difficult site from which to remove air in the case of a tube which is open at both ends. Also, tubular models of half-length which are closed at one end have this problem. To overcome this problem, the new European standard prEN867 part 5:1998 uses, in addition to a porous load, a hollow Process Challenge Device (PCD), in order to monitor air removal problems and steam penetration.

Validation of the Process of Sterilization for Hollow Instruments

The use of a process control device

The sterilization of hollow instruments (catheters, endoscopes) is difficult because it is physically difficult for steam and heat to reach all the hollow portions. This is further made difficult by presence of air bubbles, which hinder proper contact. So, to ensure sterilization of these devices the concept of process control device is used. This is nothing but a hollow instrument similar to the geometrical size and shape of the instrument to be sterilized, which is used as a control. This control also has a biological or physical indicator inserted for the purpose of validation of the loads.[9]

The proof of air removal from dead-end regions can be accomplished in three ways:

a. Thermoelectric measurement of temperature
b. Biological indicators
c. Chemical indicators that are able to differentiate between non-condensable gases and steam

The standard Bowie-Dick test pack is used to check porous loads by monitoring air removal and steam penetration of the steam steriliza-

Table 15.4: Air removal and packing of goods in different types of autoclaves. The difficulty of removing air also varies with the type of equipment to be sterilized.

Types of autoclaves	Air Removal	Air Removal	Packing of goods to be sterilized
	Poor ↓	**Easy** ↓	
1. Gravity displacement			1. Instruments (without holes and unpacked)
2. Single vacuum			2. Instruments (without holes and packed)
3. Vacuum- steam injection			3. Porous goods (e.g. cotton) –packing +/-
4. High-vacuum			4. Hollow instruments like (endoscopes) catheters- packing +/-
5. Fractionated vacuum	**Good**	**Difficult**	

tion process, while the Process Challenge Device (PCD) checks conditions of sterilization in hollow devices.

The concept of 'highest standards' and 'minimum standards'

Though the standards of care (sterilization of critical equipment) are quite clear, there are certain constraints while dealing with certain groups of equipment. A classical example is sterilization or high-level disinfection for endoscopes. They are classified as critical instruments, but many centres around the world carry out high level disinfection rather than sterilization. Why? There are a number of constraints when we talk about endoscopes:

- Expensive—smaller number of sets available, therefore when there is a high turnover of cases, it is not possible to meet the standard of sterilization.
- Heat intolerant—fear of damage to fiberoptic systems.

When the highest standards are not attainable, then the aim should be to attain at least a minimum set of standards at all times (e.g. Endoscopes should not be used without at least high-level disinfection) (Photos 15.7, 15.8).

Also, there is still a debate on the varying standards for different endoscopes depending on the site where they are used.

ANYTHING NEW IN THE OFFING?

Nowadays, operating rooms are pressurized to carry out heavier workloads, turn-over rooms with less downtime and reduce costs with little or no increase in instrument inventory. Also, there is maximal use of costly, heat-and-moisture sensitive medical and surgical devices, such as cameras, fibre optic cables and rigid endoscopes. Under such circumstances, the availability of newer and better methods of sterilization and disinfection can certainly contribute to quality patient care and ease the pressure on the OR managers and staff.

Antibiotic resistant pathogens such as VRE and MRSA are as susceptible to disinfectants as antibiotic susceptible strains. However, commonly used surface disinfectants such as phenols and quarternary ammonium compounds, while effective in eliminating these pathogens, do not have residual activity. Hence, after disinfection, surfaces may rapidly be recontaminated.

There are several newer methods of both disinfection and sterilization, cleared in 1999/2000 by the FDA (or submitted to the FDA or EPA but not yet cleared). These have the potential to improve patient care, but in general, their antimicrobial activity has not been independently validated.

A brief description of some of the newer methods of disinfection/ sterilization are given below:

Disinfectants

1. Surfacine
2. Ortho-phthalaldehyde
3. Superoxidized water

Sterilants

1. Endoclens
2. Attest
3. Sterrad 50

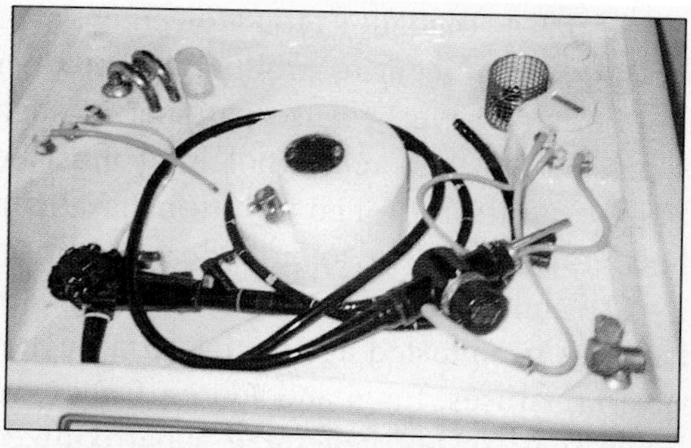

Photo 15.7: Automatic washer for endoscopes (high-level disinfection)

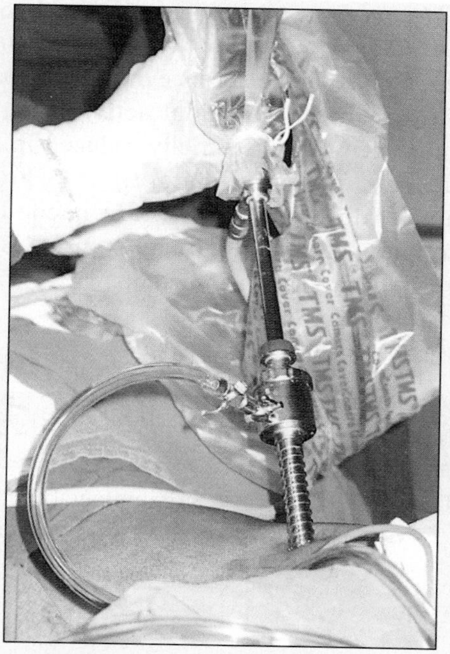

Photo 15.8: Thoracoscopy in progress

Surfacine

Surfacine is a new, persistent antimicrobial agent that may be used on animate or inanimate surfaces. It incorporates a water-insoluble antimicrobial drug compound (silver iodide) in a surface immobilised coating (a modified polyhexa-methylenebiguanide) that is capable of chemical recognition and interaction with the lipid bilayer of the bacterial outer cell membrane by electrostatic attraction. Microorganisms contacting the coating accumulate silver until the toxicity threshold is exceeded, dead microorganisms eventually lyse and detach from the surface.

This new antimicrobial drug can be applied to both animate and inanimate surfaces by dipping, brushing or spraying without prior surface treatment. The coated surfaces are resistant to biofilm formation.[10]

If this product proves to be effective and has long-term residual activity, it may be extremely useful in limiting transmission of nosocomial pathogens.

Ortho-Phthalaldehyde (OPA)

This is a new chemical sterilant solution that is clear, pale-blue with a pH of 7.5, and contains 0.55% OPA. It has demonstrated excellent microbicidal activity in in-vitro studies, even superior mycobactericidal activity compared with glutaraldehyde (efficacy test results using mycobacteria support a five-minute exposure time at room temperature for OPA with a greater than 5-log 10 reduction). There are other advantages over glutaraldehyde; it requires no activation, is not known to irritate the eyes and nasal passages, has excellent stability over a wide range of pH (pH 3-9), does not require exposure monitoring and has a barely perceptible odour. Like glutaraldehyde, it has excellent material compatibility. A potential disadvantage is that it stains proteins grey (including unprotected skin) and hence must be handled with caution. Data also indicates that OPA will last longer before reaching its minimum effective concentration limit (about 82 cycles compared to 40 of glutaraldehyde). But, OPA disposal is restricted, glycine can be used to neutralize the OPA and make it safe for disposal.[11]

Superoxidized Water

The concept of electrolyzing saline to create a disinfectant is used here because the basic materials (saline and electricity) are cheap and the end product (water) is not damaging to the environment. A commercial adaptation of this process (Sterilox) is available in the UK. The mode of action is not clear but probably relates to a mixture of oxidizing species. The main products are hypochlorous acid at a concentration of approximately 144mg/L and free chlorine radicals. This disinfectant is generated at the point of use by passing a saline solution over titanium-coated electrodes at 9 amps. The product generated has a pH of 5.0–6.5 and an oxidation reduction potential of >950mV. Equipment to produce the product may be expensive because parameters such as pH, current and redox potential must be closely monitored. The solution has been shown to be non-toxic to biological tissues.

The antimicrobial activity of this new sterilant has been tested against bacteria, mycobacteria, viruses, fungi and spores. Data have shown that freshly generated superoxidized water is rapidly effective (<2 minutes) in achieving a 5 log 10 reduction of pathogenic microorganisms (*Mycobacterium tuberculosis, M.chelonae*, poliovirus, HIV, MRSA, *E.coli*,Candida, *Enterococcus faecalis*, Pseudomonas) in the absence of organic loading. However, the biocidal activity of this disinfectant was substantially reduced in the presence of organic material (5% horse serum). Additional studies are needed to determine if this solution may be used as an alternative to other disinfectants.[12, 13]

Table 15.5: Biological indicators used in various processes

Sterilization method	Biological indicator used	Frequency of usage	Remarks
Steam (Autoclave)	*Bacillus stearothermophilus* spores	Daily	For implantables test with each load
Gaseous sterilization	*Bacillus subtilis* (Fort Detrick strain)	Daily	
Ethylene oxide (EO) or dry-heat sterilization	*Bacillus subtilis/var niger/var globigii* spore	Every load Daily	
Low temp. H_2O_2	*Bacillus subtilis* spore	Daily	
Hot air oven	Atoxigenic strain of *Clostridium tetani*	Daily	
Ionizing radiation	*Bacillus pumilis*	Daily	

Endoclens

This is a new automated endoscope-reprocessing system designed to provide rapid, automated, point-of-use chemical sterilization of flexible endoscopes and consists of a computer controlled endoscope-reprocessing machine and a new, proprietary liquid sterilant that uses performic acid. The sterilant is produced, as needed, by the machine, by automatic mixing of the two component solutions of hydrogen peroxide and formic acid. This sterilant is fast acting against spore-forming bacteria. The system's major features are an automatic cleaning process, capability to process two flexible scopes asynchronously, automated channel blockage and leak detection, filter water rinsing and scope drying after sterilization, hard copy documentation of key process parameters, user-friendly machine interface and total cycle time less than 30 minutes. The reprocessor can also be disinfected automatically to prevent infection or pseudoinfection.

During washing, enzymatic detergent is automatically dispensed, diluted with warm water (45°C), and sprayed onto the exterior of the endoscope surfaces and pumped through the endoscope lumens, with alternating pulses of compressed air to assist in removing any adhering material. The total cycle time for scope testing, washing, sterilization and drying is less than 30 minutes. Upon completion of each cycle, the reprocessor prints a hard-copy record, as well as retaining a record in memory, accessible through its floppy disk drive.

Attest Ethylene Oxide (EO) Rapid Readout

This is a new, rapid readout EO biological indicator, designed for rapid and reliable monitoring of EO sterilization. Biological monitors are always recommended because, unlike chemical indicators, they measure the sterilization process directly by using the most resistant microorganism (e.g. *B.subtilis*), not by merely testing the physical and chemical conditions necessary for the sterilization.

The new rapid readout EO biological indicator will indicate an EO sterilization process failure by producing a fluorescent change, which is detected in an auto-reader within 4 hours of incubation at 37°C, and a visual pH colour change of the growth media within 96 hours of continued incubation. The rapid readout EO biological indicator detects the presence of *B.subtilis* by detecting the activity of an enzyme present within the *B.subtilis* organism, beta-glucosidase. The fluorescence indicates the presence of active spore-associated enzyme and a sterilization process failure.[14]

The rapid readout EO biological indicator can be used to monitor 100% EO, EO-chlorofluorocarbons and EO-hydro chlorofluorocarbon mixture sterilization cycles. The self-contained design (i.e, it contains both the spore strip and growth media) of the indicator makes it easy to use in the department where the sterilizer is located. If a hospital could quarantine the load for the 4 hour readout, the need for recalls of potentially nonsterile packages and for informing physicians about the use of nonsterile medical devices could be eliminated. New indicator technologies such as the rapid readout EO biological indicators are likely to improve patient safety.[15]

Sterrad 50

This is a new hydrogen peroxide plasma sterilizer. It contains a single shelf for placement of instruments to be sterilized within a rectangular chamber. The sterilization cycle is 45 minutes, and it sterilizes even the smallest-lumened device, which is 1mm in diameter. It has two hydrogen peroxide vapor-diffusion stage-plasma cycles and is initiated by pulling a vacuum to remove air and water. A small amount of concentrated hydrogen peroxide in aqueous solution is then injected from a cassette, which is then vapourized and dispersed throughout the chamber and load. Radio waves then create an electric field, which generates a gas plasma from the hydrogen peroxide. These free radicals destroy microorganisms present on clean, dry accessible surfaces. The process is repeated and finally, the chamber is restored to atmospheric pressure by introducing filtered air.[16]

Gas Plasma Process over Ethylene Oxide

Advantages

- Shorter duration
- Aeration is unnecessary
- No toxic emissions/residues

Disadvantages

- Special adapters are required for lumened devices.
- Not suited for long narrow-lumened devices closed at one end
- Certain materials, like cellulose, instruments with bisphenol and epoxy coatings or components made of polysulphones or polyurethane, tend to absorb hydrogen peroxide, preventing the normal pressure changes during a cycle and thus aborting it.
- Requires the use of compatible packaging
- If items are not thoroughly clean and dry, the cycle will abort.

STERILIZATION PROCEDURES FOR SPECIAL ORGANISMS

Human Immunodeficiency Virus (HIV)

The AIDS-causing virus, HIV, is not a particularly resistant microorganism. Yet, it is considered in isolation because AIDS is a condition without any cure, and so prevention is the only recourse. Thus, one needs to know what measures can be adopted to inactivate the virus. It has been found that the HIV virus is inactivated by almost all the disinfectants used normally and in much lower concentrations. Thus, 25% ethanol or 1% glutaraldehyde is sufficient to inactivate this virus. Also, freshly prepared solution of 500 to 5000 ppm sodium hypochlorite (0.5%), formalin, hydrogen peroxide, ethyl/isopropyl alcohols, Lysol, NP-40 detergent, chlorhexidine gluconate and quarternary ammonium chlorides.

Legionella Pneumophila

Legionella pneumophila can cause HAI in the form of respiratory infections. The bacteria is susceptible to chlorine, heat (60^0–80^0C), ozone and UV light. It is to be remembered here that Legionella bacteria is often capable of living inside cells of Entamoeba, which in turn would affect its susceptiblity to disinfectants.

Hepatitis B Virus (HBV)

Standard sterilization and disinfection procedures for patient care equipment are adequate to sterilize or disinfect instruments or devices contaminated with blood or other body fluids from persons infected with HBV. Persons cleaning spills should wear disposable gloves and other personal protective equipment as indicated.

Slow Viruses and Prions

Prion diseases, such as Creutzfeldt-Jakob disease (CJD), represent a unique infection control problem because prions exhibit an unusual resistance to conventional chemical and physical decontamination methods. Following epidemiological studies of prion transmission, the infectivity of human tissues and the efficacy of removing microbes, recommendations have been made for prion-specific disinfection/sterilization. Such techniques however, are required only in limited settings, because blood or blood products have not been demonstrated to be vehicles for transmission.[17]

Only critical (e.g. surgical instruments) and semicritical devices contaminated with high-risk tissue (i.e., brain, spinal cord, eye) from high risk patients (e.g. with known or suspected CJD) require special treatment. Such items must be steam sterilized for at least 30 minutes, at a temperature of 132°C (121°C is not effective) in a gravity displacement sterilizer. A prevacuum sterilizer used for 18 minutes at 134°C to 138°C has also been found to be effective. Immersion in 1 N sodium hydroxide for 1 hour at room temperature followed by steam sterilization at 121°C for 30 minutes is an alternative. Non-critical items and surfaces (e.g. tables, floors) may be disinfected with either bleach (1:10 dilution) or 1 N sodium hydroxide at room temperature for 15 minutes or less. A formalin-formic acid mixture is required for inactivating infectivity in tissue samples from patients with CJD.[18]

Selection of a disinfectant depends on several factors

- Purpose for which it is used
- Properties of the disinfectant—like mechanism and spectrum of activity
- Whether the disinfectant is affected by the presence of organic matter
- Compatibility with surfaces and equipment on which it is used
- Effect on safety of personnel
- Cost factor

Points to be stressed in the use of disinfectants

1. Correct disinfectant and its optimal concentration
2. Type of container to be used
3. Frequency with which the solution is to be changed
4. Substances/ materials which will neutralize the disinfectant
5. Duration for which it must be stored. Working solutions must be prepared each day.
6. Not to mix/disinfectants/other cleaning solutions

7. Facilitate the process of disinfection by decreasing bioburden by cleaning and reduction of the organic material.
8. Adequate exposure should be ensured by allowing overnight exposure at room temperature.
9. List of risks and measures required for protection (personnel safety measures)
10. Policy to ensure that the solution continues to be effective by adding process-monitoring and chemical estimation of concentration if possible
11. Details of all precautions for use from the manufacturers while supplying the disinfectant
12. Mandatory annual review of policies
13. Training of personnel in every institution
14. Disinfection policy and the type of disinfectants/sterilants to be used by HICC
15. Choose a disinfectant for a specific purpose.
16. Should be able to destroy tubercle bacilli

STEPS FOR STERILIZATION AND DISINFECTION

1. List your equipment.
2. Classify each according to Spaulding's classification-single patient use (disposable) or reprocessable
3. Understand minimum and maximum standards. According to literature, manufacturer's recommedations, local hospital policy and cost considerations.
4. Finally, state Standard Operating Procedure (SOP) for each equipment.

1. List your Equipment (ICU, anaesthetic, surgical equipment)

Diagnostic equipment

1. Auroscope/ophthalmoscope
2. Portable ECG
3. Portable X-ray machine
4. Neuro-diagnostic equipment
5. Blood gas machine
6. Glucometer
7. Portable ultrasound machine
8. Portable ECHO machine

Procedural equipment

1. Emergency cart
2. Emergency drugs
3. Ventilators with nebulizers, humidifiers
4. Noninvasive ventilation equipment
5. High-frequency ventilators
6. Nitric oxide delivery and monitoring equipment
7. Infusion pumps
8. Defibrillators/cardiovertors
9. Portable suction

Hand ventilating assemblies

1. AMBU bags (adult, paediatric)
2. Mapleson's anaesthesia bag with circuit
3. T-piece

Monitoring equipment

1. Transducers
2. Doppler
3. Rectal thermometer
4. Glass thermometer
5. Non-invasive blood pressure monitoring equipment
6. Bed weighing scale
7. Oxygen analyzer
8. Portable monitor
9. Pulse oximeter
10. End tidal carbon dioxide monitor and connections
11. ECG machine
12. Respirator
13. Arterial pressure measurement equipment
14. Central venous pressure catheters
15. Intracranial pressure monitoring device
16. Neurophysiological monitoring equipment

Airway management equipment

1. Laryngoscope
2. Endotracheal tubes
3. Anatomical masks
4. Laryngeal masks
5. Intubating flexible scopes

Drug delivery systems

1. Nebulizers
2. Oxygen delivery devices
   - Rebreathing masks
   - Nasal cannulae
   - Non-rebreathing masks
   - Oxygen hood
   - Oxygen portable cylinders
3. Nasogastric tubes
4. Vascular access equipment
   - Inter-osseous needles
   - Multi-lumen central catheters
   - IV cannula
   - Needles and syringes

Warming and lighting equipment

1. Heating and cooling blanket
2. Overhead warmer
3. Bilirubin light (phototherapy unit)
4. Procedure light (portable)

Airway access equipment

1. Bronchoscopes
2. Gum elastic bougies

Transport equipment

Special equipment

1. Haemodialysis
2. Intra-aortic balloon pump

Chest drainage equipment

- Tray
- Bottles
- Tubes
- Wall-mounted suction and portable suction

Paediatric equipment

- Incubators—open and closed
- Cribs
- Beds
- Feeding equipment
- Bedside chair
- IV poles
- Procedure stool
- Clocks
- TV
- Toys
- Breast pump
- Infant weighing machine

Controversies in Standards Used, e.g. Laryngoscope

Laryngoscopy is an invasive procedure involving contact with blood, mucous membrane and saliva. The laryngoscope, if not cleaned and decontaminated, has the potential to transmit nosocomial infections not only to other patients but also to the user. A laryngoscope is therefore, according to the Spaulding's classification, an instrument which is categorized somewhere between a semicritical and a critical instrument, (breaches mucous membranes). Should it be 'sterilized' or just 'decontaminated' or 'disinfected' as is usually done? There is enough evidence to show that there is need for sterilization of laryngoscopes.[19-24]

1. Cultures have been grown from laryngoscopes, which include *Listeria monocytogenes* and *Pseudomonas aeruginosa.*
2. Handles are also a source of infection, as 50% of them have been tested for occult blood. This could mean HIV, HCV, HBV transmission.
3. Simple soap and water washing does not eliminate bacterial contaminants effectively.
4. Disinfecting with betadine and hibiscrub are considered unacceptable.
5. Most hospitals do not have a policy for sterilizing the laryngoscope.
6. Emerging threats such as the Creutzfeldt-Jakob disease in some countries are forcing a relook at the sterilization procedures.

There are a number of reasons for non-sterilization of the laryngoscopes:

1. Lack of awareness about infection control protocols.
2. Lack of infection control policy for anaesthetic equipment
3. Shortage of laryngoscopes. There is generally an inadequate number of laryngscopes to cope with the high turnover of cases and there is no time in between cases to adequately sterilize the laryngoscopes.
4. Fear of damage to laryngoscopes. The bulbs of the laryngoscopes undergo degradation and become dimmer with autoclaving and this leads to a fear in the minds of the anaesthesiologists that their equipment will not be replaced if damaged. There is also fear that the rubber washer in the handle may get damaged if autoclaved repeatedly.

5. Inadequate sterilization facilities or overloaded facilities. Most smaller centres do not have the facility to autoclave/sterilize equipment other than the surgical equipment.
6. Cutting costs. The cost of additional laryngoscopes, sterilizing agents and the cost of prophylactic treatment for accidental exposure are considered expensive or a waste by most hospital administrators/ managers/ heads of departments and, often, there is no fund allocated for this, unless they see a threat of litigation.
7. Use of improper methods of decontamination. This includes methods such as a betadine or a hibiscrub wash. These are ineffective in sterilizing.

Practice of cleaning and decontamination of laryngoscopes[19]

1. There should be a written-down policy for sterilizing anaesthetic instruments which is accepted by the department and the hospital infection control committee. It should include the steps of decontamination, the agents and procedures to be used and the precautions to be taken by the staff, e.g. precautions during handling of gluteraldehyde.
2. While ordering laryngoscopes, knowledge of the decontamination procedures recommended by the company should be known. E.g. the number of times the laryngoscope can be autoclaved, etc. The details of the laryngoscope (whether bulb type or the fiberoptic variety), must be known. The fiberoptic bundles do not tolerate autoclaving very well and the light gets dimmer/ degraded with repeated autoclaving. The number of autoclavings tolerated are mentioned by the manufacturer. In the bulb type, the bulb can be detached and the blade can be autoclaved. The details of decontaminating the handle also needs to be ascertained from the manufacturer. Sometimes the handle has a rubber washer which may not tolerate autoclaving. Also, they are not often watertight and the handle can get damaged due to leakage of the disinfectant into it. Presently there are companies that specify these details.
3. The decontamination procedure should begin with washing and clearing of debris and organic matter. This includes detachment of the blade from the handle before cleaning and decontamination.
4. The next step is to dry the laryngoscope for 10 minutes before subjecting it to decontamination.
5. The following are methods which can be used (varying standards), the pros and cons are discussed below:

a) Chemical methods: These can be used in high turnover theatres where autoclaving and ethyleneoxide are difficult to use due to shortage of laryngoscopes. Gluteraldehyde (2–3.2%) is the most commonly used method, although its efficacy is controversial. There is also an exposure of patients and staff to the harmful effects of residual gluteraldehyde. The most important of these are the allergies, colitis and proctitis due to gluteraldehyde in patients in whom there was improper reprocessing or removal of the disinfectant. Detailed precautions and regulations are given by OSHA for occupational health exposures. The handles with improper washers can leak and there may be internal damage to the battery holding chamber. The standard time of disinfection followed is 20–30 minutes and this is classified only as disinfection and not sterilization. Also, this process does not eliminate tubercle bacilli. An alternative method recommended is a 70% alcohol dip for an adequate period of time.

b) Autoclave: This is an effective method with a processing time of 1–2 hours. This brings in a time constraint in centres with inadequate number of laryngoscopes. It is easier in theatres with an autoclaving machine inside the theatre complex. Damage to laryngoscope fibre-optic bundles is to be taken into consideration, after a certain number of uses. Handles cannot be autoclaved unless specified by the manufacturer and this is a great disadvantage as both need to be sterilized.

c) Ethylene oxide: This needs 6–8 hours for a cycle (aeration and de-aeration). It is suitable for sterilizing the laryngoscopes overnight. Many large hospitals with an adequate stock of laryngoscopes have switched over to this method of sterilization. (40–50 laryngoscopes used daily). Since there is no pressure for time, all the laryngoscopes are 'gassed' (blades and handles) at night. This is the safest method and does not involve damage to the metal, bulb or washer.

d) Use of disposable laryngoscopes: This came along in a big way after the detection of prions (causative agents of 'mad cow disease') from the tonsillar bed. These prions are not sterilized by standard sterilizing procedures such as autoclaving and ethylene-oxide and require sodium hydroxide (NaOH) for sterilization (CDC guidelines). Disposable laryngoscopes are available from some manufacturers at an affordable price. These single-use laryngoscopes can also be used in other infective cases e.g. HIV. This would protect other patients and the staff. So, there may be a genuine cause in opting for disposable laryngoscopes in certain instances.[20-24]

Therefore, the standards to be followed in a centre need to be specified after understanding the various constraints.

CLEARLY STATE PLAN (SOP)

Specify Minimum and Maximum Standards, Specify SOPs and Validation

CRITICAL ITEMS

Item	**Recommended practice**
1. Vascular needles	Disposable
2. Catheters (CVP, arterial, Swan sheaths, Swan ganz)	Disposable
3. Regional block needles	Disposables/ ETO
4. Associated tubings and connectors	Disposable
5. Syringes	Disposable
Change over to another patient	No
6. Urinary catheters	Disposable
7. Transducers	Disposable

8. Spinal Needles	Disposable
9. Epidural Needles	Disposable
10. Epidural catheters	Disposable
11. Continuous spinal catheters	Disposable

SEMICRITICAL ITEMS

(Those that touch mucous membranes, but do not penetrate body surfaces)

Item	Recommended Practice
1. Endoscopes	As per manufacturer's guidelines.
2. Laryngoscope blades	ETO/ Autoclave/ HLD (As per manufacturer's guidelines)
3. Oesophageal temperature probe	Disposable/ ETO/ Soak in Glutaraldehyde 2% for 20 minutes (HLD) (As per manufacturer's guidelines)/ ETO

NON-CRITICAL ITEMS AND THEIR DISINFECTION METHODS

BP Cuff and Tubing

Clean with detergent disinfectant (Sterilium/ Bacillocid) at the end of the day. When visibly contaminated, wash with detergent and wipe with noncorrosive disinfecant. Periodic sterilization-weekly/ETO/chemically with glutaraldehyde after infected cases (HIV, HCV, HBsAg, *M.tuberculosis*).

Stethoscopes

Clean with detergent and wipe with noncorrosive disinfectant/ETO.

Pulse Oximeter Cables and ECG Cables

Wash/wipe clean with detergent solution after every case. For known infected case, wipe with disinfectant (Sterilium/ Bacillocid), or sterilize with ETO in chamber.

Temperature Monitor Cables/ Reusable Temperature Probes

Wash/wipe clean with detergent solution after every case. For known infected case, wipe with disinfectant (Sterilium/Bacillocid), or sterilize with ETO in chamber.

Head Rings (Rubber, Plastic)

Wipe clean after every case with bacillocid and wash with water.

Soda Lime Cannister

Clean weekly with detergent germicide. Disinfect with 2% glutaraldehyde.

Unidirectional Valves

Weekly immersion.Weekly cleaning with alcohol or detergent after disassembling.

Reservoir Bag and Non-Disposable Part

Change, if soiled, and weekly autoclave.

Disposable Breathing\Tubings (Circuits)

Ethylene Oxide/Chemical disinfection (2% glutaraldehyde)/disposed of after single use.

Anaesthetic Ventilators

High level disinfection weekly/sterlization

Anatomical Face Masks

Disposable/Glutaraldehyde 2% for 20 minutes.

Gas Cylinders

Wash with water and detergent. Wipe outer surface with disinfectant before bringing into operating room.

Ventilators

a. Use heat-moisture exchangers and bacterial filters.

b. Removable internal circuit can be autoclaved.

c. Circuits are disposable/autoclavable/ sterilizable.

d. Change circuits every 48 hours if water baths are used.

e. Change circuits weekly if heat moisture exchangers are used.

Humidifiers

a. Water vapour type: Change every 48 hours. Disinfect with alcohol.

b. Nebulizers: Sterilize/disinfect with heat, daily (as per manufacturers instruction).

Mattresses

There are different mattresses marketed to prevent pressure sores in a patient. The mattress overlay (covering) with plastic is easy to clean and decontaminate and is a one-time cost. Uncovered mattresses are difficult to clean and decontaminate. If heat intolerant, use 70% alcohol.

Air Circulating Beds

Outer surface is cleaned with chlorine releasing agent.

Air sacs cleaned—machine washed at 60°C.

Internal ducting cleaning—as per manufacturer's instructions.

Water Circulating Beds

Outer cleaning: Use chlorine releasing agent

Internal: As per manufacturer's instructions.

Monitoring Equipment e.g. Neurophysiological Monitoring

Electrode Decontamination

The general trend in most places is to use

disposable electrodes as the costs have considerably reduced. However, this may not be possible in all countries and therefore, it is important to work at protocols given by important organizations such as OSET (Organisation of Societies of EEG Technologists, France) and EPTA (Electrophysiological Technologists Association). Source of guidelines for decontamination of electrodes is adapted from 'Guidelines for infection control in the clinical neurophysiology department'. http://epta.50megs.com/resources/inf.cont.pdf by permission of the OSET executive committee.

For all recordings, use only electrodes decontaminated by the standards recommended in approved guidelines. Strict adherence to this principle will make the chances very small for any cross-infection caused by clinical neurophysiology procedures.

Routine Procedures after Use

Environmental cleaning:

All surfaces should be regularly cleaned with detergent and water. For routine disinfection of the headbox or other equipment in the vicinity of patients, use disinfectant wipes (saturated with chlorhexidine gluconate solution B.P. 2.5% v/v in industrial methylated spirit B.P. 70% v/v), or hypochlorite solution (1000 ppm, available chlorine concentration 0.1%) followed 10 minutes later by a wipe with a damp cloth. Detergent and hot water or alcohol wipes are considered to be adequate by some infection-control protocols.

Additional precautions are necessary for specific procedures and infections.

Disposable gloves should be worn for all procedures.

Pad electrodes

Should be autoclaved at 134^{0}C for 18 minutes or 6 cycles of 3 minutes each.

Surface electrode

Should be washed carefully, as previously described, to reduce the amount of particulate material. They should then be sterilized by autoclave at 134^0 C for 18 minutes or 6 cycles of separate 3 minute cycles, or a hypochlorite concentration of 25,000 ppm available chlorine for 1 hour may be used.

Needle electrodes

These must be of the disposable kind and extreme care has to be exercised in disposing them. The needles should be dropped directly into a container designed for incineration or disposed of in accordance with hazardous waste protocols.

Scarifying needles are strongly discouraged. If used, they should be disposed of appropriately.

Corneal contact electrodes

Should be disposable and destroyed after a single use.

Any other material sent for disposal should be enclosed within infectious waste bags labelled with the international biohazard symbol.

Neurodiagnostic equipment and other related instruments should be wiped with detergent and water or 70–90% ethyl alcohol. If the machine is contaminated with secretions or blood, follow the documented procedure for spills of blood or body substances.

Intraoperative Considerations[25, 26, 27]

1. All used items (laryngoscopes, Mc Gill forceps, airways, etc.) should be placed in a receptacle (tray) on the anaesthesia machine. This is to separate them from the unused items. The tray may or may not contain a detergent to prevent drying of secretions. The various items placed on the tray are washed/cleaned/disposed of/ disinfected appropriately. The tray is also cleaned and disinfected at the end of the case.
2. A clean cloth should be placed at the beginning of each case for the unused items on the anaesthesia cart, to be changed after every case. The top of the anaesthesia machine should be wiped with a detergent/disinfectant at the end of the day's work.
3. Heavy duty, fluid-resistant protective gloves should be worn by technicians while carrying out disinfection procedures. A face mask should be worn as also goggles or safety glasses for eye protection.
4. Hands must be washed immediately after cleaning.
5. Once a week the equipment should be removed from the drawers and the drawers cleaned and wiped with a cloth containing disinfectant solution or a germicidal spray.

Laundry

Hospital linen may be categorized into 'clean' (less contaminated) and dirty (contaminated/ soiled with blood, pus, urine, faeces, etc.). They should be segregated and sent to the CSSD units, where they are handled as per their status. The dirty linen need to be disinfected in hot water. Use of electrically-operated washing machines is convenient and recommended, especially for the large-sized items like bedsheets and curtains.

Central Sterile Supply Department (CSSD)

This is an important unit in the hospital which receives, stores, processes, sterilizes, distributes and controls equipment from wards, out-patient departments, operating suites and other specialized units, when there is no dedicated sterilizing units in those areas. Diet, drugs, linen, bedpans and urinals are not handled by this department. The CSSD is under the supervision of a technical officer who is responsible for its day-to-day functioning.

REFERENCES

1) Favero MS. Chemical disinfection of medical and surgical materials. In: Block SS, ed. Disinfection, sterilization and preservation. 3rd ed. Philadelphia: Lea and Febiger, 1983; 469-92.
2) Rutala WA, Stiegel MM, Sarubbi FA et al. Susceptibility of antibiotic-susceptible and antibiotic-resistant hospital bacteria to disinfectants. Infect Control Hosp Epidemiol 1997; 18: 417-21.
3) Kampf G and Wendt C. Sterilization and Use of Sterile Products. In: A Guide to Infection Control in the Hospital. An official publication of the International Society for Infectious Diseases. BC Decker Inc. 1998; 13-17.

4) Rutala WA. APIC Guidelines Committee. APIC guideline for selection and use of disinfectants. Am J Infect Control 1996; 24: 313-42.

5) Fraise AP. Choosing disinfectants. J Hosp Infect 1999; 43: 255-64.

6) Keene JH. Sterilization and pasteurization. In: Mayhall CG, ed. Hospital epidemiology and infection control. Baltimore, MD: Williams and Wilkins.1996; 937-46.

7) Kaiser U. Simple method to assess efficacy of sterilization processes for hollow instruments. Zentr Steril. Jahrgang 1999; 7: 393-395.

8) Gomann J, Kaiser U and Menzel R. Air removal from porous and hollow goods using different steam sterilisation processes. Central Service; 2001; 9: 182-186.

9) Kaiser U. Simple method to assess efficacy of sterilisation processes for hollow instruments. Zentral Sterilisation. Jahrgang, 1999; 7: 393-395.

10) Rutala WA, Gergen MF and Weber DJ. Evaluation of a new surface germicide (Surfacine) with antimicrobial persistence. Infect Control Hosp Epidemiol 2000; 21: 103.

11) Walsh SE, Maillard JY and Russell AD. Ortho-phthalaldehyde: a possible alternative to glutaraldehyde for high level disinfection. J Appl Microbiol 1999; 86: 1039-46.

12) Tanaka H, Hirakata Y, Kaku M et al. Antimicrobial activity of superoxidized water. J Hosp Infect 1996; 34: 43-9.

13) Shetty N, Srinivasan S, Holton J et al. Evaluation of microbicidal activity of a new super-oxidized water, Sterilox 2500 against *Clostridium difficile* spores, *Helicobacter pylori*, vancomycin resistant Enterococcus species, *Candida albicans* and several Mycobacterium species. J Hosp Infect 1999; 41: 101-5.

14) Rutala WA, Gergen MF and Weber DJ. Evaluation of a rapid readout biological indicator for flash sterilization with three biological indicators and three chemical indicators. Infect Control Hosp Epidemiol 1993; 14: 390-4.

15) Baird RM. Sterility assurance: Concepts, methods and problems. Chapter 16. In: Fraise AP, Lambert PA, Maillard GY. Eds. Principles and practice of disinfection, preservation and sterilization. 4th edn. Blackwell Publishing 2004; 526-539.

16) Rutala WA, Gergen MF and Weber DJ. Sporicidal activity of a new low-temperature sterilization technology: the Sterrad 50 sterilizer. Infect Control Hosp Epidemiol 1999; 20: 514-16.

17) Weber DJ, Rutala WA. Managing the risk of nosocomial transmission of prion diseases. Current opinion in Infect Dis. 2002; 15(4): 421-25.

18) Fink R. Destruction of Microorganisms. In: Liberman DF, ed. Biohazards management handbook. 2nd edition. Marcel Dekker Inc. 1995; 241-269.

19) Roberts RB. Cleaning the laryngoscope blade. Canadian Anaesthetists' Society Journal. 1973; 20: 241-4.

20) Abramson AL, Gilberto E, Mullooly V, et al. Microbial adherence to disinfection of laryngoscopes used in office practice. Laryngoscope 1993; 103: 503-8

21) Fowrekar JE. The laryngoscope as a potential source of cross-infection. J Hosp Infect. 1995; 29: 315-16.

22) Philips RA and Monaghan WP. Incidence of visible and occult blood on laryngoscope blades and handles. American Association of Nur Anesth J. 1997; 65: 241-6.

23) Skilton RWH. Risks of cross infection associated with anaesthesia; cleaning

procedures for laryngoscopes – a need for Association Guidelines? Anaesthesia 1996; 51: 512-13

24) Esler MD, Baines LC, Wilkinson DJ et al. Decontamination of Laryngoscopes: a survey of national practice. Anaesth 1999; 54: 582-98.

25) Gould GW. New and emerging technologies. Chapter 13. In: Fraise AP, Lambert PA, Maillard GY. Eds. Principles and practice of disinfection, preservation and sterilization. 4th edn. Blackwell Publishing 2004; 473-483

26) Fraise AP. Decontamination of the environment and medical equipment in hospitals. Chapter 18. In: Fraise AP, Lambert PA, Maillard GY. Eds. Principles and practice of disinfection, preservation and sterilization. 4th edn. Blackwell Publishing 2004; 563-585.

27) Underwood E. Good manufacturing practice. Chapter 21. In: Fraise AP, Lambert PA, Maillard GY. Eds. Principles and practice of disinfection, preservation and sterilization. 4th edn. Blackwell Publishing 2004; 622-640.

Chapter 16

Hospital Waste Management

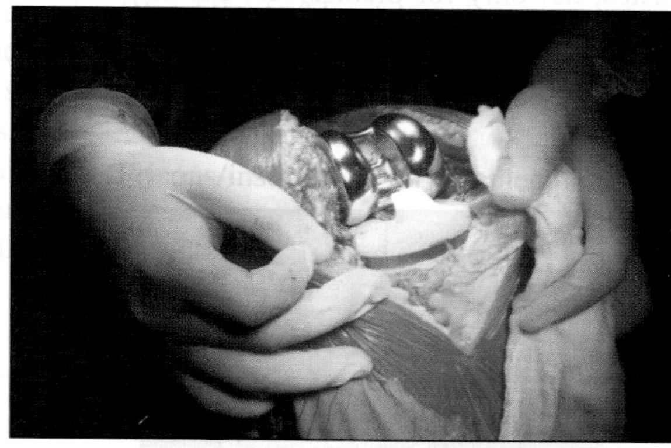

The activist is not the man who says the river is dirty. The activist is the man who cleans up the river.

—Ross Perot

Highlights

What Is Hospital/Healthcare Facility Waste?

Who or What Contributes to Wastes?

What are the Hazards to Environment and Humans due to Hospital Wastes?

Waste Management Regulation

The Principles of Effective Waste Management and Safe Waste Control

Setting up a Biomedical Waste Facility

Waste Treatment and Disposal

THE PRINCIPLES OF EFFECTIVE WASTE MANAGEMENT AND SAFE WASTE CONTROL

(FIGURE 16.2)

1. Minimize the amount of waste produced. Every effort must be made to reduce the total waste by employing more reusable items and recycling them, and by minimizing clinical waste by better segregation
2. Selection and use of materials in a judicious manner such that their disposal is possible in a safe manner
3. Using recyclable items like sterilizable glassware, stainless steel, etc.
4. Adopting a rational purchasing policy
5. Segregation of wastes in an appropriate manner
6. Appropriate management of stock

Containing Waste at the Point of Generation (Collection, Segregation and Storage)

(Photos 16.1, 16.2, 16.3)

Waste segregation is the key to waste management and helps in various ways. Waste has to be segregated into different colour-coded bags, which are also labelled with a biohazard symbol. This can be facilitated by having proper SOPs and training the healthcare workers in the whole process. The process of segregation takes into account the source, the type of disposal and the type of disinfection. Segregation is carried out inside the operating room/laboratory/intensive care/blood bank. It prevents danger to other workers and simplifies transport and disposal. The statutory

Waste generator

↓

Segregation

↓

Collection

↓

Packaging

↓

Transport

↓

Storage

↓

Treatment

↓

Disposal

↓

Maintain records/returns/accidents/follow-ups

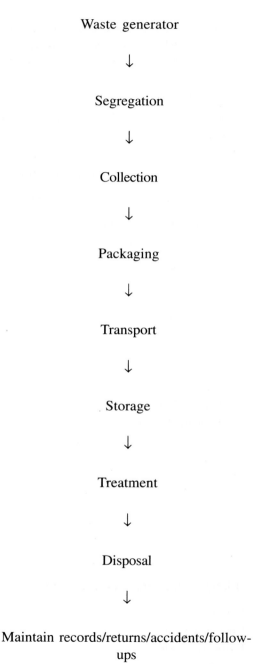

Figure 16.2: Steps of waste management

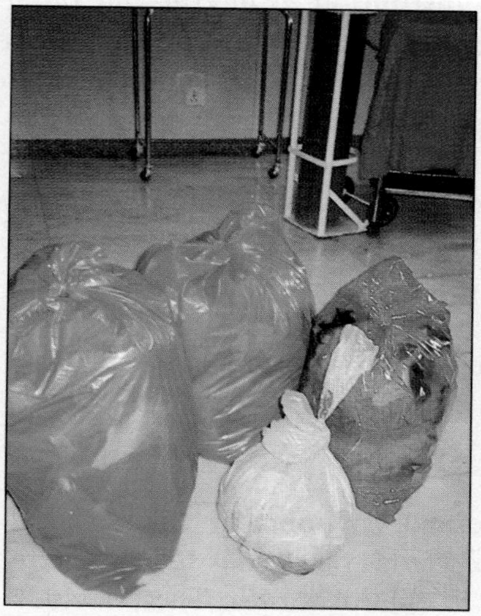

Photo 16.2: Segregation of waste into appropriate bags at source is an important step followed by sealing of bags before transport.

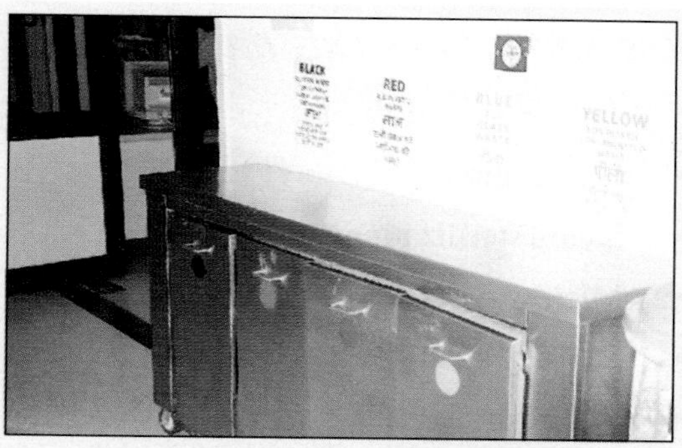

Photo 16.3: Segregation of waste in the wards

guidelines by the national board of pollution control must be followed meticulously.[5]

Waste collection must be carried out with care and with appropriate personal protective equipment. Healthcare workers who are involved in this must be educated, protected, adequately treated in case of injuries and vaccinated.

Healthcare facilities need also to be aware of the possible contamination of reusable infectious waste containers with microorganisms capable of causing nosocomial infections in patients who are compromised.[6]

SETTING UP A BIOMEDICAL WASTE FACILITY

Biomedical waste should not be generated without authorization.

All institutions generating biomedical waste should install an appropriate facility in the premises or set up a common facility in accordance with the directions given by the appropriate national authority for the purposes of granting authorization for collection, reception, storage, treatment and disposal of biomedical waste and to implement biomedical waste management rules of 1998.

Minimum on-site safety requirements for an Effluent Treatment Plant (ETP) to be set up in a hospital should also conform to strict guidelines and regulations, e.g.

- Use two lagoons (minimum) and a soil filtration bed, if no sewage treatment is to be carried out.
- Isolate enteric fever patients and disinfect excreta.
- Do not discharge chemicals and pharmaceutical items to the sewer.
- Never use hospital sewage for agriculture.
- Do not discharge to natural waters.
- Infiltrate through porous soil in small rural establishments.[7]

WASTE TREATMENT AND DISPOSAL

(FIGURE 16.3)

The Central Pollution Control Board (CPCB) in India is a national body that lays down guidelines for waste disposal by hospitals and other healthcare institutions. For example, they have set the safety limits for a water body as follows:

pH range: 6.5–9.0

Suspended solids: 100 mg/L

Oil/grease: 10 mg/L

BOD: 30 mg/L

Bioassay test: 90% survival of fish after 96 hours in 100% effluent

SEGREGATION AND COLLECTION

Pre-treatment of waste: This is done to disinfect the waste and render it non-infectious. It also reduces the bulk and facilitates transport and storage. The waste is made unrecognizable for aesthetic reasons and recyclable items are made usable.[8]

Note: It may not always be possible to assign a category to the waste item. There are some wastes that can fall into more than one category. E.g. radioactive sharps, plastic IV tubes with cytotoxics. Such wastes need to be treated first for the hazardous component and then treated as infectious metal sharps, glass, etc., and disposed of accordingly.[9]

According to CPCB, it is the responsibility of the waste 'generators' and 'operators' to make sure all waste is disposed of in a hygienic way. This is done by segregation of the waste at the source of generation itself, viz., the OTs, ICUs, wards, labour rooms, laboratories, etc. It is also very important for every institution to devise and implement an integrated biomedical waste management plan for the disinfection and treatment of the segregated waste. This is achieved in a sequential manner as shown in figure 16.2 (Of course, the first step towards handling wastes is to minimize its production as much as possible).

What are the Waste Disposal Methods Available?

(Table 16.1)

Concern for environment pollution and obligation towards society has led to several measures to control wastes. These include infectious waste incineration, water and waste water treatment plants, air pollution control equipment and lately, the microwave disinfectant system for bio-medical waste.[8, 10]

The various methods presently available include[9, 10]

- Incineration
- Steam sterilization/autoclave
- Microwaving
- Sanitary landfill
- Deep burial

Incineration refers to the process by which the waste is burnt or reduced to ashes at high temperatures. Any healthcare institution which has over 250 beds needs to have an on-site incinerator.[11] The incinerator must be located within the premises of the hospital in a convenient area, away from the main hospital, the wards and the OTs. It can be of two types: a common incinerator that is shared by two or more institutions or the individual incinerator, catering to one institution.

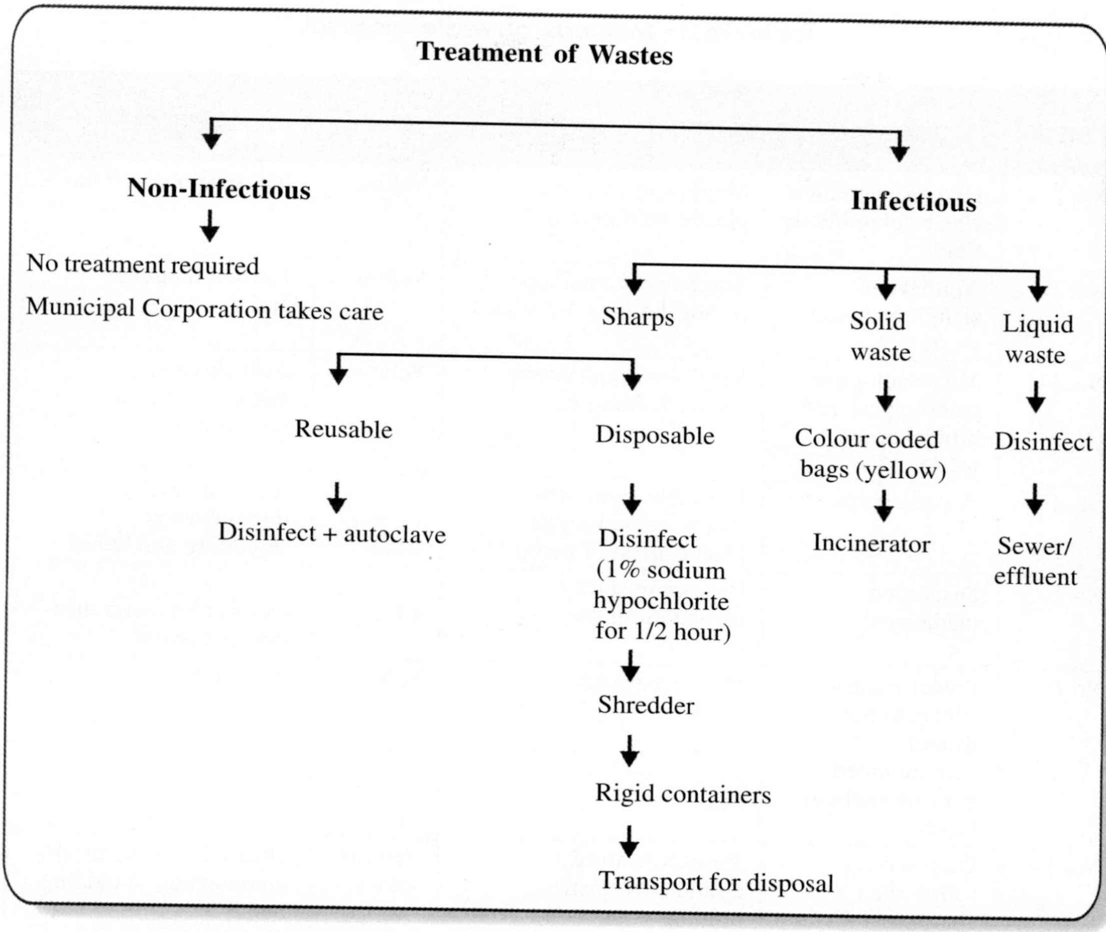

Figure 16.3: Treatment of wastes (also see Table 16.1)

The principal factors that should be considered when incinerating infectious wastes are: a) variation in waste composition, b) waste feed rate, c) combustion temperature.

The temperatures attainable in an incinerator vary between 750°C and 1050°C. Waste is burnt in the primary chamber at 800–850°C and the volatile gases emitted are again burnt in the secondary chamber at 1050°C. The cycle time for the entire operation is one hour. It is absolutely necessary to maintain these high temperaures followed immediately by quenching with water, otherwise toxic gases will be emitted.

Plastics must never be burnt in an incinerator, especially the chlorinated ones, which release toxic carcinogenic gases such as dioxins and furans.

Workers handling wastes and transporting them to the incinerator site must take

Table 16.1: Methods of waste disposal

Waste category	Waste class	Type of container	Colour coding	Treatment/Disposal option
No. 1	Human anatomical waste, blood/body fluids	Single-use containers/ plastic holding bags	Yellow	Incineration/deep burial
No. 2	Animal and slaughter house waste	Single use containers/ plastic holding bags/sacs	Yellow	Incineration/deep burial
No. 3	Microbiological, pathological and biotechnology waste.	Single-use containers/ plastic holding bags	Yellow	Autoclaving/ microwaving and incineration
No. 4	Waste sharps	Reusable/single-use sturdy containers of plastic, glass or metal	Blue	Autoclaving/ microwaving/ shredding and burial
No. 5	Discarded medicines	Re-usable/sturdy cardboard/glass/plastic	Blue	Destruction/neutralization and burial
No. 6	Soiled wastes (linen, cotton, gauze) contaminated with blood/body fluids	Plastic bags/sacs	Yellow	Incineration
No. 7	Disposables (other than sharps)	Re-usable/sturdy containers/plastic holding bags	Yellow/ Black	Disinfection-chemical/ autoclaving, shredding, burial
No.8	Infectious plastics like gloves, IV sets, tubings, catheters etc.	Plastic sturdy bags	Red	Autoclaving/ hydroclaving/ microwaving/ chemical treatment/ shredding/burial
No. 9	Liquid wastes	NA	NA	Chemical treatment and discharged into drains, if drains are connected to terminal treatment plants
No. 10	Non-infectious general waste incinerator ash	Plastic sturdy bags	Black	Municipal dump
No. 11	Chemical wastes, cyotoxic drugs	Sturdy containers/ plastic holding bags	Black	Burial/disposal in secured landfill

adequate precautions like wearing gloves, masks, goggles, etc.

The incinerator user must follow the CPCB guidelines for the same.

Incinerator ash must be removed periodically and dumped in sanitary landfills well away from the main city.

The operation and maintenance of an incinerator requires skilled personnel and proper care.

Microwave: Specially useful for non-incinerable bio-medical waste. The system employs strategically positioned twin magnetron assembly that generates microwave energy, which effects intermolecular heating within waste placed in microwave-proof moulded container.

Deep Burial: Towns having a population of less than five lakhs are permitted to use deep burial as an option for treating their infectious wastes.

The deep burial pit must be about 6.5 feet (2 metres) deep, and every time wastes are put into it, it must be covered with a layer of soil. When the pit is three-fourths full, lime is added and again covered with soil. The pit should be protected with a mesh cover to prevent entry of animals and birds.

Common waste treatment facility: This facilitates the safe collection, transportation, treatment and disposal of biomedical waste by an entepreneur, a cooperative or the government on a pay-and-use basis. Such facilities are usually established on the outskirts of the city and the wastes collected from different healthcare institutions are brought to the facility for treatment and disposal in a cold storage van.

Hazards of not complying with biomedical waste management rules

- The administrator is punishable with imprisonment for a term, which may extend up to five years or a fine which may extend to Rs. 1 lakh or both.
- If failure of compliance continues, an additional fine of up to Rs. 5000 for each day of failure to comply may be imposed after the conviction for the first such failure or contravention.
- If failure of compliance continues beyond a period of one year, the person shall be punishable for a term (imprisonment), which may extend up to 7 seven years.

Monitoring of waste disposal methods

- Use of biological indicators, e.g. resistant bacterial spores
- Use of chemical indicators

Do's and Don'ts for Clinical Practice

A doctor who is generating the waste is himself responsible for safe disposal of it. He should not mix infectious and non-infectious waste and must follow the use of colour-coded bags for segregation. He should always observe standard precautions during invasive procedures like contact with blood, body fluid and tissue.[12]

Do's for hospital waste management

- Segregate waste at the point of generation

- Collect waste in colour-coded bags
- Train all HCWs in waste disposal
- Decontaminate all gloves, sharps and plastic waste
- Shred plastic waste
- Incinerate body parts, animal carcasses, blood-soaked dressings
- Autoclave blood bags, blood soaked dressings, cultures and biotechnology waste
- Use recyclable/reusable items as far as possible
- Cover all waste collection containers
- Transport waste through covered trolleys
- Provide protective wear to transporters and handlers
- Immunize all waste handlers

Don'ts for handling and disposal of hospital waste

- Never mix the infectious with the non-infectious waste.
- Do not throw sharps in the trash or into non-puncture-proof containers/bags.
- Never recap the needles or bend or break needles by hand.
- Do not fill the waste container to more than three-fourths of its capacity.
- Do not allow unauthorized persons access to waste collection/storage areas.
- Do not use open buckets for infectious waste or sharps
- Do not incinerate plastic waste

Do's and Don'ts for chemical treatment

Do's

- Do treat sharps and infected plastic ware with chemicals.[13]
- Do use 1% hypochlorite or equivalent disinfectant. Proper concentration is essential.
- Do ensure all surfaces come in contact with chemical (including lumen).
- Do let the contact time be at least 30 minutes.
- Do change chemical solutions frequently (with every shift).
- Do handle with gloves and mask. Wear apron and boots if splashing is expected.

Don'ts

- Do not chemically treat incinerable waste

Keeping Track (Records)

The State Pollution Control Board requires that a report be made, which includes the various categories of waste generated, as also the quantity generated daily on an average. The air and water forms are also to be filled. Records related to generation, collection, reception, storage, transportation, treatment, disposal and/or any form of handling of biomedical waste are subject to inspection and verification at any time. Any accident occurring at any institution or at the treatment/disposal site should be recorded in the stipulated form. Payment of authorization fee should be prompt and regular.[14] When wastes are managed efficiently, there are several benefits the institution enjoys:

- Reduced incidence of hospital acquired infections
- Rag pickers and other miscreants are discouraged and hence fewer dangers to community health
- Several occupational hazards are minimized.
- Reduction in the cost of infection control, the benefits of which can be reaped by putting money to better use[14]

Definitions of Relevant Terms

Airborne waste: Particles and gases discharged in the air by way of an incinerator stack or a facility exhaust fan

Liquid waste: Waste in liquid form from hospitals that may contain microbiological pathogens, hazardous chemicals, pharmaceuticals or radioactive isotopes. These should conform to the standards laid down.

Solid waste: Items contaminated with blood and other body fluids, cotton, dressings, plaster casts, linen, bedding and other items

Infectious waste: Waste that is positively identified as having the capability of transmitting infection

Isolation waste: All waste generated by a patient who has been placed on isolation precaution

Biohazard waste (biomedical waste) (BMW): Often used synonymously with infectious waste. Such waste may be found in research or clinical laboratories, as well as biological defence installations. Also includes waste from microbiology and biotechnology laboratories. Sometimes called as Regulated Medical Waste (RMW).

Potentially infectious waste (PIW): 'Potential' for transmitting infections. This term is used synonymously with 'infectious waste'.

Pathological waste: Waste from pathological services—tissue, gross specimen and limbs

Chemical waste: Liquid and solid chemicals used in production of biologicals, chemicals generated from laboratories, solvents, disinfectants, surfactants, insecticides, pesticides and contaminated containers. These should be pretreated and discharged into drains. The solids should be disposed of in secured landfills. Their containers should be mutilated and disposed of to discourage their reuse for storing water or food

Cytotoxic waste: Includes anti-neoplastic drugs, which inhibit cell growth and multiplication. Catatonics cannot be dispensed of in bulk quantities in incinerators, although small quantities can be incinerated or sterilized and landfilled in engineered landfills.

General waste: Waste categories such as those emanating from office and food services which present no potential hazard and require no special handling procedures. These may be dry (e.g. paper, plastic packaging and metal containers) or wet (leftover food, vegetable/fruit peels, meat, fish, floor sweepings, etc). These are neither infectious nor contaminated and hence can be segregated and recycled. The wet type can be planned for careful composting and manure formation.

Medical waste: Waste generated by a medical facility (not synonymous with potentially infectious waste)

Regulated Medical waste: Waste generated from medical facility, subject to regulation (radioactive, chemical, potentially infectious)

Sewage: General term used to refer to all waste discharged into sanitary services

Radioactive waste: Waste generated in radiotherapy units and radiological departments. The Bhabha Atomic Research Centre (BARC) lays down regulations for such waste disposal. The radioactive waste must be stored in lead containers until 10 times the half-life is over before disposing. Expired radioactive needles like cobalt needles used in cancer therapy can be returned to BARC in appropriate containers. Liquid radioactive waste can be discharged into the drains after the half-life is over.

Anatomical waste: Human tissues, organs and body parts

Segregation: It is the separation of waste into different categories and the treatment of each category appropriately to ensure complete sterilization and recycling.

Animal waste: Animal tissues, organs, body parts, carcasses used for experiments in research, veterinary hospitals, colleges and animal houses

Waste sharps: Needles, syringes, scalpels, blade, broken glass, etc.

Metal Sharps Manager: Device for separating the needles from syringes. It has a protected opening for dropping the blades, canula, needles and scalpels. The machine mutilates and sterilizes all metal sharps with dry heat in a hot air oven.

Needle cutter: It is a mechanical device consisting of a container with a blade. The blade cuts the nozzle of the syringe and also the base of the needle, thus ensuring that both the needle and the syringe are mutilated and hence cannot be reused. Care should be taken to minimize the production of aerosols/droplets during the cutting procedure.

Needle destroyer: A device with an exposed filament wherein the circuit is completed when a needle is inserted. This generates a high temperature electric arc which burns the needle. There is also a cutter to cut the nozzle of the syringe.

Plastic shredder: A device which mechanically mutilates disposable syringes and other disinfected plastic items into small unrecognizable pieces.

Microwave: Here, high frequency microwaves cause molecules within the waste to vibrate, generating heat from within. This heat is sufficient to ensure that all microbes are killed. Microwaves are introduced in special treatment chambers which evenly heat the waste to temperatures between 97°C and 100°C. The residence time is 45 mins.

Incinerator: Incineration refers to the process by which the waste is burnt or reduced to ashes. The device which performs this function is called an incinerator.[11]

Autoclave: A device for sterilizing items. The principle of autoclave is the use of steam under pressure. Gravity flow autoclaves do not include a vacuum cycle to purge the autoclave of air before sterilization whereas the pre-vacuum ones do. If the temperature achieved is 135°C, the residence time should be 30 mins, and if the temperature achieved is 121°C, the residence time should be 45 mins.

Effluent Treatment Plant (ETP): Treats liquid waste generated as a result of laboratory services, washing, cleaning, disinfection. The following processes are used:

- Pre-chlorination
- Grease-trapping
- Sedimentation
- Sand filtration
- Post-chlorination
- Oxidation

Waste water treated in this manner can be used for irrigating gardens.

Hydroclave: Offers a remarkably simple, affordable and proven medical waste treatment process that achieves high waste sterility at a very low treatment cost.

Advantages:

1. Totally sterilizes the waste (not just disinfection)
2. Treats all infectious waste, even bulk, and liquid and pathological wastes
3. There is complete waste dehydration, even of liquid waste
4. Handles large weight and there is volume reduction of waste
5. It is a low temperature steam process
6. There are no harmful emissions
7. Very low operating costs

It consists of a sturdy container with powerful rotators to mix the waste and break it into pieces. Steam fills the double wall (jacket) of the vessel and heats the vessel interior.

REFERENCES

1) Rutala WA and Mayhall CG. SHEA position paper: medical waste. Infec Cont Hosp Epidemiol 1992; 13: 38.
2) Ayliffe GAJ. Clinical waste: how dangerous is it? Current opinion in Infectious Diseases 1994; 7: 499-502.
3) Hedrick ER. Infectious waste management: Will science prevail? Infect Cont Hosp Epidemiol. 1989; 9: 488-490
4) Moritz JM. Current legislation covering clinical waste. J Hosp Infect 30 (suppl): 1995: 521-530.
5) Rutala W: Management of infectious waste by US hospitals. JAMA , 1989; 262(12): 1635-40.
6) Neely AN, Maley MP and Taylor GL. Investigation of single-use versus reusable infectious waste containers as potential sources of microbial contamination. Am J Infect Control. 2003; 31(1): 13-7.
7) Daschner FD and Dettenkofer M. Protecting the patient and the environment – new aspects and challenges in hospital infection control. J Hosp Infect 1997; 36: 7-15.
8) Boyland JL and Liberman DF. Infectious/ Medical Waste Management. In: Liberman DF, ed. Biohazards management handbook. 2nd edn. Marcel Dekker Inc. 1995; 275-309.
9) Blenkharn JI. The disposal of clinical wastes. J Hosp Infect. 1995; 30 (Suppl): 514-520.
10) Collins CH. Decontamination. Chapter 7. In: Laboratary acquired infections. 3rd edn. Butterworth Heinemann 1993; 121-33.
11) US environment protection agency. Medical waste management and disposal. Chapter 6. In: Medical waste treatment methods. Noyes Data Corporation 1991; 108-20
12) Kim KM, Kim MA, Chung YS et al. Knowledge and performance of the universal precautions

by nursing and medical students in Korea. Am J Infect Control. 2001; 29 (5): 295-300.

13) Hatcher IB. Reducing sharps injuries among healthcare workers: a sharps container quality improvement project. Jt Comm J Qual Improv. 2002; 28 (7): 410-4.

14) Bradley CR. Treatment of laundry and clinical waste in hospitals. Chapter 19. In: Fraise AP, Lambert PA, MaillardGY. Eds. Principles and practice of disinfection, preservation and sterilization. 4th edn. Blackwell Publishing 2004; 586-594

Chapter 17

Microbial Pathogens

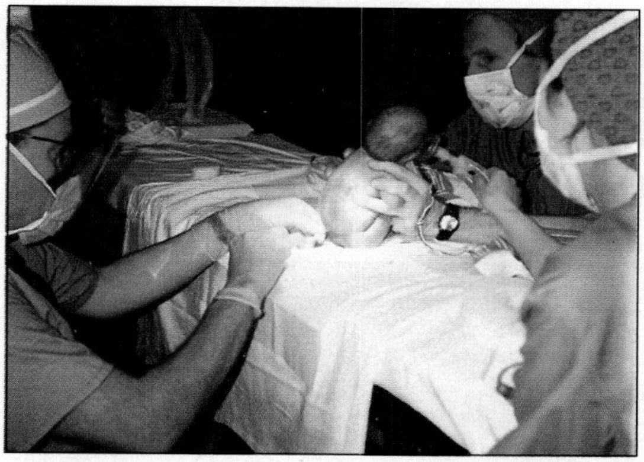

The principal element in biosafety is the inculcation of sound microbiological practices in both microbiologists and non-microbiologists.

—Dr J. E. M. Whitehead

Highlights

Bacteria
Bacteria of Special Relevance in the Hospital Setting
VISA (GISA)
MRSA
Vancomycin-Resistant Enterococcus (VRE)
Drug-Resistant *Streptococcus Pneumoniae* (DRSP)
Multi-Drug-Resistant Tuberculosis (MDR-TB)
Coagulase Negative Staphylococcus (CoNS)
Viruses
Fungal Infections
Parasites
Prions
Quick Glance

INTRODUCTION

HAI-causing pathogens are organisms which are quite the same as those causing community acquired infections. The big difference here is that the nosocomial pathogens are mostly the ones that have acquired resistance to several of the antimicrobial drugs used in routine practice (Photo 17.1). That is why special strategies are adopted in the prevention, diagnosis, management and treatment of infections caused by these pathogens as compared to community acquired ones.

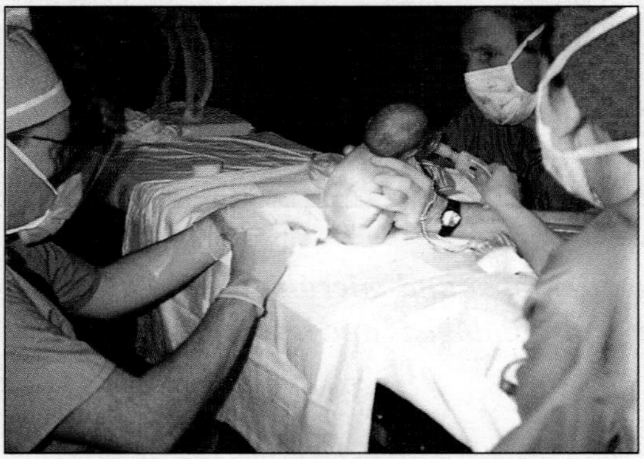

Photo 17.1: Spinal anaesthesia in a preterm neonate. Specific procedure and specific sites may carry unique infective risks.

Why Learn about HAI Pathogens?

A knowledge of HAI pathogens has the following advantages:

a. Facilitates accurate identification and thus assists diagnosis
b. Helps formulate preventive methodologies
c. Leads to specific/correct treatment
d. Aids in containment of outbreaks by adoption of preventive measures (like specific transmission-based precautions, vaccines and immune sera)
e. Facilitates surveillance, screening and early reporting of changes in susceptibility patterns and antimicrobial resistance to conventionally used drugs
f. Streamlines sample collection strategies, e.g. deciding when to culture surfaces, walls, etc. in OTs, ICUs and other key areas
g. Helps in tracing sources of infections: Epidemiological studies for typing of organisms
h. Allows participation in Internal and External Quality Assurance Programmes

Role of the Microbiology Laboratory

The microbiology laboratory plays a crucial role in the management of these infections and helps to make special changes in the diagnosis, monitoring and treatment of HAI. It contributes in:

1. Accurate identification of organisms
2. Timely reporting of laboratory data
3. Providing support for investigations
4. Offering recommendations for routine performance and periodic sampling of personnel and environment, e.g.
   a. Monitoring of steam sterilization (ethylene-oxide sterilizers, dry-heat sterilizers)
   b. Elective environmental monitoring (surveys for specific problems of patient infection or educational services)
   c. Sampling of infant feed formulas or high-risk hospital prepared products

d. Specifying procedures not recommended for routine monitoring
   - Routine cultures of patients or hospital personnel
   - Routine cultures of commercial products labelled as sterile
   - Routine testing of disinfectants and sterilants
   - Routine culture of blood units
   - Routine monitoring of disinfection process for respiratory therapy equipment[1]

Organisms causing HAI include the following:

Bacteria

Viruses

Fungi

Protozoa

Helminths

Prions

BACTERIA

Gram-Positive Cocci

***Staphylococcus aureus*:** This bacteria is shed from skin, perineum and nares. The presence of skin lesions leads to an increased spread in the hospital set-up.

***Streptococcus pyogenes*:** It is commonly shed from upper respiratory tract by the acts of coughing, sneezing or singing.

Streptococcus pneumoniae: It is usually an endogenous infection and isolation of patient is not necessary except for the first 1–2 days of treatment. Gram's stain of the sputum is a simple but important exercise in establishing the diagnosis. Nowadays, development of resistance to penicillin and other groups of drugs has increased the mortality. An effective way to prevent this condition would be to protect the host (especially elderly patients) with a polyvalent vaccine.

Other Gram-positive bacteria include Enterococcus spp and Coagulase negative Staphylococcus (CoNS), (which are opportunistic pathogens).

Gram-Negative Cocci

These are relatively rare in hospitals, e.g. *Neisseria meningitidis* is commonly a community acquired infection and can spread when a patient is admitted to a hospital. Therefore, the first 48 hours of treatment often requires isolation of the patients. For staff who are closely associated with the patient, a course of prophylactic antibiotics is recommended. A vaccine is also available for this infection.

Gram-Negative Bacilli

The introduction of penicillin saw a decrease in the Gram-positive infections and an emergence of Gram-negative infections. E.g. *Pseudomonas aeruginosa*—a common cause of infection in patients with undefended tissue, as in burns. Here, the spread is more by contact than by air route. Patient isolation and other routine precautions may be necessary. *Escherichia coli, Klebsiella, Proteus spp, Enterobacter spp, Serratia marcescens* are some of the members of Enterobacteriaceae family that may be implicated in the hospital set-up, especially in the nurseries and paediatric wards.

Non-Fermenting Gram-Negative Bacilli

Acinetobacter— A point worthy of mention here is that *Acinetobacter baumannii* is a mildly virulent organism that becomes resistant to antimicrobials. It causes outbreaks of nosocomial infections in ICUs and burn units, thus making it necessary to focus on methods of transmission and multi-disciplinary measures aimed at eliminating it from the ICU and burn units. Because of multiple antibiotic resistance, strict contact isolation, cohorting and aseptic techniques should be the primary modes of containment.

Legionella pneumophila —Legionellosis (Legionnaire Disease) is an acute, pneumonia-like illness caused by *Legionella pneumophila*, with a case fatality rate around 12% in hospitalized patients.[1]

Mycobacterium tuberculosis

In many countries tuberculosis is of paramount public health importance. Closed settings, congestion and overcrowding seem to favour its spread. Thus, the hospital is likely to provide a flourishing environment for growth and spread of *Mycobacterium tuberculosis*, unless adequate precautions are taken.

> Remember—very few bacilli are required for tuberculosis transmission. Open cases of tuberculosis with sputum smear positive status are a threat and require isolation.

The patterns of infections in the hospital arena have been changing due to the introduction of antibiotics and the development of resistance. A clinician should be aware of the drug-resistant bacteria, the diagnostic methods and the strategies to control and manage these bacteria. Knowing the patterns of infection and resistance is the basis of empirical antibiotic prescription strategies. Several drug-resistant bacteria are in the reckoning nowadays, including MRSA, MRCoNS, VRE, VISA, VSSA, VRSA, GISA, MDR-TB, ESBL third-generation cephalosporin-resistant *Enterobacteriaceae*, and imipenem-or ciprofloxacin-resistant *P. aeruginosa* and *A. baumannii* and the like. These are commonly seen to be hospital strains, but are of great concern because they are threatening to spill over into the community, which would be disastrous, and compromise the antimicrobial therapy (see Chapter 19).

BACTERIA OF SPECIAL RELEVANCE IN THE HOSPITAL SETTING

Since the introduction of penicillin, more than half a century ago, the β lactams have remained the largest antibiotic class of clinical relevance. They comprise four major families: the penicillins and their derivatives, the cephalosporins, the carbapenems and the monobactams. These antibiotics continue to be chemically modified in order to alter their antimicrobial activity.

There are three known mechanisms of resistance to β lactams:

1. Reduced affinity of drug targets (Penicillin Binding Proteins) due to a substitution (occurs in both Gram-positive and Gram-negative organisms).
2. Alteration in outer membrane permeability leading to block in passage to β lactams (down regulation of an outer membrane porin confers resistance to imipenem in Pseudomonas). This occurs in Gram-negative bacteria.

3. Production of β lactamases that inactivate drug through hydrolysis of the β lactam ring. (Occurs in both Gram-positive and Gram-negative bacteria especially *Klebsiella pneumoniae*).

1. Extended Spectrum Beta Lactamases (ESBL)

The β lactamases can be encoded by genes on chromosomes or plasmids. In the latter case, they can be readily transferred to other bacteria. One of the most common forms of antimicrobial resistance is produced through the actions of β lactamases, enzymes which hydrolyze the β lactam ring of beta-lactam antibiotics like Penicillins. Initially, extended spectrum cephalosporins, such as the third generation cephalosporins, were thought to be resistant to hydrolysis by β lactamases (especially those produced by enteric bacilli such as *E coli* and *Klebsiella*). However, in the mid 1980s, it became evident that a new type of β lactamase was being produced by *Klebsiella spp* and in some cases by *E coli,* that could hydrolyze even the extended spectrum cephalosporins.[2] These new beta-lactamases have been collectively termed the 'extended spectrum β lactamases' (ESBLs).[3] β lactamase inhibitors such as clavulanic acid, tazobactam and sulbactam do not inhibit these extended spectrum β lactamases sufficiently. Monobactams such as aztreonam are also inactivated. Recently, it has been discovered that the cephamycins (cefoxitin, cefotetan, moxalactam) have diminished activity against the ESBL producing bacteria.[4] More troubling is the observation that resistance to non β lactams is associated with ESBLs. Equally disturbing is the fact that ESBLs are carried on plasmids (extrachromosomal genetic material), which can be transferred to other bacteria.

Thus, ESBL producing bacteria include those which are resistant to not only penicillin group of drugs, but also to an extended spectrum of antimicrobials. Such ESBL strains are so far only described in Gram-negative bacteria, most commonly Klebsiella sp, (predominantly *Klebsiella pneumoniae*), and *Escherichia coli,* although they have been described in almost all members of Family Enterobacteriaceae.[5]

ESBL producing strains have been isolated in clinical practice, from abscesses, blood, catheter tips, lung, peritoneal fluid, sputum and throat culture.[6-7]

There Are Three Categories of ESBLs

1. Bush class A beta-lactamases

These are resistant to penicillins, narrow spectrum cephalosporins, the oxyimino-containing cephalosporins (like cefotaxime and ceftazidime), many extended spectrum cephalosporins and monobactams (like aztreonam). But the beta lactamase inhibitors like clavulanic acid, sulbactam and tazobactam generally inhibit these ESBL producing strains.

2. Bush class B beta-lactamases

These include metaloproteases, which are capable of hydrolyzing carbapenems such as imipenem and meropenam. In addition to carbapenems, the bacteria are resistant to other beta-lactams and beta-lactamase inhibitors, with the exception of aztreonam.

3. Bush class C beta-lactamase

Enzymes are primarily chromosomal rather than plasmid-mediated. The most prevalent enzyme in this group which is found among the Enterobacteriaceae and *P. aeruginosa* is Amp C. Class C beta-lactamases are resistant to beta-lactamase inhibitors and occur at a high frequency among *Enterobacter cloacae*, and result in resistance to all beta-lactams except carbapenems.

Incidence of ESBLs

In the United States from 1990 to 1993, a survey of the intensive care units (ICUs) of 400 hospitals recorded an increase from 3.6% to 14.4% in ESBL producing strains of *Klebsiella spp.*[3, 8] By 1994 the Center for Disease Control and Prevention, National Nosocomial Infections Surveillance System (NNIS) reported that 8% of *Klebsiella spp* had ESBLs with producers predominantly from a few large centers.[5, 7] In Europe as of 1995, ESBLs occur in 20%–25% of *Klebsiella spp* from patients in ICUs, although they have been found in up to 30%–40% in France.[9]

Rates vary greatly worldwide and within geographic areas and are rapidly changing over time.

How Are ESBLs Acquired?

Resistant strains are generally found post treatment with broad-spectrum cephalosporins or through acquisition of a resistant strain via nosocomial transmission. Medical use of antibiotics can considerably accelerate the selection pressure for diversification and dissemination of mutant extended-spectrum beta-lactamases.

Diagnosis of ESBLs

An observation of increasing rates of treatment failure with extended-spectrum cephalosporins should arouse suspicion of an ESBL.

Laboratory diagnosis: Detection of ESBL producing GNBs remains a challenge for the microbiology laboratory because routine methods for monitoring a decrease in susceptibility to oxyimino-cehalosporins and aztreonam have not been sensitive enough to detect ESBL producing strains. Minimum Inhibitory Concentrations (MIC) may be raised only slightly and fail to reach the level of the accepted breakpoint for resistance. The importance of routinely screening all isolates with extended-spectrum cephalosporins, not just those isolates resistant to narrower spectrum cehalosporins was recommended by the National Committee for Clinical Laboratory Standards (NCCLS) in 1999.[10]

The current NCCLS recommendations for detection of ESBLs in *Klebsiella spp. and E. coli* includes an initial screening test with any two of the following beta-lactam antibiotics: cefpodoxime, ceftazidime, aztreonam, cefotaxime, or ceftriaxone. Isolates exhibiting a MIC >1microg/ml should be confirmed phenotypically using ceftazidime plus ceftazidime/clavulanic acid, cefotaxime plus cefotaxime/clavulanic acid. A three two-fold concentration decrease in a MIC for either antimicrobial agent tested in combination with clavulanic acid versus its MIC when tested alone should be considered an ESBL producer.[11]

Transmission

Known risk factors for colonization and/or

infection with organisms harboring ESBLs include:

- admission to an intensive care unit
- recent surgery
- instrumentation
- prolonged hospital stay
- Antibiotic exposure, especially to extended-spectrum beta-lactam antibiotics. Use of extended-spectrum antibiotics exerts a selective pressure for emergence of ESBL producing GNBs. The resistance plasmids can then be transferred to other bacteria, not necessarily of the same species, conferring resistance to them. The lower digestive tract of colonized patients is the main reservoir of these organisms.[12-13] Gastrointestinal carriage can persist for months.
- Nursing home patients are more likely to be treated empirically with antibiotics, and thus on admission to a hospital to be more likely to possess an ESBL producing strain.[8, 10]
- Patient to patient transmission of ESBL producing GNBs occurs via the hands of hospital staff. It is known that ESBL producing strains can survive in the hospital environment.
- Hospitalized patients
- Nosocomial infections in patients occur through the administration of extended spectrum betalactam antibiotics or transmission from other patients via healthcare workers.
- Healthcare workers may become colonized with resistant strains via exposure to patients or other healthcare workers.

Prevention

- Spread of ESBL producing GNBs can be controlled by good infection-control practices, especially by good hand-washing technique and antibiotic manipulation and restriction to control ESBL outbreaks.
- Improved laboratory detection and reporting of ESBL producing strains is needed. Laboratories should test for susceptibility of all *K. pneumoniae* and *E. coli* isolates to extended-spectrum antibiotics by both screening and confirmatory tests as recommended by NCCLS guidelines.
- Monitoring and control of usage of extended-spectrum cephalosporins and regular surveillance of antibiotic resistance patterns as well as efforts to decrease use as empirical therapy is an indicated protocol. Termination of the use of ceftazidime as a monotherapy has helped in controlling outbreaks. The other effective strategy has been the encouragement of the use of penicillins or other class of antibiotics.
- Treatment: With the production of ESBLs, and hence resistance to extended spectrum cephalosporins, with no effective strategy, only two approaches show promise:

a. Use of Carbapenems like imipenem and meropenem

b. Combination of β lactams and β lactamase inhibitors. E.g., Piperacillin/tazobactam.

AmpC BETA LACTAMASES (ESAC)

In the process of evolution, bacteria have acquired well-developed mechanisms to ward

- Transport all specimens in double bags.
- Further information can be obtained through the CDC's Hospital Infection Program, National Center for Infectious Diseases (404) 639-6413 or http://www.cdc.gov/ncidod/hip/vanco/vanco.htm
- Vancomycin use should be limited to situations in which it is absolutely indicated. Guidelines have been published by the Hospital Infection Control Practices Advisory Committee.[23]
- Surveillance should be performed in patients with documented MRSA infections, especially if they have received long-term vancomycin therapy with additional emphasis in the Haemodialysis (HD) and Continuous Ambulatory Peritoneal Dialysis (CAPD) populations.
- Laboratories should monitor heterogenous MRSA populations (i.e., increased MIC).
- Drain, clean and disinfect water supplies periodically. Clean the water containers. Maintain hot water systems at higher temperatures (above 50°C). Use sterile water and not tap water for respiratory therapy devices.

Situation When Vancomycin Is Not Recommended

- Routine prophylaxis for surgical patients without allergy to beta lactam antibiotics, low birth-weight infants, dialysis patients, patients with neutropenia, patients with central venous catheters

3. MRSA AND *CLOSTRIDIUM DIFFICILE*[24-28]

(TABLE 17.1)

Methicillin-resistant *Staphylococcus aureus* and *Clostridium difficile* colonization are increasingly common in elderly patients, and are associated with cephalosporin or prolonged aminopenicillin courses and can be transmitted by direct contact. Management is by side-room isolation. Ward closure may sometimes be required to contain outbreaks. Enhanced infection-control policies are required, like emphasis on hand-washing, cephalosporin restriction, seven-day time limits on antibiotics and feedback of infection rates. Standardization of sampling techniques and laboratory methodology are indispensable for a correct HAI diagnosis. These measures have been shown to reduce the incidence of *Clostridium difficile* and MRSA significantly.[27]

4. VANCOMYCIN RESISTANT ENTEROCOCCUS (VRE)

Modify and abstracted from hicpac recommendation http://www.cdc.gov/ncidodvancom.htm dated: 10.09.2000

Guidelines for Preventing the Spread of VRE (Adapted from HICPAC) Source of Guidelines

It has been shown that VRE epidemics have the ability to influence the epidemiology of other nosocomial pathogens, especially MRSA, when infection-control measures are exhausted.

Table 17.1: Methods for susceptibility testing of *Staphylococcus aureus*

Method	MRSA	GISA	Comment
Microdilution broth	+++	+++	Incubate for full 24 hours.
Agar dilution	+++	+++	
Agar screening plates	+++	+++	
E test	++	+++	
Disc diffusion	++	0	Some MRSA strains may not be detected; fails to detect GISA strains
Automated (24 hour)	++	++	Some systems may report GISA isolates as having MICs of 4–6 ug/ml
Automated (3 hour)	++	+	Not reliable for detecting GISA

+ = somewhat useful, ++ = useful, and +++ = very useful

Situations in which the use of vancomycin is appropriate or acceptable

a. For treatment of serious infections due to ß-lactam-resistant Gram-positive microorganisms. Clinicians should be aware that vancomycin may be less rapidly bactericidal than ß-lactam agents for ß-lactam-susceptible Staphylococcal species.

b. For treatment of infections due to Gram-positive microorganisms in patients with life-threatening allergy to ß-lactam antimicrobials

c. When antibiotic-associated colitis (AAC) fails to respond to metronidazole therapy or if AAC is severe and potentially life-threatening

d. Prophylaxis, as recommended by the American Heart Association, for endocarditis preceding/during certain procedures involving patients at high risk for endocarditis

e. Prophylaxis for major surgical procedures involving implantation of prosthetic materials or devices, e.g. cardiac and vascular procedures and total hip replacement, at institutions with a high rate of infections due to methicillin-resistant *Staphylococcus aureus* (MRSA) or methicillin-resistant *S.epidermidis* (MRSE)

Situations in which the use of vancomycin should be discouraged

a. Routine surgical prophylaxis other than in a patient with life-threatening allergy to ß-lactam antibiotics

b. Empiric antimicrobial therapy for a febrile neutropenic patient when an infection is unconfirmed. However, if there is strong evidence at the outset that the patient has an infection due to gram-positive microorganisms (e.g. inflamed exit site of Hickman catheter) and MRSA is endemic in the hospital, vancomycin may be indicated.

c. Treatment in response to a single blood culture positive for coagulase-negative Staphylococci (if other blood cultures drawn in the same time frame are negative, or if contamination of the blood culture is likely). Because contamination of blood cultures with skin flora, e.g. *S.epidermidis*, may lead to vancomycin being administered to patients inappropriately, phlebotomists and other personnel who obtain blood cultures should be trained properly to minimize microbial contamination of specimens.

d. Continued empiric use for presumed infections in patients whose cultures are negative for ß-lactam-resistant gram-positive microorganisms

e. Systemic or local (e.g. antibiotic lock) prophylaxis for infection or colonization of indwelling central or peripheral intravascular catheters

f. Selective decontamination of the digestive tract

g. Eradication of MRSA colonization

h. Primary treatment of antibiotic-associated colitis (AAC)

i. Routine prophylaxis for very-low-birth-weight infants

j. Routine prophylaxis for patients on continuous ambulatory peritoneal dialysis or hemodialysis

k. Treatment (chosen for dosing convenience) of infections due to ß-lactam-sensitive Gram-positive microorganisms in patients with renal failure

l. Use of vancomycin solution for topical application or irrigation or for pre-transplant gut decontamination

Educational programme

Information about VRE and other antibiotic-resistant organisms and their potential impact: Special emphasis should be placed on providing continuing education programmes to the medical, nursing, pharmacy, and administrative staff. Information about the epidemiology of VRE, risk to patients, and VRE's impact on antimicrobial prescribing practices and on hospital and financial resources should be emphasized.

Enhancing the Detection and Reporting of VRE in the Microbiology Laboratory

The ability of the microbiology laboratory to accurately identify Enterococcus species and detect vancomycin resistance is an integral component in recognizing the emergence of VRE colonization and infection in healthcare facilities. Cooperation and communication between the laboratory and those responsible for infection control is equally important.

Identification of Enterococcus species

A system for presumptive identification of enterococci on primary isolation media is required in the microbiology laboratory. For laboratories not familiar with identifying VRE, additional tests for motility and pigment production may be required to distinguish *E. gallinarum* and *E. casseliflavus* from *E. faecium* and *E. faecalis*. For those laboratories not familiar with these methods or if financial resources do not permit such identification, a mechanism should be in place for the prompt referral of organisms to provide an appropriate level of identification with a rapid turnaround time.

Susceptibility testing

Routine testing depends on local surveillance and jurisdictional practices. Laboratories should ensure that a mechanism is available to determine vancomycin resistance and high-level resistance to penicillin and aminoglycosides of isolates from blood and all other clinically important samples. If resources do not permit routine testing of isolates, then periodic surveys of antimicrobial susceptibility to vancomycin should be done, the frequency determined by the local/provincial epidemiologic patterns of VRE. Reliable methods such as agar dilution or broth microdilution, rather than automated or disc diffusion testing must be used.

Confirmatory testing: If VRE is isolated from clinical specimens, the guidelines presented below should be followed. It is important to emphasize that if VRE is found from one body site it can be assumed to be present in multiple body sites. Often, vancomycin resistance is detected before speciation is complete. It is important that species identification and vancomycin resistance are confirmed.

Susceptible - MIC <= 4 μg/mL

Intermediate - MIC 8-16 μg/mL

Resistant - MIC >= 32 μg/mL

(Requires immediate infection-control notification)

During performance of confirmatory susceptibility tests, ICT and appropriate patient care personnel should be notified regarding the presumptive identification of VRE. The infection-control practitioner should assess whether isolation is required until species identification and vancomycin resistance is confirmed. This preliminary report should be followed by the (final) result of the confirmatory test.

Routine surveillance procedures for detecting VRE where VRE has not been previously detected

Antimicrobial susceptibility survey of clinical isolates: Laboratories should routinely screen for vancomycin resistance in all clinically significant enterococcal isolates obtained within the facility from any body site. Susceptibility tests performed only on enterococci recovered from sterile body sites would detect only a small number of clinical VRE isolates.

Culture survey of stools or rectal swabs in tertiary medical centres and other hospitals with many critically ill patients at high risk of VRE infection or colonization (e.g. intensive care units, oncology units, transplant patients), can detect the appearance of VRE. Faecal screening is recommended even when VRE infections have not been identified clinically, because gut colonization may occur in patients in a facility before infections are identified. The frequency and intensity of surveillance should be based on the size of the population at risk, the specific hospital unit(s) involved, the prevalence of VRE in the area and the cost-benefit ratio of screening.

Screening procedures for detecting VRE when a first isolate of VRE has been detected

The finding of a first isolate of VRE should prompt faecal screening (stool survey or rectal swabs) for the identification of other colonized patients in an effort to establish the optimal and timely application of isolation precautions and control measures. It must be emphasized that the use of screening surveys are merely a tool to elucidate the epidemiology of VRE within a given ward, patient population or facility and are not considered a mandatory component of an infection-control programme. The optimal timing and extent of screening procedures remain unknown. Currently, there are no data available on cost-effectiveness. Consideration of patient populations, risk factors for acquisition of VRE, and the costs and resources available within the facility must be taken into account when implementing screening procedures. As a minimum, stools or perirectal swabs may be obtained from roommates and other close contacts of patients found to be newly colonized with VRE. Additional screening of patients in the same ward or unit may also be considered. In outbreak situations, it may be necessary to screen patients outside of the ward to avoid missing colonized patients. The utility of massive screening efforts directed at all possible contacts, entire healthcare facility patient populations and staff, is unknown at this time and such efforts are not currently recommended.

Infection-control precautions to prevent the transmission of VRE in the healthcare setting

The infection-control practitioner or other responsible individual must be aware that there are several *Enterococcus* species. However, *E. faecalis* and *E. faecium* represent the species most often associated with disease and nosocomial transmission. Laboratories unfamiliar with speciation and susceptibility testing of enterococci may not correctly differentiate *E. faecalis* and *E. faecium* from other VRE that do not warrant the same infection-control precautions. Practitioners must confirm that their laboratory uses methods that will reliably identify these other species of Enterococcus (e.g. *gallinarum, casseliflavus*) that are intrinsically resistant to low levels of vancomycin. *Enterococcus gallinarum* and *E. casseliflavus* are less likely to be pathogens, their resistance has never been observed to transfer to other bacteria, and they do not require isolation, as do other VRE. If the laboratory identifies a VRE, the practitioner must confirm that it has been identified to species level, by a reference laboratory, if necessary. VRE isolates should be confirmed as such by laboratories experienced in enterococci identification and genotyping.

The presence of any isolate of VRE other than *E. gallinarum* and *E. casseliflavus* (VRE positive) from a single patient should receive prompt attention by infection-control team or other responsible personnel, and the ensuing guidelines should be initiated.

Note: *Enterococcus faecium* can be transmitted by electronic thermometers.

5. DRUG-RESISTANT *STREPTOCOCCUS PNEUMONIAE* (DRSP)

In 1981, the myth that *Streptococcus pneumoniae* is susceptible to all antimicrobial drugs was shattered, when Hungary reported a 47% resistance to Penicillin, as against 38% in 1979, and 20% in 1975. In 1989, Spain became the first Western country to declare an unexpected rise in the rate of isolation of drug resistant *Strep. pneumoniae* (44%). Following close on this was Brazil and Mexico with a frequency of 10–20% resistance.

Further, in Europe, the overall increase in Penicillin resistance has been from 10.4%–24.9%. In USA too, there has been a marked increase in penicillin-resistant strains from 5.6% to 12.3% between 1992 and 1995.

In India too, the first documented evidence of the existence of drug resistant *Strep. pneumoniae* was in 1995. A high level of resistance to penicillin was found in 8% of strains, while 14% showed intermediate resistance. By 1999, several states reported penicillin resistance—Indore (66.7% Intermediate and 3.3% frank resistance), Hyderabad (32% intermediate and 12% frank resistance), Chandigarh (63% intermediate resistance) and Mumbai (7.7% intermediate and 5.8% frank resistance).

The above facts only highlight the truth that drug prescription must be made with caution and after performance of a susceptibility test prior to prescription as far as possible.

Measures to combat this problem would be:

a. Wherever possible assign separate waiting and care areas(wards/rooms) to patients with acute chest infections.

b. Wear gloves and gowns and observe all Standard Precautions when handling patients with acute respiratory infections.

c. Disposal of secretions and other wastes must be meticulous.

d. Administer polyvalent pneumococcal polysaccharide vaccine to adults and children above two years of age with risk factors for invasive disease.

e. Monitor prevalence of DRSP strains in hospital and, if increased, serotype strains to detect clusters of cross infection. If an outbreak is documented, infected patients should be nursed in isolation with barrier precautions.

6. MULTI-DRUG-RESISTANT TUBERCULOSIS (MDR-TB)

MDR-Tuberculosis: MDR strains refer to those strains of tubercle bacilli that are resistant to the two most important drugs used in the treatment regimens (viz, INH and Rifampicin), with or without resistance to other ATT agents. MDR-TB is threatening to undo all that was ever achieved in the control of tuberculosis, and make the tubercle bacilli invincible, if not acted upon at once. MDR-TB in HIV patients has recently been shown to be associated with nosocomial spread to patients and HCWs in the hospital set-up. If this deadly combination is not broken up promptly, mankind may well be set back a hundred years in time!

Prevention and control

- Perform drug susceptibility tests in *M.tuberculosis* isolates
- Ensure patient compliance in treatment
- Always opt for a combination drug regimen and never a single drug regime

7. COAGULASE NEGATIVE STAPHYLOCOCCUS (CONS)

Although CoNS is a part of the normal flora in skin and other parts of the body, infections due to this have been increasingly reported, particularly in cases of prosthetic implant surgery, vascular catheterization, leukemia, and in premature neonates. Resistance to various antimicrobials are also on the rise, and hence it is important to perform susceptibility testing for *S. epidermidis*, whenever it is established as the causative organism.

VIRUSES

The viral infections that commonly spread in the hospital are:

Exanthematous Disease

Paediatric wards may be specially prone to spread infections like chicken pox, measles, Herpes virus infections, human parvovirus B19 infections and Rubella. These are spread through respiratory secretions and skin lesions. Less common causes are haemorraghic fevers.

Respiratory Tract Infections

Infections among staff and patients may be caused by Influenza virus, Respiratory Syncytial Virus (RSV), Adenovirus, Parainfluenza virus, Enteroviruses, and Rhinoviruses. In such conditions, isolation should be considered.

Other Viruses Found in Respiratory Secretions

Cytomegalovirus, Epstein Barr Virus, Herpes simplex, HHV-6, Measles virus, Mumps virus, Rubella virus, Pox virus and Varicella zoster virus.

Gastrointestinal Infections

These are caused by enteroviruses, adenoviruses, rotaviruses, astroviruses, coronaviruses and hepatitis A and E viruses. Transmission is mainly by the faeco-oral route. Viral diarrhoeas are less commonly spread in hospitals, but can occur.

Blood-borne Diseases

Most important among these are infections due to Hepatitis B and C viruses and Human Immuno-deficiency Virus (HIV) (Tables 17.2, 17.3, 17.4).

HEPATITIS B VIRUS (HBV)

This virus is the causative organism of Hepatitis B infection. Its surface antigen, also known as the Australia antigen, is detected in the serum for diagnosis. Man is the only natural host in this highly infectious viral disease of the liver which may progress to chronic liver disease, liver cirrhosis or even hepatocellular carcinoma. The virus is at least a hundred times more infectious than HIV. The incubation period is long (40–180 days) and extrahepatic manifestations may be seen. 5–10% of acute Hepatitis B cases are followed by chronic disease, which may be either chronic persistent or chronic active liver disease. The latter may progress to cirrhosis and primary hepatocellular carcinoma.

It is a DNA virus with three antigenic components—the outer coat contains the surface antigen (HBsAg), the inner core contains the hepatitis core antigen (HBcAg), and the 'e' antigen is associated with the viral core (HBeAg). While all the three antigens are immunogenic and elicit antibody production, the HBcAg cannot be detected in serum, as it is found only in the hepatocytes. Chronic carriers are those who test positive for HBsAg for more than six months (about 5–10% of infected individuals).

The routes of transmission of HBV include sexual route or contact with infectious blood by various modes. The virus has been detected in blood and also a wide variety of body fluids like semen, saliva, vaginal secretions, sweat and tears. The most important method for diagnosis of HBV infection is detection of the serological markers. An effective vaccine is available for Hepatitis B infection.

Table 17.2: Comparison of hepatitis viruses A, B, C, D, E

	HAV	HBV	HCV	HDV	HEV
Virus type	RNA	DNA	RNA	Defective RNA	RNA
Virus group	Enterovirus-72 (Picorna virus) (Hepatovirus)	Hepadnavirus	Flavivirus (Hepacivirus)	Deltavirus (Dependovirus)	Calcivirus
Modes of infection	Faeco-oral	Percutaneous, vertical, sexual	Percutaneous	Percutaneous	Faeco-oral
Infective material	Faeces	Blood, blood products, semen, vaginal secretions, sweat, saliva, urine, breast milk, bile	Blood, Blood products, Semen, Vaginal Secretions	Blood	Faeces
Age affected	Mostly children	Any age	Adults	Any age	Young adults
Incubation period	2–6 wks	1–6 mths	2 wks–5 mths	1–6 mths	2wks–2 mths
Onset of illness	Acute, mild and self-limiting	Insidious, occasionally severe	Insidious. moderate to severe	Insidious, occasionally severe	Acute, mild
Laboratory Diagnosis	IgM antibody in serum during early infection and IgG later.	HBsAg in blood	Antibody detection by ELISA. PCR and bDNA assay useful	IF detection of antigen in liver cell nuclei	

Table 17.2: (Contd.)

Treatment	Symptomatic	Interferon with Lamivudine, Famcyclovir are all of some benefit	Interferon and Ribavirin		
Carrier state	Nil	5–10% of adults 30% children 90% neonates. Types- Super carriers, simple carriers	Present1–20% world wide.	Nil (only with HBV)	Nil
Oncogenicity	Nil	Present	Present	Nil	Nil
Prevalence	Worldwide	Worldwide	Worldwide	Certain endemic areas	Only develop-ing countries
Mortality	<0.5%	0.5–2.0%	0.5–1%	-	-
Specific prophy-laxis	Immunoglo-bulin and vaccine	Immunoglobulin (HBIG- 300–500 i.u IM) and Recombinant vaccine. Gluteal injection not recommended as it may result in poor immune response. 3 doses at 0,1 and 6 months	Nil	HBV vaccine	Nil
Remarks	Infectious hepatitis Subclinical infections common -Low mortality -No extrahuman source	Dane particle is the complete virus, while Australia antigen is the hepatitis B surface antigen. In neonatal infections, strong chance of oncogenicity- serum hepatitis- transfusion	Commonest cause of post transfusion hepatitis in developed countries. Seen only in humans. High mutability	Mediterranean countries, N. Europe, Central and N. America. Co-infection and super-infection possible	Asia, Africa, Central America Can be severe in pregnancy

Table 17.2: (Contd.)

	can spread in hospital set-ups with over-crowding, poor sanitation, contaminated food or water	hepatitis-extrahepatic complications can occur, the only human cancer that is vaccine-preventable. Relatively heat-stable virus. Viable at room temperature for long periods. Hypochlorite and 2% glutaraldehyde inactivate the virus. Natural infection occurs only in humans. In some countries like the UK, carriers are barred from invasive medical practice and also not permitted to be medical students			

Table 17.3: Serological markers of Hepatitis B and their significance

If the patient has		Clinical State	Infectivity
ANTIGEN	ANTIBODY		
HBsAg + HBeAg	Anti HBc IgM	Acute HBV infection	Highly infectious
HBeAg +/-	Anti HBc IgM Anti HBe +/-	Early acute infection	Infectious
HBsAg + HBeAg	Anti HBc IgG	Late chronic infection Carrier state	Highly infectious
HBsAg	Anti HBc IgG Anti HBe +/-	Late chronic infection Or Carrier state	Of low infectivity
-	Anti HBc IgM Anti HBs +/- Anti HBe +/-	Past infection	Very low or not infectious
-	Anti HBs +		Immune following HBV vaccine

Table 17.4: Some common viruses and organs affected

	Other viruses and their sites of infection in the body					
	Blood	Lungs	Heart	Brain	Liver	Skin
CMV	+	+	+	+	+	+
Epstein–Barr	+	+	+	+	+	+
HSV - 1		+		+	+	+
HHV 6	+	+		+		+
HHV 8						+
HBV					+	
HCV					+	

Diagnosis

Antigen detection

Antibody response

Electron microscopy

Virus isolation

Polymerase Chain Reaction

Hepatitis C virus

Responsible for 16% of acute hepatitis cases in a CDC sentinel study (1982–1993). Incubation period is 2–26 weeks. Clinical illness occurs in 30–40% patients but only 20–30% patients will develop jaundice. The risk of a healthcare worker acquiring infection after percutaneous exposure with an infected needle is estimated to be in the range of 1.8% (range 0–7%) and only one case has been reported by a conjunctival splash. Progression may take 20, 30 or 40 years.

Diagnosis:

Antigen detection

Antibody response

Electron microscopy

Virus isolation

Polymerase Chain Reaction

There are two approved therapies for chronic hepatitis

Interferon

Interferon plus ribavirin

HIV

Causative organism is a retrovirus, which encodes its genetic information in RNA and uses a unique viral enzyme called reverse transcriptase to copy its genome into DNA, which is then integrated into the host cell genome as a provirus. HIV infection produces dysfunction of both the cellular and humoral components of immunity. It has a prolonged period of latency. Seroconversion leads to infection and later to full blown AIDS with symptoms. There may be a gap of 8–10 years from the time of exposure to a stage of disease.

HIV seropositive persons are commonly prone to the following infections:

Persistent Fever due to Mycobacterium, cytomegalovirus, Histoplasmosis, Listeria or Salmonella.

GI infections due to CMV, Cryptosporidium, Salmonella, Shigella, Campylobacter, Adenovirus, *Giardia lamblia.*

Pulmonary infections due to *P. carinii*, CMV, Cryptococcus, *H. capsulatum, Toxoplasma gondii,* Streptococcus, *M. tuberculosis, Legionella pneumophila*

CNS infections-*T. gondii*, Papovavirus

Risk factors for transmission in a hospital setting: Contact with secretions, infected needles, mother to child.

Diagnosis of HIV infection:

1. Virus isolation: time consuming and laborious.
2. Serological determination of anti-HIV antibodies by screening/ELISA/confirmation is by Immunofluorescence (IF), Radio Immuno Precipitation (RIP) or Western Blot (WB)

FUNGAL INFECTIONS

(TABLE 17.5)

Candida spp and *Aspergillus* spp are the most common fungal causes of HAI. The others include *Fusarium* and *Trichosporon.* Candida has been found to be the fourth most common agent to be found in the blood, following *Staph. aureus, S. epidermidis* and *Enterococcus*. Almost two thirds of the fungal infections are associated with central venous catheters and the same proportion in ICU.

The conditions in which the patients are susceptible to fungal infections include leukaemia, lymphomas, bone marrow or solid organ transplants, diabetes, severe burns, premature births, chemotherapy, immunosuppressive drugs, broad spectrum antibiotics and prolonged hospitalization. The incidence of candidaemia is higher in the critical care units than in other parts of the hospital. Aspergillus spp. are common fungi found in the hospital set-up along with Candida spp. especially in Cardiac surgery units and immunocompromised hosts.

I Colonization

II Infection
- a. Suppurative peripheral thrombophlebitis
- b. Fungaemia

Spread
- a. By contact—fomites and infected personnel
- b. Hyperalimentation: seen to be a major risk factor for fungaemia
- c. Endogenous-spread from colonized areas from the same patient.

Mortality: Crude mortality seen in NISS for fungaemia is 55% and attributable mortality is 38%. Fungaemia has been found to be an independent predictor of mortality wherein 29% patients with fungaemia may die, whereas the mortality is only 17% in non-fungal pathogens causing blood stream infections.

Laboratory diagnosis: Blood culture for fungi is advocated for suspected blood stream infections with fungus. One has to carefully rule out contaminants in these cases, by doing repeat/ multiple cultures wherever possible.

Table 17.5: Some common fungi/parasites and organs affected

Blood	Lungs	Heart	Brain	Liver	Skin
C. albicans	+	+		+	+
H. capsulatum	+	+			+
C. neoformans	+	+		+	+
T. gondii		+	+	+	
S. stercoralis		+			
P. falciparum	+				
T. cruzi			+		

Relatively newer methods, including serological tests like LAT, ELISA, IFA and molecular methods / PCR may be relied upon wherever such facilities are available.

Resistance and susceptibility testing: Nowadays, it is necessary to do an antifungal susceptibility test for fungi, as fluconazole and ketoconazole resistance levels are on the rise. Other antifungal agents that can be tested for susceptibility include Amphotericin B, Clotrimazole, Itraconazole and Miconazole. A new antifungal agent is available as an IV infusion in treatment of invasive aspergillosis in patients who are refractory to or intolerant to other antifungal therapies—Capsofungin acetate—a semi synthetic lipopeptide (echinocandin) compound.

PARASITES

These are not as important as the bacterial infections. Many of the community acquired parasitic infections can also be encountered in the hospital set-up. These include protozoal diseases, such as Amoebiasis, giardiasis, toxoplasmosis and nematodal infections such as round worm infestation, hook worm and other worm infestations.

PRIONS

These are proteinaceous infectious particles implicated in several slow virus infections, of which the bovine spongiform disease ('mad cow disease') is an example. Originally a disease of the sheep, this agent has jumped species to cows and then to humans—and is now transmitted to other humans either by eating infected beef or from usage of infected equipment such as the tonsillectomy equipment. The infection manifests after many years (long incubation). These agents have a predeliction for the CNS and are eventually fatal. The immune response is generally poor or absent. These agents are highly resistant to normal methods of disinfection and sterilization. Recommendations for sterilization to destroy these agents include the use of NaOH or autoclaving at 134°C for 20 minutes. Otherwise, the best option would be to use disposable instruments for these patients.

QUICK GLANCE

MRSA

How does it occur?

Prolonged admission

Prolonged course of Beta-lactams or other antimicrobials

Prolonged stay in ICU

Prolonged contact with colonized in-patients

Mechanism

- Intrinsic methicillin resistance encoded by the mec gene
- Acquired or borderline resistance (BORSA), due to hyper-production of penicillinase
- Methicillin-intermediate *S aureus.* (MISA)

Therapy: Drug of choice for MRSA treatment is a parenteral glycopeptide like Vancomycin or Teicoplanin. Borderline resistant strains can be treated with high-dose cloxacillin.

Prevention and control

Surveillance: Laboratory-based surveillance using NCCLS method of testing

- A record of MRSA patient details
- Routine screening of in-patients not recommended except during suspected outbreaks (sample from anterior nares)
- Patients with MRSA tend to remain colonized for long. So, data of such patients can be retained. In the event of re-admission, appropriate measures can be taken at once.

Isolation of MRSA patient is the ideal method. If isolation facilities are not available, then cohorting all MRSA patients in the same room may be followed.

If this too is impracticable, barrier precautions to be followed (except in patients with MRSA respiratory infections and open wounds, where isolation is necessary).

Management of Colonizers

Decolonization therapy is not recommended except during outbreaks.

HCWs who are carriers of MRSA are to be treated only if persistent carriers or colonized in skin lesions or dermatitis. Treatment of nasal carriers is with topical Mupirocin. If that fails, use oral agents like Rifampicin, Trimethoprim/Sulphamethoxazole, Minocycline or Ciprofloxacin.

Treat infected patients with parenteral glycopepetide (vancomycin or teicoplanin)

VRE

Risk factors

- Underlying disease of patients
- Length of hospital stay
- Prior surgery
- Renal insufficiency
- ICU admission
- Catheterization (urinary or vascular)
- Broad spectrum antimicrobial therapy or vancomycin therapy

Mode of acquisition of VRE

- Patient-to-patient transfer

- Contaminated equipment
- Food chain

Treatment option

- Teicoplanin may be used if the organism is susceptible
- Combination of Penicillin, Ampicillin or a glycopeptide with an aminoglycoside for synergistic activity
- Chloramphenicol may be tried
- Quinipristin/Dalfopristin (this is not active against *E. faecalis*)
- For UTI, Nitrofurantoin or quinolones

Prevention and control of VRE

1. Prudent use of Vancomycin
2. Education and updates of status
3. Laboratory surveillance—by susceptibility surveys of isolates from stools or rectal swabs

Policy

- Notify appropriate staff
- Isolate or cohort colonized patients
- Try to use disposable materials in patient care
- Screen patients sharing room with colonized patients
- Keep records of colonized or infected patients in case of readmission.

ESBL

Prevention and control

- Termination of empirical Ceftazidime monotherapy helps control outbreaks
- Use contact or barrier precautions
- Gradually try and change the antimicrobial policy of the institution and discourage the use of cephalosporins
- Encourage the use of penicillins or other classes of drugs
- Early detection and prompt containment

Treatment of ESBL infections

Imipenem is the most effective drug against ESBL.

REFERENCES

1) C D Alert. Monthly Newsletter of the National Institute of Communicable Diseases, DGHS, Govt. of India. February 1998. Vol. 2: Issue 2.
2) Katsanis GO, Spargo J, Ferraro MJ et al. Detection of *Klebsiella pneumoniae and Escherichia coli* strains producing extended-spectrum beta-lactamases. J Clin Microbiol 1994; 32: 691-696.
3) Tenor FC, Mohammed MJ, Gorton TS et al. Detection and reporting of organisms producing ESBLs: Survey of laboratories in Connecticut. J Clin Micro 1999; 37: 4065-4070.
4) Moland ES, Sanders CC and Thomson KS. Can results obtained with commercially available MicroScan panels serve as an indicator of beta-lactamase production among *Escherichia coli and Klebsiella* isolates with hidden

resistance to extended-spectrum cephalosporins and aztreoman? J Clin Microbiol 1998; 36:2575-2579.

5) Babay HA. Detection of extended-spectrum beta-lactamases in members of the family Enterobacteriaceae at a teaching hospital, Riyadh, Kingdom of Saudi Arabia. Saudi Med. J 2002; 23(2): 186-90.

6) D'Agata E, Venkataraman L, DeGirolami P et al.The molecular and clinical epidemiology of enterobacteriaeae producing extended-spectrum beta-lactamase in a tertiary care hospital. J Infect 1998; 36: 279-85.

7) Quinn JP. Clinical significance of extended-spectrum beta-lactamases. Eur J Clin Microbiol Infect Dis. 1994; 13 (Suppl): 39-42.

8) Monnet D, Jay C, Edwards J et al and the National Nosocomial infections Surveillance (NNIS) System. Transmission of extended spectrum beta-lactam resistant *Klebsiella neumoniae* among hospitals in the United States, abstr. J38 in Program and Abstracts of the 34th International conference on Antimicrobial Agents and Chemotherapy. American Society for Microbiology, Washington, DC 1994.

9) Livermore DM. Beta-lactamases in laboratory and clinical resistance. Clin Micro Review 1995; 8: 557-584.

10) Emery CL and Weymouth LA. Detection and clinical significance of extended-spectrum beta-lactamases in a tertiary care medical center. J Clin Micro 1997; 35: 2061-2067.

11) Naumovski L, Quinn JP, Miyashiro D et al. Outbreak of ceftazidime resistance due to a novel extended-spectrum beta-lactamase in isolates from cancer patients. Antimicrob Agents Chemother 1992; 36:1991-1996.

12) Burwen DR, Banerjee SN and Gaynes RP. The National Nosocomial Infection Surveillance System. Ceftazidime resistance among selected nosocomial gram-negative bacteria in the United States. J Infect Dis 1994; 170: 1622-1625.

13) Massova I and Mobashery S. Kinship and diversification of bacterial penicillin-binding proteins and beta-lactamases. Antimicrob Agents Chemother 1998; 42: (Minireview)1-17.

14) Rice L. Evolution and clinical importance of Extended Spectrum Beta Lactamases.Chest. 2001;119: 391S-396S.

15) Reduced susceptibility of *Staphylococcus aureus* to vancomycin – Japan, 1996. MMWR 1997; 46:624-6.

16) *Staphylococcus aureus* with reduced susceptibility to vancomycin – United States, 1997. MMWR 1997; 46: 765-6.

17) Update: *Staphylococcus aureus* with reduced susceptibility to vancomycin - United States, 1997. MMWR 1997;46:813-15.

18) *Staphylococcus aureus* with reduced susceptibility to vancomycin – Illinois, 1999. MMWR 2000; 48: 1165-67.

19) Sieradski K, Roberts RB, Haber SW et al. The development of vancomycin resistance in a patient with methicillin-resistant *Staphylococcus aureus* infection. NEJM, 1999; 340: 517-523.

20) Smith TL, Pearson ML, Wilcox KR, et al. Emergence of vancomycin resistance in *Staphylococcus aureus*. NEJM. 1999; 340: 493-501.

21) Tenover, F.C. Implications of vancomycin-resistant *Staphylococcus aureus*. J Hos Infect, 1999; 43: S3-S7.

22) Recommendations for preventing the spread of vancomycin resistance: recommendations of the Hospital Infection Control Practices Advisory Committee (HICPAC). MMWR 1995; 44(RR-12): 1-13.

23) Interim Guidelines for prevention and control of Staphylococcal infection associated with reduced susceptibility to vancomycin. MMWR 1997; 46: 626-8, 635.

24) Vriens M, Blok H, Fluit A et al. Costs associated with a strict policy to eradicate methicillin-resistant *Staphylococcus aureus* in a Dutch University Medical Centre: a 10-year survey. Eur J Clin Microbiol Infect Dis. 2002; 21(11): 782-6.

25) Fitzpatrick F, Murphy OM, Brady A et al. A purpose built MRSA cohort unit. J Hosp Infect. 2000; 46(4): 271-9.

26) Bartley PB, Schooneveldt JM, Looke DF et al. The relationship of a clonal outbreak of Enterococcus faecium van A to methicillin-resistant *Staphylococcus aureus* incidence in an Australian hospital. J Hosp Infect. 2001; 48(1): 43-54.

27) Norazah A, Lim VKE, Rohani MY et al. A major Methicillin-resistant *Staphylococcus aureus* clone predominates in Malaysian hospitals. Epidemiol Infect. 2003; 130: 407-411.

28) Stone SP, Beric V, Quick A et al. The effect of an enhanced infection-control policy on the incidence of *Clostridium difficile* infection and methicillin-resistant *Staphylococcus aureus* colonization in acute elderly medical patients. Age Ageing. 1998; 27(5): 561-8.

Chapter 18

Clinical Practice Guidelines

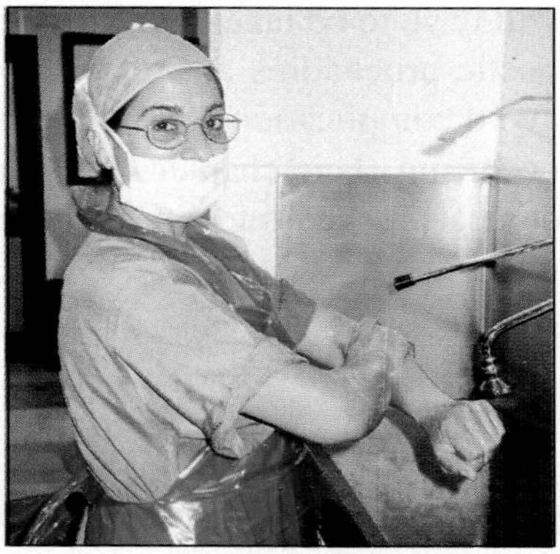

The highest reward for a man's toil is not what he gets for it, but what he becomes by it.

—John Ruskin

Highlights

Clinical Practice Guidelines

HAI-Related 'Process of Care'

Use of Guidelines for HAI Control

Urinary Tract Infections (UTIs)

Surgical Site Infections (SSIs)

Hospital Acquired Pneumonia

The Surviving Sepsis Campaign Guidelines for Septic Shock

The Neutropenic Patient

INTRODUCTION

Clinical management of HAI basically consists of Diagnosis, Treatment and Prevention. These measures must go hand in hand and do not necessarily follow in a rigid sequence. For example, it may often be necessary to start the treatment even as the diagnostic procedures are on. So also, preventive measures will have to be taken while treatment or diagnostic procedures are underway, in order to avoid complications and adverse events from occurring. This chapter highlights the use of clinical practice guidelines for clinical management.

Critical Points in the 'Process of Care'

Providing immediate care
↓
Making a presumptive diagnosis
↓
Ordering investigations
↓
Interpretation of results
↓
Undertaking invasive procedures
↓
Treatment: Supportive and specific
↓
Ward management
↓
Continued care till patient is fit for discharge
follow-up care
(prevention at every step)

CLINICAL PRACTICE GUIDELINES[1-4]

A Clinical Practice guideline constitutes a plan for managing a clinical problem based on evidence whenever possible and on consensus in the absence of evidence. A practice guideline could apply to all aspects of the clinical process of care. It is an important tool in guiding individual and collective practices and therefore is important in making practice standards uniform (decreased variation; see quality management).

In addition, these must be combined with guidelines for other areas such as environmental hygiene, antibiotic prescribing, waste management, sterilization and disinfection and existing statutory regulations (which are discussed in their respective chapters), for improved outcomes.

Evidence-based guidelines

Guidelines are subject to change due to emerging evidence and must be reviewed on a regular basis. Organizations can adopt the entire set of guidelines or a part of it (bundle). An organization must ensure implementation of the entire bundle for better results rather than random application of individual guidelines.

Consensus-based guidelines

Practices such as sampling methods for nosocomial pneumonias, septic shock, ARDS are consensus-based guidelines. As extremely expensive therapeutic modalities are emerging and are aggressively touted by manufacturers, these consensus-based guidelines help in selecting diagnostic and therapeutic strategies and guide us on when they should be applied and therefore prevent misuse of diagnostic and therapeutic modalities and risk of litigation. Relevant modifications may be made by national and state guideline setting bodies to suit their circumstances.

HAI-RELATED 'PROCESS OF CARE'

Screening for Communicable Disease

Screen all non-trauma triage patients (point of first contact) with a purpose to identify all individuals who present with symptoms suggestive of an infection or communicable disease.[1] Remember that a community acquired infection has the potential to become a rapidly spreading HAI, e.g. SARS. It is also mandatory to check for infection if the patient is being shifted from another healthcare facility. Relevant clinical details, date and time of onset, clinical symptoms, signs, information about treatment, history of travel abroad, details of visits to a healthcare facility, history of operations, procedures carried out in the past, transfusions, details of allergies to drugs, are all relevant points to note. This action serves two purposes:

1. Diagnosis of an infective problem and taking necessary steps in preventing further spread of an infective condition
2. Deciding whether the infection in question was acquired in the community or in a healthcare facility[5]

Clinical Diagnosis

Differentiating between infective and non-infective causes of the patients' signs and symptoms is the first step to establishing a definitive diagnosis.

When investigating nosocomial infections, one must keep in mind that several noninfectious causes of fever exist in hospitalized patients that do not necessarily have a microbial aetiology. These include:

1. Drug fever (quite common with phenytoin, H_2 blockers, antibiotics like sulphonamides)
2. Phlebitis
3. Tissue necrosis following surgery
4. Trauma
5. Burns
6. Haematomas
7. Pancreatitis
8. Atelectasis
9. Acalculous cholecystitis

Though bacterial infections are the commonest, it is important to understand that other organisms such as viruses, fungi, protozoa and prions can also cause infections.

The importance of differentiating nosocomial and community acquired infections is that the organisms may be different (resistant strains are more prevalent in the hospital setup). The pathogenesis and the empirical treatment strategies may also be different.[5] For example, the strategies for management of community acquired pneumonia and nosocomial pneumonia are completely different.

Laboratory Diagnosis

(Figure 18.1)

The laboratory has to be equipped to perform tests that will yield reproducible, reliable, accurate and speedy results. Expectations from the laboratory include:

- Adequate sampling methods
- Appropriate transport of specimens
- Performance of general tests

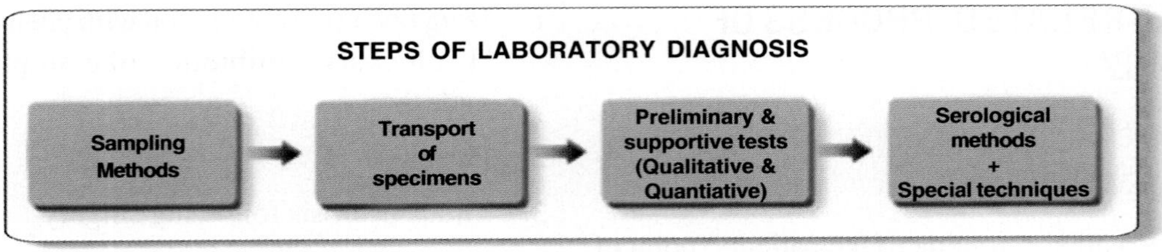

Figure 18.1: Steps of laboratory diagnosis

- Differentiating between colonization and infection
- Performance of specific/special tests under certain circumstances
- Follow qualitative and quantitative diagnostic criteria for that particular disease. Supportive laboratory data

Prevention of HAI

This needs understanding of the pathophysiology of the disease (HAI) and its relation to patient groups or populations. Certain groups of patients are at a greater risk due to certain factors, which can be grouped into host, device, personnel or procedure-related factors. Preventive strategies are developed keeping the following factors in mind.

A. Host-related factors

Age

Underlying illnesses: COPD, Diabetes mellitus, depressed consciousness, surgery, malnutrition

Drug history, vaccination status, PEP

Factors predisposing to colonization

B. Device-related factors

C. Personnel or procedure related factors

D. Special clinical settings

(Burns, transplant units, the oncology unit, neonatal and paediatric units, etc.). Many oncology patients have altered neutrophil counts, which has a direct impact on the body's ability to fight off infection. Oncology patients are particularly prone to infection with opportunistic organisms[6] (organisms that are ubiquitous in the environment but cause problems in severely immunocompromised patients like aspergillus, viruses like cytomegalovirus, herpes virus, etc.). This is one reason stem cell/ bone marrow transplant units have special ventilation systems (all the rooms are at positive pressure, so the air flows from the room into the hall). This is specifically designed to keep airborne pathogens out of the patient rooms. Children, especially premature infants have immature host defences and are at greater risk of infection.[7] As with the adults, use of mechanical ventilation, invasive lines and nutrition concerns can increase infection rates. Adherence to aseptic technique, hand hygiene practices, care for invasive lines and ventilator care can do much to reduce the incidence. Several other objectives should be kept in mind:

- The removal of invasive devices as quickly as possible
- Restriction of visitors to children's ICUs, during seasonal outbreaks of respiratory viruses,which can reduce exposure to these community viruses

- Vigilance of HCWs in observing visitors with signs of infections
- Education of visitors and staff on the importance of hand hygiene

Preventive vaccination

Preventive vaccines should be considered in specific age groups, high risk categories, immunocompromised state and for post exposure prophylaxis.[8]

E.g. pneumococcal vaccine, diphtheria toxoid, typhoid vaccine, mumps vaccine, influenza vaccine.

Post-exposure prophylaxis

It is important to have protocols for the prophylaxis after exposure. Incident monitoring is important (e.g. needle-stick injury) and a cell to advice the requisite investigations and the drugs to be administered soon after the exposure (antimicrobials, vaccines, sera). These have to be available within the organization. It is also important that the management or administration of the organization is fully involved and accountable for provision of the requisite drugs. Smaller hospitals and nursing homes must be able to contact state level or national level bodies for advice.[9]

Supportive Management

Patients with severe nosocomial infections may display varying degrees of organ failure and may require support such as ventilation in respiratory failure, vasopressors in septic shock, and various other forms of organ support such as dialysis. This is not specific treatment.

Preventing the effect of mediators

A number of effects are the end result of a cascade of mediators, which are triggered off in response to the infection. These mediators are cytokines, arachidonic acid metabolites and other mechanisms. A number of treatment modalities are targeted at these mechanisms. Hence the management is multipronged, targeting different mechanisms. It is recommended that the clinical process of care be guided by evidence-based guidelines and consensus committee reports for uniformity of practice and judicious use of newer drugs and management modalities. These recommendations are dynamic and change from time to time with changing evidence, introduction of newer modalities and concepts.

Antimicrobial Therapy

Treatment policy

The strategies for antimicrobial therapy of HAI are different from those of community based infections. This is discussed in greater detail in the chapter on antimicrobial therapy.

Empirical treatment

The organisms grown in the ICU are surveyed and antibiotics are chosen according to local patterns. The treatment schedule advocated by some standard national/international body or society, like the American Thoracic Society may be locally adapted and followed.

Specific treatment

This is instituted when culture and sensitivity results are available. Invasive diagnostic sampling followed by rapid testing with specific therapy is advocated by some European centres without use of empirical therapy. (Fig. 18.2)

Surgery

Surgical treatment is to remove the focus of infection and is referred to as source control. This includes:

Drainage

Collection of pus in any cavity such as a joint, thorax, abdomen or an organ.

Debridement

Examples include diffuse infections such as necrotizing fascitis, pancreatic necrosis and intestinal infarction.

Device removal

Examples include infected catheters, endotracheal tubes, contraceptive devices.

Definitive control

E.g. amputation for clostridial myonecrosis.

USE OF GUIDELINES FOR HAI CONTROL

(FIGURE 18.2)

Guidelines should form the basis of clinical practice in the control of HAI. There are guidelines for every step in the process of care. When guidelines are modified or specified for local use by organizations, they become protocols. Four important HAIs have been discussed—urinary tract infections, catheter-related infections, surgical site infections and nosocomial pneumonias. The source of the guidelines have been mentioned in each section. It must be understood that there may be differences in guidelines given by various bodies for the same problem. Therefore, it is important to know your local and international guidelines.

Guidelines for practice patterns in ICU infections and post-operative infections are given by bodies such as CDC, Atlanta, USA or Health Department, UK.

When a guideline is framed, it is important to mention the grade of evidence by which it is backed. At the 'Centre for Disease Control and Prevention (CDC)', evidence-based recommendations were developed by Hospital (now Healthcare) Infection Control Practices Advisory Committee (HICPAC) in 1994-95. Systematic reviews and meta-analysis have been conducted by others since the publication of HICPAC guidelines in an attempt to identify reported outcomes clearly linked to evidence. These guidelines are available on the internet. http://www.cdc.gov/ncidod/hip/guide/guide.html

Bundling or Grouping of Recommendations

Each recommendation is important. But if a number of recommendations are implemented together then they become even more effective. Each unit, organization or department can select its own bundles (group of guidelines), by consensus (multidisciplinary approach) and implement them. This has been found to yield better results.

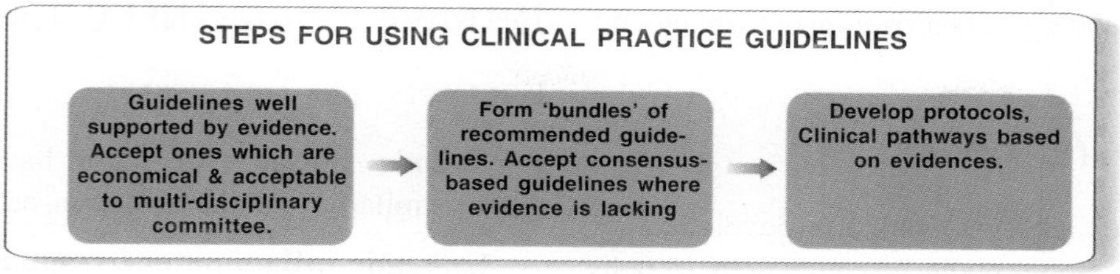

Figure 18.2: Steps of using clinical practice guidelines

URINARY TRACT INFECTIONS (UTIs)

Aetiology of UTI

The most commonly isolated bacteria is *Escherichia coli*. Other common nosocomial pathogens are *Pseudomonas aeruginosa, Klebsiella pneumoniae, Proteus mirabilis, Staphylococcus epidermidis, Staphylococcus aureus*, Enterococci, *Corynebacterium jeikeium,* Group D Streptococci and Candida species.

Normal host defences against UTI include an unobstructed urethra, the voiding process and normal bladder mucosa. These are bypassed by the insertion of a urinary catheter, and its manipulation provides a conduit for organisms to reach the bladder. Factors that predispose to infection include catheterization and its duration, errors in catheter care, microbial colonization of drain bag, specific disease states that predispose patients to infection (i.e., diabetes mellitus or anatomic abnormalities), female patient, catheter placement other than for surgical or output measurement and an abnormal creatinine level.

Incidence of Nosocomial UTIs

UTI is the commonest type of nosocomial infection, accounting for 40%–80% of all infections in hospitals. Catheter-associated HAI are estimated to cause one death per 1000 episodes. There is a greater risk for UTI with increased duration of catheterization. The prevalence of asymptomatic bacteriuria is 15% in patients catheterized for less than 30 days and 90% for patients catheterized for more than 30 days.[10, 11, 12]

A number of guidelines have been recommended by various bodies and in addition there is an attempt to reduce incidence by other methods such as engineering controls.

Laboratory Diagnosis of UTI[13-19]

The CDC and NNIS define UTI (Significant bacteriuria) as $>10^5$ colony forming units (CFU) with 1 or 2 microorganisms. The Maki definition of UTI is $>10^3$ CFU with 1 or 2 organisms. These definitions are applicable to acute care. Quantitative counts are a load on the laboratory services and many laboratories are not able to achieve the recommended standards. They adopt semiquantitative methods. However, these methods are not as accurate as the quantitative methods.

In chronic care situations significant bacteruria should be dealt with on an individual basis. To treat or not to treat is the question in these cases of bacteruria in the absence of bacteremia or absence of symptoms as in cases of long standing catheterization or sympathetic bladders.

Source of Guidelines

Guidelines are systematically developed by various national bodies/organizations to help clinical decision making. The guidelines given in Tables 18.1 to 18.4 have been modified and abstracted from 'Guidelines for preventing infections associated with the insertion and maintenance of short-term indwelling urethral catheters in acute care' developed by department of health, UK, published in *Journal of Hospital Infection* (2001) 47 (supplement): S 39-S 46.

These guidelines have been laid down for preventing infections associated with the insertion and maintenance of short-term in-dwelling urethral catheters in acute care. These recommendations are divided into four distinct interventions (Tables 18.1 to 18.4).

Grading of Evidence, Department of Health, UK is as follows

Category 1: Generally consistent findings in a range of evidence derived from a majority of acceptable studies.

Category 2: Evidence based on a single acceptable study, or a weak or inconsistent finding in multiple acceptable studies.

Category 3: Limited scientific evidence that does not meet all criteria of 'acceptable studies' or an absence of directly applicable studies of good quality. This includes published expert opinion derived from systematically retrieved and appraised professional, national and international guidelines.

INTRAVASCULAR INFECTIONS

Concepts and Definitions

Bacteremia: Presence of viable bacteria in blood (similarly viremia, fungemia, etc.).

Systemic inflammatory response syndrome (SIRS): Systemic inflammatory response can occur to a variety of insults including infection, ischaemia, multiple trauma and tissue injury, haemorrhagic shock, immune-mediated organ injury and exogenous administration of inflammatory mediators, such as tumour necrosis factor or other cytokines.[20] SIRS is manifested by (but not limited to):

- Temperature higher than 38°C
- Heart rate more than 90/min
- Respiratory rate more than 20/min
- WBC count > $12x10^9$/l, < $4x10^9$/l or >0.1% immature (band) forms

Sepsis: Systemic response to infection. This response is identical to SIRS except that it must result from infection.[21]

Severe sepsis: Sepsis associated with organ dysfunction, perfusion abnormalities or hypotension. Perfusion abnormalities may include, but are not limited to, lactic acidosis, oliguria and acute alteration in mental status. Hypotension is defined as systolic blood pressure < 90 mm Hg or reduction of >40 mm Hg from baseline in the absence of another known cause of hypotension.

Septic shock: Sepsis with hypotension (as defined above), despite adequate fluid resuscitation, in conjunction with perfusion abnormalities (as defined above). Patients receiving inotropic or vasopressor agents may not be hypotensive when perfusion abnormalities are

Table 18.1: Clinical practice guidelines: urinary tract infections

Intervention 1 (Assessing the need for catheterization)		
Issue	**Recommendation**	**Evidence**
Catheterization	Use indwelling catheters only after considering alternative methods of management	Category 3
Continuing catheterization	Review patient clinical status regularly	Category 3

Table 18.2: Clinical practice guidelines: urinary tract infections

Intervention 2 (Is one catheter better than the other?)		
Type of Catheter	**Recommendation**	**Evidence**
Choice of catheter material	Will depend on clinical experience, patient assessment and anticipated duration of catheterization	Category 3
Catheter size and Balloon size	Select the smallest gauge that will allow free urinary outflow. A catheter with a 10ml balloon should be used. Urological patients may require larger gauge sizes and balloons	Category 3

Table 18.3: Clinical practice guidelines: urinary tract infections

Intervention 3 (Catheterization is a skilled aseptic procedure.)		
Issue	**Recommendation**	**Evidence**
Asepsis during insertion	Ensure that healthcare personnel are trained and competent to carry out urethral catheterizations	Category 3
Clean the urethral meatus	Prior to the insertion of the catheter	Category 3
Use an appropriate lubricant	Use a single use catheter to minimize urethral trauma and infection	Category 3

Table 18.4: Clinical practice guidelines: urinary tract infections

Intervention 4 (Catheter maintenance: leave the closed system alone)		
Issue	**Recommendation**	**Evidence**
Urinary drainage system	Connect in-dwelling urethral catheter to a sterile closed system	Category 3
The connection between the catheter and urinary drainage bag	Ensure that the urinary system is not broken except for good clinical reasons, e.g. changing the bag in line with the manufacturer's recommendation	Category 3
Manipulating a patient's catheter	Decontaminate hands and wear a new pair of clean, non-sterile gloves before and decontaminate hands after removing the gloves	Category 3
Obtaining urine samples	Obtain from a sampling port using an aseptic technique	Category 3
Positioning urinary drainage bags	Position below the level of the bladder on a stand that prevents contact with the floor. When such drainage cannot be maintained, e.g. during moving and handling, clamp the urinary drainage bag tube and remove the clamp as soon as dependant drainage can be resumed.	Category 3
Emptying the drainage bag	Empty frequently enough to maintain urine flow and prevent reflux. Use a separate and clean container for each patient and avoid contact between the urinary drainage tap and container.	Category 3
Adding antiseptic or antimicrobial solutions into urinary drainage bags	Not recommended	Category 1
Changing catheters unnecessarily or as part of routine practice	Not recommended	Category 3
Maintaining meatal hygiene	Routine personal hygiene is all that is needed.	Category 1
Bladder irrigation, instillation and washout	Not recommended, does not prevent catheter-associated infection	Category 2

measured, yet may still be considered to have septic shock (see survival sepsis campaign).

Multiple organ dysfunction syndrome (MODS): Presence of altered organ dysfunction in acutely ill patient, such that homeostasis cannot be maintained without intervention. Primary MODS is a direct result of well-defined insult in which organ dysfunction occurs early and can be directly attributable to insult itself. Secondary MODS develops as a consequence of host response and is identified within the context of SIRS.

Colonized catheter: growth of >/= 15 colony-forming units (semi-quantitative culture) or $>10^3$cfu (quantitative culture) from a proximal or distal catheter segment in the absence of accompanying clinical symptoms.

Exit-site infection: Erythema, tenderness, induration or purulent discharge within 2cm of the skin at the exit site of the catheter.

Pocket infection: Erythema and necrosis of the skin over the reservoir of a totally implantable device, or purulent exudate in the subcutaneous pocket containing the reservoir.

Tunnel infection: Erythema, tenderness and induration in the tissues overlying the catheter and > 2cm from the exit site.

Catheter-related blood stream infection (CR-BSI): Isolation of the same organism (i.e., identical species, antibiogram) from a semi-quantitative or quantitative culture of a catheter segment and from the blood (preferably drawn from a peripheral vein) of a patient with accompanying clinical symptoms of BSI and no other apparent source of infection. In the absence of laboratory confirmation, defervescence after removal of an implicated catheter from a patient with BSI may be considered indirect evidence of CR-BSI.

Infusate-related blood stream infection: Isolation of the same organism from infusate and from separate percutaneous blood cultures, with no other identifiable source of infection.

Laboratory Diagnosis[22-27]

1. **Sample through CVC**: If the ratio of quantitative culture between CVC sample versus peripheral blood sample is 10:1 or more, it is indicative of CVC-related sepsis. Only a few laboratories quantify the number of organisms as this is a time-consuming exercise.
2. **Distal tip culture:** Here, the distal tip of the catheter is rolled across the culture plate. Detection of more than 15 colony-forming units is indicative of infection. This is called the Roll-plate technique.
3. **Catheters flushed** with broth to determine the numbers of organisms attached to the inner surface have found >1000 CFU of bacteria associated with bacteremia.
4. **Endo-luminal brush:** A recently developed method to determine catheter-related sepsis is the use of an endoluminal brush designed to sample the lumen and the distal tip of the CVC in situ. Its value in the clinical situation is still under investigation.

Source of Guidelines of Catheter-Related Infections

The source of clinical pratice guidelines given in Tables 18.5 to 18.13 are modified and abstracted from http://www.cdc.gov/ncidod/dhqp/gl_intravascular.html (MMWR recommendations and reports Vol. 51, number RR-10).

These guidelines focus on providing evidence-based recommendations for preventing hospital-acquired infections associated with the use of central venous catheters in patients who are four years of age or older.

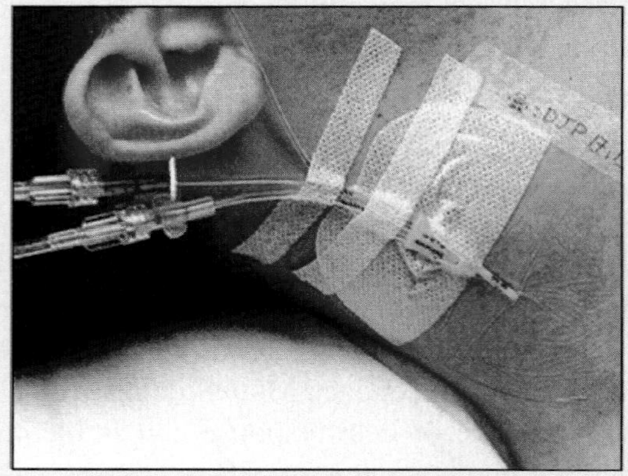

Photo 18.1: Transparent dressing helps detect early signs of infection (Courtesy 3M India Ltd.)

Grading of evidence

Category IA: Strongly recommended for implementation and strongly supported by experimental, clinical or epidemiologic studies.

Category IB: Strongly recommended for implementation and supported by some experimental, clinical or epidemiological studies, and a strong theoretical rationale.

Category IC: Required by state or federal regulations rules or standards.

Category II: Suggested for implementation and supported by suggestive clinical or epidemiologic studies or theoretical rationale.

Unresolved Issue: Represents an unresolved issue for which evidence is insufficient or no controversy regarding efficacy exists.

These recommendations are divided into various categories or intervention groups.

Selection of Catheter Type

(Table 18.5) (Photo 18.1)

Selecting the right catheter for the right patient can minimize the risk of infection. Different types of CVC are available i.e., may be an important determinant in the risk of infection, there is inconclusive evidence as of now, and hence cannot be drawn as a conclusion.

Selection of Site

(Table 18.6)

It is based on:

1. Patient-specific factors (e.g. pre-existing catheters, anatomic deformity, bleeding diathesis, some types of positive pressure ventilation)
2. Relative risk of mechanical complications (e.g. bleeding, pneumothorax, thrombosis).
3. The risk of infection

CVC are generally inserted in the subclavian, jugular or femoral veins, or peripherally inserted into the superior vena cava by way of the cephalic and basilar veins of the antecubital space.

Aseptic Technique During Catheter Insertion: Cutaneous Antisepsis

Using optimum aseptic technique during CVC placement will significantly reduce the risk of infection. Studies examined by HICPAC concluded that if maximal barrier precautions were used during CVC insertion, catheter contamination and subsequent CR-related infections could be significantly minimized.

Infections can be minimized by a good catheter and catheter site care because the catheter hub and connection port are common portals of infection.

Antibiotic prophylaxis is unnecessary. Prophylactic administration of systemic antimicrobials had previously been used to reduce the incidence of CR-BSI, but scientific studies by HICPAC on the efficacy of this practice were inconclusive. Also, it is felt that such prophylaxis may select for resistant microorganisms, particularly those resistant to Vancomycin.

Catheter Site Care and Surveillance

(Tables 18.7 to 18.11)

Cutaneous antisepsis is essential before insertion of catheter (Category IA). This may be done with 70% alcohol, 10% povidone iodine, or 2% tincture iodine before catheter insertion.

When tincture of iodine is used, it must be cleaned with alcohol prior to insertion of catheter (category II). Dressing with a sterile gauze or transparent dressing must be used to cover the catheter insertion site (category IA). Replace gauze or dressing when the dressing becomes loose, dampened or soiled (category IB). Avoid touching or soiling the catheter when it is replaced (category IA).

Antibiotic-Coated Catheters

A new technology that safely inhibits the growth of bacteria, yeast and other organisms from the surface of catheters is that of the silver zeolite antimicrobial. Silver ions are known to restrict and inhibit the growth of damaging microorganisms from taking hold on the surfaces. Thus, when the catheters are coated with silver ions, these ions are slowly released over the life of the product and they have a harmful effect on bacteria and other microorganisms. Antibiotic locks are, however, not routinely recommended. (Category II)

Selection and Replacement of Intravascular Devices

Select the device/catheter according to patient requirement (category IA). This must pose the lowest risk (assess cost benefit ratio) and lowest cost. Remove when clinical use is over (category IA).

Replacement of IV Fluids and Administration Sets

(Tables 18.12, 18.13, 18.14)

An extension is considered a part of the vascular device, and this is replaced when the vascular device is replaced (Category II). The administration sets consist of the portion entering fluid container to the vascular device or the extension.

SURGICAL SITE INFECTIONS (SSIs)

Source of guidelines

The guidelines for surgical site infections given in Tables 18.15 to 18.20 are modified and abstracted from CDC, HIPAC (USA) guidelines for prevention of surgical site infections, 1999. http://www.cdc.gov/ncidod/dhqp/guidelines/SSI.pdf,www.cdc.gov/mmwr/pdf/rr5011.pdf (MMWR April 23, 1999/48 (15);

316). SSIs can become a mammoth problem for ICU patients who may have more drains than the patients elsewhere. To reduce the risk of complications, medical staff should adhere to recommended practices regarding care.[28, 29] Since these patients usually cannot ambulate as early, the risks for complications increase. Dominant factors that contribute to a rising incidence of nosocomial infections include the increasing number of patients with immunocompromised status, high frequency of invasive procedures and extensive use of broad spectrum antibiotics.[30, 31]

Criteria for Defining a Surgical Site Infection (SSI) as given by CDC, HICPAC

I. Skin and subcutaneous tissue SSI

Infection occurs within 30 days after the operation and infection involves only skin or subcutaneous tissue and at least one of the following:

a. Purulent discharge
b. Organisms isolated from fluid or tissue from incision site

Table 18.5: Clinical practice guidelines: catheter-related infection

Type of Catheter	Recommendation	Evidence
Having one or more lumens	HICPAC states that clinicians often preferred multi-lumen CVC because they permitted the concurrent administration of various fluids and medications and haemo-dynamic monitoring among critically ill patients. The conclusions were: Use a single-lumen catheter unless multiple ports are essential for the management of the patient. If total parenteral nutrition is being administered, use one central venous catheter or lumen exclusively for that purpose	IB
Impregnated with antimicrobial or antiseptic agents or heparin, one is the chlorhexidine and silver sulphadiazine catheter and the other is the antiseptic agent (silver ions) bonded with the polyurethane	The use of an antimicrobial impregnated central venous catheter for adult patients who require short term (<10 days) central venous catheterization and who are at high risk for CR-BSI can be considered.	IB
Cuffed and designed to be tunnelled (having totally implantable ports)	It is advisable to use a tunnelled catheter or an implantable vascular access device for patients in whom long-term (>30 days) vascular access is anticipated.	II

Table 18.6: Clinical practice guidelines: catheter-related infection

Selection of Site	Recommendation	Evidence
In selecting an appropriate insertion site	Assess the risks for infection against the risk of mechanical complications	IA
Subclavian site	Unless medically contraindicated, use this in preference to the jugular or femoral sites for non-tunnelled catheter placement	IA
Site for Swan-Ganz catheter	No recommendation	Unresolved Issue

Table 18.7: Clinical practice guidelines: catheter-related infection

Insertion of Catheter	Recommendation	Evidence
Use optimum aseptic Barriers (Maximum Barriers)	A sterile gown, gloves and a large Sterile drape—Recommended	IA
Skin Preparation	HICPAC guideline developers regarded skin cleansing/antisepsis of the insertion site as one of the most important measures for preventing CR-infection	IA
Contact Time	Allow the antiseptic to dry before inserting the catheter. Clean the skin site with an alcoholic chlorhexidine gluconate solution prior to CVC insertion	IB
Agents	Use an alcoholic povidone-iodine solution for patients with a history of chlorhexidine allergy. Study revealed that 2% aqueous chlorhexidine sensitivity was superior to either 10% povidone-iodine or 70% alcohol for preventing CVC and arterial CR-infections	IA
Use of organic solvents, e.g. Acetone	Do not apply acetone or ether to the skin before catheter insertion —Not recommended	IA
Antimicrobial ointment	Do not routinely apply to the catheter placement site prior to insertion	IA

c. At least one of the signs of infection: Pain or tenderness, localized swelling, redness, or heat and superficial incision is deliberately opened by the surgeon, unless incision is culture negative

d. Diagnosis of superficial skin infection by the surgeon or attending physician

Do not report the following conditions as SSI

a. Stitch abscess

b. Infection of episiotomy or newborn circumcision site

c. Infected burn wound

d. Infected SSI that extends to fascial and muscular layers

II Deep incisional SSI

Infection that occurs within 30 days after the operation, and if no implant is left in place or within one year if implant is in place and the infection appears to be related to the opera-

Table 18.8: Clinical practice guidelines: catheter-related infection

Catheter and catheter site care	Recommendation	Evidence
Access	Before accessing the system, disinfect the external surfaces of the catheter hub and connection ports with an aqueous solution of chlorhexidine gluconate or povidone-iodine, unless contraindicated by the manufacturer's recommendations	IA
Cover the catheter site (dressing)	Use either a sterile gauze or transparent dressing (healed tunnelled catheters may not need dressing)	IA
Replacement of dressing	It must be replaced when the dressing becomes damp, loosened or soiled or when inspection of the insertion site is necessary	IB
Antimicrobial ointment	Do not apply to CVC insertion sites as part of routine catheter site care	IA
Routine flushing of indwelling central venous catheters	With an anticoagulant unless advised otherwise by the manufacturer. Preventing catheter thrombosis and maintaining catheter patency will minimize opportunities for infection	II

Table 18.9: Clinical practice guidelines: catheter-related infection

Catheter and tubings replacements	Recommendation	Evidence
Catheter replacement	Do not routinely replace non-tunnelled CVC as a method to prevent catheter-related infection.	IB
Guide wire replacement at same site	Use guide wire assisted catheter exchange to replace a malfunctioning catheter, or to exchange an existing catheter if there is no evidence of infection at the catheter site or proven CR-BSI.	IB
In proven CR infection	Do not use guide wire assisted catheter exchange for patients with CR-infection. If continued vascular access is required, remove the implicated catheter, and replace it with another catheter at a different insertion site.	IB
Suspicion of CR infection	If CR-infection is suspected, but there is no evidence of infection at the catheter site, remove the existing catheter and insert a new catheter over a guide wire; if tests reveal CR-infection, the newly inserted catheter should be removed and, if still required, a new catheter inserted at a different site.	II
Non-tunnelled CV catheters	Do not routinely change	IA
Peripherally inserted catheters	No recommendation	Unresolved issue
Totally implantable device	No recommendation	Unresolved issue
Pulmonary artery catheters	5 days	IB
Arterial catheter introducer	5 days	IB
Inserted in emergency	No recommendation	Unresolved issue
Replacement of tubing	Replace all tubing when the vascular device is replaced.	IA
Regular replacement of stopcocks	Replace intravenous tubing and stopcocks no more frequently than at 72-hour intervals, unless clinically indicated.	IA
Tubings used for blood	Replace intravenous tubing used to administer blood, or lipid transfusions blood products, or lipid emulsions at the end of the infusion or within 24 hours of initiating the infusion.	IB

tion and infection involves deep soft tissues (e.g. fascial and muscular layers) of the incision and at least one of the following:

a. Purulent drainage from the deep incision and not from the organ/space component of the surgical site

b. A deep incision spontaneously dehisces or is deliberately opened by the surgeon when the patient has at least one of the following signs and symptoms: Fever (>38^{0}C), localized pain, or tenderness, unless site is culture-negative.

c. Diagnosis of an SSI made by a surgeon or attending physician

III. Organ/Space SSI

Infection occurs within 30 days after the operation if no implant is left in place or within one year if implant is in place and the infection appears to be related to the operation and involves any part of the anatomy (organ or spaces) other than the incision, which was opened or manipulated during an operation and at least one of the following:

a. Purulent discharge

b. Organism isolated

c. Abscess seen in organ/space on direct examination/histopathology/radiologic examination

Table 18.10: Clinical practice guidelines: catheter-related infection

Catheter site care	Allowable period	Category of evidence
Catheter-site care	If multi-lumen catheters are used designate one lumen for parenteral nutrition.	II
Flush solutions, anticoagulants and other IV additives	Routinely flush (except Groshongs) with anticaogulant.	IB
Cutaneous antisepsis and antimicrobial ointments	Do not apply ointment.	IB
	Do not apply acetone or ether.	IA
Additional guideline for prevention of infection- a) Dialysis catheters b) Umbilical catheters c) Arterial systems	Are given by the CDC	
Antimicrobials routinely (Prophylaxis) before insertion or during insertion of catheter	Do not administer systemic antimicrobials to prevent catheter colonization or blood stream infection.	IA

d. Diagnosis of an organ/space SSI made by a surgeon or attending physician

Surgical Wound Classification/ Grading (CDC, HICPAC)

Class 1/Clean

An uninfected operative wound in which no inflammation is encountered and the respiratory, alimentary, genital or uninfected urinary tract is not entered. In addition, clean wounds are primarily closed and, if necessary, drained with a closed drainage. Operative incisional wounds that follow non-penetrating (blunt) trauma should be included in this category if they meet the criteria.

Class II/Clean-contaminated

An operative wound in which the respiratory, alimentary, genital, or urinary tracts are entered under controlled conditions and without unusual contamination. Specifically, operations involving the biliary tract, appendix, vagina and oropharynx are included in this category, provided no evidence of infection or major breach in technique is encountered.

Class III/Contaminated

Open, fresh, accidental wounds. In addition, operations with major breaks in sterile technique (e.g. open cardiac massage) or gross spillage from the intestinal tract and the incisions in which acute, non-purulent inflammation is encountered are included in this category.

Class IV/Dirty-infected

Old traumatic wounds with retained devitalized tissue and those that involve existing clinical infection or perforated viscera. This definition suggests that organisms causing postoperative infection were present in the operative field before the operation.

Surveillance of SSI

For inpatient case-finding (including readmissions), use direct prospective observations, indirect prospective detection, or a combination of both direct and indirect methods for the duration of patient's hospitalization. Category IB

When post-discharge surveillance is performed for detecting SSI following certain operations (e.g. CABG), use a method that accomodates available resources and data needs. Category II

For outpatient case-finding , use a method that accomodates available resources and data needs. Category IB

Assign the surgical wound classification upon completion of an operation. A surgical team member should make the assignment. Category II

For each patient undergoing an operation chosen for surveillance, record those variables shown to be associated with increased risk of SSI, e.g. Surgical wound class, ASA (American Society of Anesthesiology) class, and duration of operation Category IB

Periodically calculate operation-specific SSI rates stratified by variables shown to be associated with increased risk of SSI (e.g. NNIS risk index). Category IB

Report appropriately stratified, operation-specific SSI rates to the surgical team members. The optimum frequency and format for such rate computations will be determined by stratified case-load sizes (denominators) and the objectives of local, continuous quality improvement initiatives. Category IB

No recommendation to make available to the infection-control committee coded surgeon-specific data. Unresolved issue

HOSPITAL ACQUIRED PNEUMONIA

This is the second most common hospital acquired infection (20%). It is a disease with a high crude mortality of 50%, and an attributable mortality of 27–33% with an odds ratio of 4.25. It increases the length of stay and the cost of treatment.[32-36]

Epidemiology of SSI

Causative organisms

More than 70% are bacterial, viruses are the

Table 18.11: Clinical practice guidelines: catheter-related infection

General CDC Recommendation for intravenous device use:		
Issue	**Recommendation**	**Evidence**
Healthcare worker education and training	Recommended	1A
Surveillance for catheter insertion	Express data as the number of catheter -related infections or catheter-related bloodstream infections (CR-BSI) per 1000 catheter days	1B
Insertion site for tenderness through in-out dressing	Daily	1B
Visually inspect the catheter site for signs of local or blood stream infection	Daily	1B
	Record date and time of catheter insertion	1B
Routine Surveillance culture of patients or devices	Do not routinely perform surveillance	1B
Hand-washing. During catheter insertion and care	Recommended	1A
While changing dressings on intravascular devices	Wear gloves	1B
Use of sterile versus non-sterile clean gloves during dressing changes	There is no recommendation	Unresolved issue

Table 18.12: Clinical practice guidelines: catheter-related infection

Replacement of IV fluids and Administration Sets		
Issue	**Recommendation**	**Evidence**
Type of administration set	**Frequency of replacement**	**Category of evidence**
IV sets, stopcocks	72-hr intervals	Category IA
IV sets for blood /blood products	24 hrs	Category IB
Fluid	**Hang time**	**Category of evidence**
Crystalloids, non-lipid TPN	72 hrs	Category II
Blood and blood products	4 hrs	Category II
Lipid containing TPN	24 hrs	Category IB
Only lipid solutions	12 hrs	Category IB
Access to injection ports	Clean with 70% alcohol or povidone iodine before accessing.	Category IA

(TPN = Total Parenteral Nutrition)

Table 18.13: Clinical practice guidelines: catheter-related infection

Preparation of IV fluids/admixtures		
Issue	**Recommendation**	**Evidence**
Preparation of fluids in pharmacy	Use laminar flow hood, check before use	IB
Checking of container, fluids, etc.	Turbidity/cracks particulate matter. Date of expiry	IA
Use of additives/medications	Single-dose vials—Recommended	II
Multidose vials	Refrigerate Cleanse diaphragm Use sterile device and discard if contaminated	IA
In-line filters for routine use	Not recommended	IA
Intravenous therapy personnel	Recommended	IB
Use of needleless devices	No recommendation	Unresolved issue
Prophylactic antibiotics during insertion	Not recommended	

Table 18.14: Clinical practice guidelines: catheter-related infection

Selection of Central Venous Catheters and Arterial Catheters	Recommendation	Evidence
Single lumen vs multiple lumens	Single lumen catheters are preferable unless multiple ports are essential for patient management	IB
For patients needing long term catheters (>30 days)	Peripheral central venous catheters, tunnelled (Hickman or Broviac) or an implantable catheter are preferable	IA
Antiseptic or antimicrobial-coated catheters	May be used in patients with high incidence of infection in spite of barrier precautions	II

Table 18.15: Clinical practice guidelines: Surgical Site Infection (SSI)

Pre-operative Preparation and status		
Issue	**Recommendation**	**Evidence**
Remote site infections	Treat prior to elective operations.	Category IA
Hair at or around incision	Do not preoperatively trim/shave unless it interferes with the operative area.	Category IA
	Remove hair immediately before surgery.	Category IA
Control blood sugar levels	Recommended	Category IB
Preoperative tobacco use	Stop 30 days before surgery	Category IB
Blood products	Do not withhold to prevent SSI	Category 1B
Bathe/shower antiseptic agent	At least the night before operation	Category IB
Washed/cleaned site of incision	Before antiseptic skin preparation	Category IB
Skin preparation	Use an appropriate antiseptic agent Preoperative skin antiseptic application in concentric circles moving toward the periphery.	Category IB Category II
Area of application of antisepsis	Large enough to extend the incision and create new incisions/drain sites	Category II
Preoperative stay	Should be as short as possible	Category II

Table 18.16: Clinical practice guidelines: Surgical Site Infection (SSI)

Issue	Recommendation	Evidence
If patient is on preoperative steroid	There is no recommendation to taper or discontinue systemic steroid before elective operation (when medically permissable)	Unresolved issue
Nutritional support for surgical patients	There is no recommendation to enhance solely as a means to prevent SSI	Unresolved issue
Preoperatively apply mupirocin to nares	No recommendation to provide measures that enhance wound space oxygenation to prevent SSI	Unresolved issue

cause in 20% cases, the rest comprise fungi and others.

Bacteriological profile in a major hospital ICU in northern India

Pseudomonas aeruginosa	40.24%
Acinetobacter spp.	30.02%
Klebsiella spp.	8.92%
Staphylococcus spp.	4.14%
E.coli	3.37%
Streptococcus spp.	1.24%
Enterococcus spp.	1.86%
Candida spp.	1.45%

(Muralidhar V et al. JACP. 1996)

Diagnosis

A presumptive clinical diagnosis of nosocomial pneumonia is generally made if a patient develops progressive pulmonary infiltrates associated with fever, leucocytosis and purulent tracheal secretion. Each of these signs and symptoms have a high sensitivity but low specificity because of other conditions which mimic each of these findings. For example, a number of conditions can cause a pneumonia-like picture on x-ray. Clinical diagnosis of pneumonia can lead not only to an error in diagnosis but also an improper selection of antibiotics. Improper treatment with antibiotics, in turn, contributes to an increased fatality. On the other hand the patient's survival may improve if pneumonia is correctly diagnosed and treated. To increase the specificity of diagnosis it is important to combine proper sampling methods and microbiological analysis (qualitative and quantitative) of a sample derived from the lower respiratory tract (avoiding contamination of the colonized bacteria in the upper airway and the tube).

Diagnostic methods for nosocomial pneumonia: Specificity increases from 1 to 4 and hence 4 is ideal

1. Clinical criteria alone
2. Clinical + Radiological

Table 18.17: Clinical practice guidelines: Surgical Site Infection (SSI)

Barrier precaution, surgical scrub, attire, infected personnel		
Issue	**Recommendation**	**Evidence**
Surgical attire and drapes	Wear a surgical mask that fully covers the mouth and the nose when entering the operating room if an operation is about to begin or already underway, or if sterile instruments are exposed. Wear the mask throughout the operation.	Category IB
	Wear a cap or hood to fully cover hair on the head and face when entering the operating room.	Category IB
Shoe covers for the prevention of SSI	Do not wear	Category IB
	Wear sterile gloves if a scrubbed surgical team member. Put on gloves after donning a sterile gown.	Category IB
	Use surgical gowns and drapes that are effective barriers when wet (i.e. materials that resist liquid penetration).	Category IB
	Change visibly soiled scrub suits that are contaminated, and/or penetrated by blood or other potentially infectious material.	Category IB
Hand/forearm antisepsis for surgical team members	Nails should be kept short. No artificial nails should be worn.	Category IB
	Preoperative surgical scrub should be performed for at least 2–5 minutes using an appropriate antiseptic.	Category IB
	After surgical scrub, the hands should be kept up and away from body, so that water runs from the tips of the fingers toward the elbows. Hands are dried with a sterile towel. Sterile gowns and gloves are worn.	Category IB
	Before the first surgical scrub of the day, the inner side of each fingernail is cleaned.	Category II
	Hand or arm jewellery should not be worn.	Category II
	There is no recommendation on the wearing of nail polish	Unresolved issue

Table 18.17: (Contd.)

Management of infected or colonized surgical personnel	Surgical personnel who have signs and symptoms of a transmissible infectious illness should report conditions promptly to their supervisory and occupational health service personnel.	Category IB
Policies	Well-defined policies should be formulated concerning patient-care responsiblities when personnel have potentially transmissible infectious conditions. These policies should govern: a) personnel responsibility in using health service and reporting illness b) work restrictions c) Clearance to resume work after an illness that required work restriction. The policies should also identify persons who have the authority to remove personnel from duty.	Category IB
Skin lesions	Personnel having draining skin lesions should have their cultures taken. Meanwhile, they should be excluded from duty till they receive adequate therapy.	Category IB
	It is not necessary to exclude surgical personnel who are colonized with organisms such as *Staph. aureus* (nose, hands or other body site) or Group A Streptococcus, unless such personnel have been linked epidemiologically to dissemination of the organism in the healthcare setting.	Category IB

3. Clinical + Radiological + noninvasive sampling + Microbiological (qualitative + quantitative)
4. Clinical + Radiological + invasive sampling + Microbiological (qualitative + quantitative)

Sampling techniques used for diagnosis of nosocomial pneumonia

- Broncho alveolar lavage (BAL)
- Protected specimen brush (PSB)
- Non-bronchoscopic BAL (telescoping plugged catheter)
- Non directed BAL
- Tracheal aspirate
- Needle aspiration
- Transtracheal Biopsy
- Surgical (thoracoscopic/open) biopsy

Table 18.18: Clinical practice guidelines: Surgical Site Infection (SSI)

Cleaning and draping, Surgical skin preparation, Asepsis and Surgical technique		
Issue	**Recommendation**	**Evidence**
Placing intravascular devices (e.g. central venous catheters), spinal or epidural anaesthesia catheters, or when dispensing and administering intravenous drugs	Adhere to the principles of asepsis	Category IA
Sterile equipment and solutions handling tissues	Assemble immediately prior to use. Gently, maintain effective haemostasis, minimize devitalised tissue and foreign bodies (i.e. sutures, charred tissues, necrotic debris), and eradicate dead space at the surgical site.	Category II Category IB
Surgical site heavily contaminated	Use delayed primary skin closure or leave an incision open to heal by secondary intention (e.g. Class III or IV).	Category IB
Drainage	If necessary, use a closed suction drain. Place the drain through a separate incision distant from the operative site. Remove the drain as soon as possible.	Category II
	Protect an incision that has been closed primarily with a sterile dressing for 24–48hrs post-operatively	Category IB
Post-operative incision-care	No recommendation to cover an incision closed primarily beyond 48 hrs or on the appropriate time to shower or bathe with an uncovered incision	Unresolved issue
Dressing changes	Wash hands before and after any contact with surgical site. When an incision dressing must be changed, use a sterile technique.	Category IB Category II
Education	Educate the patient and family regarding proper incision care, symptoms of SSI and the need to report such symptoms.	Category II

Table 18.19: Clinical practice guidelines: Surgical Site Infection (SSI)

Engineering and environmental prevention	Recommendation	Evidence
Positive-pressure ventilation	Maintain in the operating room with respect to the corridors and adjacent areas.	Category IB
Air changes per hour	Maintain a minimum of 15 air changes per hour, of which at least 3 should be fresh air.	Category IB
Filtration of air	Filter all air, re-circulated and fresh, through the appropriate filters as per American Institute of Architects recommendation.	Category IB
Direction of flow	Introduce all air at the ceiling, and exhaust near the floor.	Category IB
UV radiation	Do not use in the operating room to prevent SSI.	Category IB
Movement into operating room	Keep operating room doors closed except as needed for passage of equipment, personnel and patient.	Category IB
Ultraclean air	Consider performing orthopaedic implant operations in the operating rooms supplied with ultraclean air.	Category II
Number of personnel	Limit to necessary personnel entering the operating room.	Category II
Visibly soiled surfaces	When visible soiling or contamination with blood or other body fluids of surfaces or equipment occurs during an operation, use EPA-approved hospital disinfectant to clean the affected areas before the next operation.	Category IB
Special cleaning or closing of OR	Do not perform special cleaning or closing of operating room suite or individual operating rooms for infection control.	Category IB
Tacky mats	Do not use at the entrance to the operating rooms for infection control	Category IB
Terminal cleaning	Wet vacuum the operating room floor after the last operation of the day or night with an EPA-approved hospital disinfectant.	Category II

Table 18.19: (Contd.)

Equipment cleaning (Between cases)	No recommendation on disinfecting environmental surfaces or equipment used in operating rooms between operations in the absence of visible soiling	Unresolved issue
Routine microbiological sampling of the operating room environmental surfaces or air	Do not perform routine sampling of the operating room. Only as part of an epidemiological investigation	Category IB
Sterilization of surgical equipment	Sterilize all surgical equipment according to published guidelines	Category IB
	Use flash sterilization only for patient care items that will be used immediately (e.g. to reprocess an inadvertantly dropped instrument). Do not flash sterilize for reasons of convenience or to save time.	Category IB

Guidelines for PSB techniques

- Perform suction through the endotracheal tube prior to bronchscopy.
- No suction is performed while introducing the bronchoscope.
- No lidocaine is injected through the suction channel of the bronchoscope.
- The bronchoscope tip is advanced into the involved area as seen on a chest x-ray.
- The inner cannula is protruded to eject the gelatin plug into the bronchus while keeping the tip of the protected brush in the field of vision.
- The inner cannula containing the brush is then advanced into a bronchial segment leading into the involved area.
- The brush is then advanced out of the inner catheter and turned several times to obtain a specimen.
- After sampling, the brush is retracted into the inner cannula, and the inner cannula into the outer cannula and then the entire bronchoscope is removed.
- The outer sheath is cleaned with 70% alcohol, cut with sterile scissors, and discarded.
- The brush is then readvanced, cut with sterile wire clippers into a container with one ml of sterile saline.
- The specimen should be sent for quantitative culture within 15 minutes.

Guidelines for BAL technique

- Perform suction through the endotracheal tube prior to bronschoscopy.
- No suction is performed while introducing the bronchoscope.
- No lidocaine is injected through the suction channel of the bronchoscope.

Table 18.20: Clinical practice guidelines: Surgical Site Infection (SSI)

Treatment Antimicrobial prophylaxis	Recommendation	Evidence
Prophylactic antibiotics	Administer only when indicated and select it based on its efficiency against common pathogens causing SSI for a specific operation and published recommendations.	Category IA
	Administer the initial dose timed such that the bactericidal dose of the prophylactic concentration of the drug agent is established in the serum and tissues when the incision is made. Maintain therapeutic levels of the agent in the tissues and serum throughout the operation and until, at most, a few hours after the incision is closed in the operating room.	Category IA
Before colorectal operations	In addition to the above points, mechanically prepare the colon by use of enemas and cathartic agents. Administer non-absorbable oral antimicrobial agents in divided doses on the day before the surgery.	Category IA
For high-risk caesarean section	Administer the prophylactic agent immediately after the umbilical cord is clamped.	Category IA
	Do not routinely use antimicrobial prophylaxis.	Category IB

- The bronchoscope is wedged in the segmental bronchus of the lobe that is affected.
- Three aliquots of 40ml sterile saline are infused through the working channel of the bronchoscope.
- Suction is applied and the first aliquot is discarded or saved as bronchial lavage.
- The second and third aliquots of aspirate are saved as bronchoalveloar lavage.
- The specimen should be sent for quantitative culture within 30 minutes.

The optimal strategy for sampling remains controversial [37-46]

The controversy is between invasive versus noninvasive sampling. The advantages of invasive sampling with bronchoscopic methods such as protected specimen brush (PSB) and broncho-alveolar lavage (BAL) is the high sensitivity and specificity. The disadvantages are the morbidity of the invasive procedure e.g. trauma, pneumothorax, hypoxemia, etc. expertise required and the cost of the equipment. Some centres in Europe recommend an invasive sampling with isolation of the organism as a prerequisite for diagnosis and treatment and change of treatment. Proponents of the empirical treatment state that bronchoscopic methods are not only costly and time consuming, but there is also a delay in getting the results.

Microbiological analysis should not be only qualitative (mentioning only the type of bacteria) because this does not distinguish between contamination, other infections (such as the tracheo-bronchitis) and pneumonia. To draw a distinction, the bacterial load in terms of colony forming units (CFU)/ml or the bacterial index should be known. It is also important to have an established threshold for the quantitative value derived to have a higher specificity.

Guidelines for quantitative diagnostic criteria for the diagnosis of nosocomial pneumonia[47-62]

Commonly Used Quantitative Thresholds for Diagnosis of VAP

Endotracheal	10^6/cfu/ml
Non-Bronchoscopic BAL	10^6–10^7 cfu/ml
Bronchoscopic Alveolar Lavage (BAL)	10^3 cfu/ml
Protected Specimen Brush (PSP)	10^4 cfu/ml
Sputum/ET aspirate	10^6 cfu/ml[11]

Policy on Preventive Measures and Evidence-Based Guidelines

(Tables 18.21, 18.22, 18.23)

To prevent, it is important to understand risk factors, pathogenesis, important host-related risk factors and preventive factors given in the tables below.

Treatment

De-escalation therapy

Guidelines for empirical antibiotic prescribing in the initial treatment of VAP (American Thoracic Society).

Guidelines for specific antibiotic treatment and subsequent modification of treatment.

Selective digestive decontamination

This is still not recommended by the CDC, Atlanta, due to lack of evidence on the effects on mortality.

THE SURVIVING SEPSIS CAMPAIGN GUIDELINES FOR SEPTIC SHOCK

(TABLE 18.24)

The management of intensive care infections are difficult because till now there was no consensus on the treatment modalities and interventions practised across nations and continents. The Surviving Sepsis Campaign and evolution of consensus based guidelines is targeted at bringing in uniformity, acceptance of a core set of recommendations (bundle) based on evidence. The optimum treatment of severe sepsis and septic shock is dynamic and evolving and the current set of recommendations is a starting point. The impact of the recommendations on outcomes will be formally assessed and updated annually and even more rapidly as new knowledge becomes available.

Table 18.21: Clinical Practice guidelines: Hospital Acquired Pneumonia

Pathophysiology and Preventive Strategies	
Flora from stomach contents	Prevention of regurgitation by positioning, overdistention, overfeeding
Loss of fibronectin in the orophryngeal secretions	Colonization of lower respiratory tract
Bacterial translocation from the gut	Avoid ischemia, hypotension

Source of guidelines for preventive measures[37-46]

The prevention guidelines given in Table 18.22 to 18.23 have been modified and abstracted from http://www.cdc.gov/mmwr/preview/mmwrhtml/rr5303a1.htm (March 26, 2004/53 (RR03); 1-36); 'Guidelines for preventing health care associated pneumonia, 2003' developed by CDC, HICPAC. These are generally divided into Host, Device and Ventilator associated risk factors by the CDC.

Table 18.22: Clinical Practice guidelines: Hospital Acquired Pneumonia

Device-Associated Risk Factors and Preventive Measures	Recommendation	Evidence
Enteral feeding	Verify tube placement	IB
	Use sterile water	NS
	Use orogastric tube if possible	NS
	Position patient at 30–40^0	IB
	Remove residual feeds	IB
Oxygen delivery	Change tubings between patients	IB
Invasive devices	Appropriate cleaning and sterilization	IA
Spirometer	Clean, sterilize/disinfect between patients	IB
Temperature/O_2 sensor	Clean, sterilize/disinfect between patients	IB
Resuscitation bag	Clean, sterilize/disinfect between patients	IA
Bronchoscope	Judicious use	NS
Tracheostomy care	Aseptic technique while changing tube	IB
Cross infection	Education/training/surveillance/handwashing/	IA

Table 18.23: Clinical Practice guidelines: Hospital Acquired Pneumonia

Device ventilator-associated Risk factors	Recommendations and preventive measures	Evidence
Endotracheal intubation	Sterile technique/optimal cuff pressure/ Aspirate subglottic secretions before deflation	IB
	CASS (continuous aspiration of subglottic secretions)	NR
	Oral intubation	NR
	Semirecumbent position	IB
Ventilator circuit	Do not change < 48 hrs	IA
	Drain/discard the condensate away from patient	IB
	Use heat moisture exchanger	NR
In-line medication	Disinfect nebulizers between treatments/sterilize between patients	IB
Tracheal suction catheter	Aseptic technique	IA
HME filter vs heated humidifiers	No recommendation	IB
HME filter Change	Not more frequently than 48 hrs	
	Sterile single-use catheter	IA
	Closed-circuit tracheal suction catheter	NR

Grading System (Survival Sepsis Campaign)[63]

Grading of recommendations

A= Supported by at least two level I investigations

B= Supported by one level I investigation

C= Supported by level II investigations only

D= Supported by at least one level III investigation

E= Supported by level IV or V evidence

Grading of Evidence (Survival Sepsis Campaign)

(Table 18.24)

1. Large, randomized trials with clear-cut results; low risk of false positive (alpha) error or false negative (beta) error.
2. Small, randomized trials with uncertain results; moderate to high risk of false positive (alpha) and/or false negative (beta) error.
3. Nonrandomized, contemporary controls
4. Nonrandomized, historical controls and expert opinion

Table 18.24: Clinical practice guidelines: Septic shock

The surviving sepsis campaign guidelines for management of septic shock		
Issues	**Recommendations**	**Evidence**
Initial resuscitation	Goal directed therapy	Grade B
Diagnosis	Blood cultures	Grade E
Antibiotic therapy	Start within first hour	Grade E
	Empirical therapy	Grade E
Vasopressors	Fluid challenge—yes	Grade E
	Low mean pressure despite fluids	Grade D
	Norad or dobutamine—yes	
	Dopamine for renal protection— no	Grade B
	Arterial line—yes	Grade E
Ionotropic support	Low cardiac output despite fluids—dobutamine	Grade A
Steroids	Hydrocortisone—for 7 days—yes in shock	Grade C
Human Recombinant Activated Protein C	In organ failure with no contraindications—yes	Grade C
Blood products	Blood—Hb less than 7 gm%	Grade B
	Erythropoietin only in renal failure induced anaemia	Grade B
	Fresh Frozen Plasma (FFP)—yes in active bleeding or for invasive procedures	Grade E
	Antithrombin administration—no Platelets	Grade B

5. Case series, uncontrolled studies, and expert opinion

THE NEUTROPENIC PATIENT

Treatment of a neutropenic patient is a medical emergency. The risk of infections is greatly increased if the absolute neutrophil count (ANC) falls below $1000/mm^3$. The risk increases exponentially when the ANC falls below $500/mm^3$. If the count is less than $100/mm^3$ the risk of bacteremia is more than 20%. The definition of fever in these patients is a single rise of oral temperature over 38.3^0C or 101^0 Farenheit.

Clinically significant infections in neutropenic patients are caused by the following organisms:

Staphylococcus: Not fulminant but with high morbidity. Associated with the use of intravenous catheters

Streptococcus viridans: Fulminant, fatal with associated shock and ARDS.

Very virulent and destruction is proteolytic degradation and utilization of glycoproteins.

Gram-negative infections: They vary in the severity of the presentation.

Pseudomonas aeruginosa: Most feared infection.

Fungal infections

There has been a change in pattern of fungal infections. The Candidal infections have been taken over by Aspergillosis. In these patients the increase in the fungal infections has given rise to changed strategies in managing them. Antifungal prophylaxis may be considered in patients with a low ANC count.

Selection of antimicrobials in neutropenic patients

1. Prophylaxis with a single agent can be attained with ceftazidime, ciprofloxacin or Imipenem.

These are not effective against MRSA. If methicillin resistance is suspected, then vancomycin or teicoplanin may be added.

Combination of aminoglycoside with an antipseudomonas beta lactam agent may also be useful.

If patient is in shock, change or add to the initial regime as follows:

- If the infection is catheter related, vancomycin may be added.
- If the patient has signs of gastrointestinal source then metronidazole may be added.
- Empirical antifungal agents must be considered when the fever does not respond to conventional strategies.

No specific duration is recommended for therapy. Continue treatment till the counts come above 500/mm.[3]

REFERENCES

1) Masterson RG and Teare EL. Clinical Governance and infection Control in the United Kingdom. J Hosp Infect. 2001; 47: 25-31.

2) Farrington M and Pascoe G. Risk management and infection control – time to get our priorities right in the United Kingdom. J Hosp Infect. 2001; 47: 5-24.

3) Fisher RB and Dearden CH. Improving the care of patients with major trauma in the accident and emergency department. Br Med J 1990; 300: 1560-3.

4) West KH. Inter-departmental Infection Control Measures. In: Infection Control in the Emergency Department. Rockville: Aspen Publishers, Inc. 1988; 21-119.

5) Woodhead M, Torres A. Definition and classification of community-acquired and nosocoimial pneumonia. Eur Respir Man 1997; 3:1-12.

6) Rengelhart S, Krizek L and Glasmacher A. *Pseudomonas aeruginosa* outbreak in a haematology-oncology unit associated with contaminated surface cleaning equipment. J Hosp Infect. 2002; 52(2): 93-8.

7) Zafar AB, Sylvester LK and Beidas SO. *Pseudomonas aeruginosa* infections in a neonatal intensive care unit. Am J Infect Control. 2002; 30(7): 425-9.

8) Laney M and Bayley EW. Incidence of adult immunization for influenza and pneumonia in a preadmission testing unit. J Perianesth Nurs 2002; 17(5): 325-26.

9) Practice recommendation for Healthcare Facilities Implementing the US Public Health Service Guidelines for Management of Occupational Exposures to Bloodborne Pathogens.Morbidity and Mortality Weekly Report (MMWR) Recommendations and Reports. June29,2001 / Volume 50 / No.RR-11

10) Sobel, JD and Kaye D. Urinary tract infections. In: Mandell GL, Bennett JE and Dolin R (Eds.), Principles and practices of infectious diseases. Churchill Livingstone. Philadelphia, PA: 5th edn. 2000; 73: 805.

11) Valenti WM and Reese RE. Genitourinary tract infections. In: Reese RE and Douglas RG, eds. A practical approach to infectious diseases. Boston, MA: Little, Brown.1983; 491-526.

12) Stamm WE. Catheter-associated urinary tract infections: Epidemiology, pathogenesis, and prevention. Am J Med, 1991; 91(Suppl. 3B): 65S-71S.

13) Maki DG, Knasinski V, Halvorson KT et al. A prospective, randomized, investigator-blinded trial of a novel nitrofurazone-impregnated urinary cathether {abstract M49}. Infect Control Hosp Epidemiol 1997; 18 (Suppl): 50

14) Darouiche RO, Smith A, Hanna H et al. Efficacy of antimicrobial-impregnated bladder catheters in reducing catheter-associated bacteriuria: a prospective, randomized multicenter clinical trial. Urology. 1999; 54: 976-81.

15) Lundeberg T. Prevention of catheter-associated urinary tract infections by use of silver-impregnated catheters {letter}. Lancet 1986; 1: 1031.

16) Liedberg H, Lundeberg T, Ekman P. Refinements in the coating of urethral catheters reduce the incidence of catheter-associated bacteriuria. An experimental and clinical study. Eur Urol 1990; 7: 236-40.

17) Liedberg H and Lundeberg T. Prospective study of incidence of urinary tract infection in patients catheterized with bard hydrogel and silver-coated catheters or bard hydrogel-coated catheters {abstract 405A}. J Urol 1993; 149.

18) Maki DG, Knasinski V, Halvorson K et al. A novel silver-Hydrogel impregnated indwelling catheter reduces CAUTIs: a prospective double-blind trial {abstract}. In Programs and abstracts of the Society for Healthcare Epidemiology in America Annual Meeting; April 5-7, 1998; Orlando, Florida.

19) Platt, R., Polk, B. F., Murdock, B. et al. Risk factors for nosocomial urinary tract infection. Am J Epidemiol 1986; 124: 977-985.

20) Ferrari AM. A strategy for the management of hospitalized children with acute lower respiratory infections. Rev Saude Publica. 2002; 36(3): 292-300.

21) Manieu LM. Prediction of nosocomial sepsis in neonates by means of a computer-weighted bedside scoring system (NOSEP score). Crit Care Med 2000; 28(6): 2026-29

22) Mermel LA, Farr BM, Sherertz RJ et al. Guidelines for the management of intravascular catheter-related infections. J Intraven Nurs. 2001; 24(3): 180-205.

23) Nhenberg G, Biot. Prevention of infections transmitted by intravascular devices (catheters implanted sites). Rev Pneumol Clin. 2001; 57(2): 101-12.

24) Maki DG, Weise CE and Sarafin HW. A semiquantitative culture method for identifying intravenous catheter related infection. N Eng J Med 1977; 296: 1305-1309.

25) Cleri DJ, Corrada ML and Seligman SJ. Quantitative culture of intravenous catheters and other intravenous inserts. J Inf Dis 1980; 141:781-786.

26) Markus S and Bunday S. Culturing in-dwelling central venous catheters in situ. Infect Surg 1989; 5: 157-162.

27) Buxton AE, Highsmith AK, Garner JS et al. Contamination of Intravenous Infusion Fluid: Effects of changing administration sets. Annals of Internal Medicine. 1979; 90: 764-768.

28) Cruse PJ and Foord R.A five year prospective study of 23, 649 surgical wounds. Arch Surg 1973; 107: 206-210.

29) Cruse PJ and Foord R. The epidemiology of wound infection: a 10-year prospective study of 62, 939 wounds. Surg Clin North Am 1980; 60: 27-39.

30) Public health focus: surveillance, prevention and control of nosocomial infections. Morb Mortal Wkly Rep 1992; 41: 783-787.

31) Emmerson AM, Enstone JE, Griffin M et al. The second national prevalance survey of infections in hospitals – overview of results. J. Hosp. Infect 1996; 32: 175-190

32) Horan TC, Culver DH, Gaynes RP et al. Noscomial infections in surgical patients in the United States, January 1986–June 1992. National Nosocomial Infection Surveillance (NNIS) system. Infect Control Hosp Epedemiol 1993; 14:73-80.

33) Hayley Culver DH, White JW. The efficacy of infection surveillance and control programmes in US hospitals. Am J Epidemiol 1985;121: 182-205.

34) Fagon JY, Chastre J, Vuagnat A, et al. Nosocomial pneumonia and mortality among patients in Intensive Care units. JAMA 1996; 275; 886-869.

35) Prod'hom G, Leuenberger P, Koerfer J et al. Nosocomial pneumonia in mechanically ventilated patients receiving antacid ranitidine, or sucralfate as Prophyplaxis for stress ulcer. A randomized controlled trial. Ann Intern Med 1994; 120:653-662.

36) Cook DJ, Walter SD, Cook R J et al. Incidence of and risk factors for ventilator-associated pneumonia in critically ill patients. An Intern Med 1998; 129: 433-440.

37) Rello J, Gallego M, Mariscal D et al. The value of routine microbiological investigation in ventilator associated pneumonia. Am J Respir Crit Care Med 1997; 156: 196-200.

38) Kollef MH and Wad S. The influence of mini -BAL cultures on patient outcome implications for the antibiotic management of ventilator-associated pneumonia. Chest 1998; 113: 412-420.

39) Fagon JY, Chastre J, Wolff M et al. Invasive and noninvasive strategies for management of suspected ventilator-associated pneumonia. Ann Intern Med 2000; 2: 621-630.

40) Rello J, Quintana E, Ausina V et al. Incidence, aeitology and outcome of nosocomial pnemonia in mechanically ventilated patients. Chest.1991; 100: 439-444.

41) Rello J, Diaz E, Roque M et al. Risk factors for developing pneumonia within 48 hrs of intubation. Am J Respir Crit Care Med 1999; 59: 1742-46.

42) Craven DE and Steger KA. Nosocomial pneumonia in mechanically ventilated adult patients: epidemiology and prevention. Semin Respir Infect 1996; 11:32-53.

43) Celis R, Torres A, Gatell JM et al. Nosocomial Pneumonia. A multivariate analysis of risk and prognosis. Chest 1988; 93:318-324.

44) Torres A, Aznar R, Gatell JM et al. Incidence, risk, and prognostic factors of nosocomial pneumonia in mechanically ventilated patients. Am Rev Respir Dis 1990; 14:523-528.

45) Campbell GD, Nieder MS, Broguhton WA et al. Americal Thoracic Society. Hospital acquired pneumonia in adults: Diagnosis, assessment of severity, initial antimicrobial therapy, and preventive strategies. Crit Care Med 1995; 53:1711-25.

46) Baker AM, Meredith JW and Haponik EF. Pneumonia in intubated trauma patients. Microbiology and outcomes. Am J Respir Crit Care Med 1996; 153: 343-349.

47) Joines RN and Pfaller MA. Bacterial resistance: A worldwide problem. Diagn Microbial Infect Dis 1998; 31:379-88.

48) Huxley EJ, Viroslav J, Grey WR et al. Pharyngeal aspiration in normal subjects and in patients with depressed consciousness. Am J Med 1978; 64:564-568.

49) Cunnion K, Weber DJ, Broadhead WE et al. Risk factors for nosocomial pneumonia: comparing adult care population Am J Resp Crit Care Med 1996; 153:157-162.

50) Mahul PH, Auboyer C, Jospe R et al. Prevention of nosocomial pneumonia in intubated patients: respective role of mechanical subglottic secretions drainage and stress ulcer prophylaxis. Internsive care Med 1992; 18: 20-25.

51) Adair CG, Gorman SP, Feron BM et al. Complications of endotracheal biofilm for ventilator-associated pneumonia. Intensive Care Med 1999; 25: 1072-1076.

52) Jacobs SR, Chang W, Lee B et al. Continuous enteral feeding : a major cause of pneumonia among ventilated intensive care unit patients. Parenteral nutrition 1990; 13:353-356.

53) Fagon JY and Chastre J. Nosocomial pneumonia. In: Grenvik A, Ayres SM, Holbrook PR, Shoemaker WC, eds. Text book of Critical Care. 4th edn. WB Saunders Co. 2000; 464-676.

54) Rello J, Ollendrof DA, Oster G et al. For the VAP Outcomes Scientific Advisory Group. Epidemiology and outcomes of ventilator-associated pneumonia in a large US database Chest 2002; 122: 2115-2121.

55) Craven DE, Kunches LM, Kilinski V et al. Risk factors for pneumonia and fatality in patients receiving mechanical ventilationn. Am Rev Respir Dis 1986; 133: 792-796.

56) Fagon JY, Chastre J. Domart Y et al. Nosocomial pneumonia in patients receiving continuous mechanical ventilation : Prospective analysis of 52 episodes with use of a protected specimen brush and quantitative culture techniques. Am Rev Respir 1989; 139: 877-884.

57) Trivedi T, Shejale SB and Yeolekar ME. Nosocomial pneumonia in medical intensive care unit. J Associ Physicians India 2000; 48: 1070-1073.

58) Vincent JL, Bihari DH, Suter PM et al. The prevalence of nosocomial infection in intensive care units in Europe: results of the European prevalence of Infection in Intensive Care (EPIC) study. JAMA 1995: 274: 639-644.

59) Chevret S, Hemmer M, Carlet J et al and the European cooperative Group on Pneumonia. Incidence and risk factors for pneumonia acquired in intensive care. Med 1993; 19: 256-264.

60) Singh N, Rogers P, Atwood CW et al. Short-course empiric antibiotic therapy for patients with pulmonary infiltrates in the intensive care unit. Am J Respir Crit Care Med 2000; 162: 505-511.

61) Waterer GW. The diagnostic dilemma in suspected ventilator-associated pneumonia. Chest 2003; 123: 335-337.

62) Kollef MH. The prevention of ventilator-associated pnuemonia. N Eng J. Med 1999; 340: 8:627-634.

63) Delkinger RP. Carlet JM, Masur H et al. Surviving Sepsis campaign guidelines for management of severe sepsis and septic shock. Crit Care. Med. 2004; 32(3): 858-873.

Chapter 19

Prescribing Practices and Antibiotic Policy

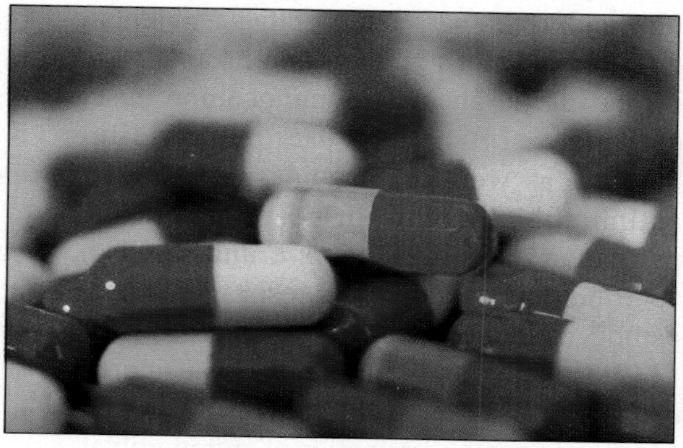

No branch of therapeutics depends so heavily on the laboratory as antimicrobials, particularly antimicrobial chemotherapy. The prescriber lacking such help has been described as a mariner without chart or compass.

—L. P. Garrod

Highlights

Guidelines and Treatment Algorithms Given by Important Bodies

Policy on Resistant Microorganisms

Antibiotic Prescribing and Appropriate Use of Antimicrobials

Restrict Use of Certain Antimicrobials

Effective Preventive Measures (Practice Guidelines)

Prompt Diagnosis

Administrative and Managerial Interventions

Development of Newer and Novel Strategies

Inappropriate Use of Antimicrobials in Animal Husbandry

Antimicrobial Abuse and Its Implications

INTRODUCTION

The emergence of resistance to antimicrobial agents is a global public health problem, particularly in pathogens causing nosocomial infections. Antimicrobial resistance results in increased illness, deaths and healthcare costs. The distribution of resistant pathogens causing nosocomial infections changes with time and varies between hospitals and among different locations in the same hospital. The increasing number of immunocompromised patients and increased use of indwelling devices, as well as the widespread use of antimicrobial agents in hospital settings, particularly in intensive care units (ICUs), contribute to antimicrobial resistance among pathogens in the hospital set-up.[1-3]

Hospitals worldwide are facing an unprecedented crisis due to the increasingly rapid emergence and dissemination of antimicrobial-resistant microorganisms. The situation is particularly alarming in countries where there is unrestricted sale of 'over the counter' (OTC) antibiotics. According to CDC, nearly 50 million of the 150 million outpatient prescriptions for antibiotics are unnecessary. This frightening scenario is not restricted to bacteria alone. Even fungi and viruses are capable of developing resistance to antifungal and antiviral agents respectively. Resistance has also increased in ICUs leading to very resistant HAIs. This high incidence of reduced antimicrobial susceptibility suggests that more effective strategies are needed to tackle this problem.[4]

At an institutional and management level, antimicrobial resistance can have a significant impact on the ability of hospitals to maintain services, since cohorting of patients and ward closures from outbreaks add to continuing bed shortages and waiting lists, and drug resistance is likely to feature prominently in audits related to these themes in the near future.

Over the past two decades, organisms resistant to multiple drugs have emerged, thereby threatening to send us hurtling back to the preantibiotic era. The link between antibiotic use (at times even abuse), sensitivity profile of microorganisms and nosocomial infections demands the inclusion of an antibiotic policy in the infection-control programme of every healthcare institution because emergence of resistant and opportunistic organisms is directly related to antibiotic usage and can vary significantly over time.

There are several factors, singly or collectively responsible for the emergence of microorganisms resistant to multiple drugs. (Fig. 19.1)

1. Modern hospitals with their aggregation of susceptible, often 'immunocompromised' patients and the increasingly invasive diagnostic and therapeutic techniques promote opportunistic pathogens, which in turn give rise to more scope for development of resistant microorganisms.
2. Failure to follow basic infection-control procedures, thus lead to dissemination of the resistant strains in the hospital set-up
3. Excessive and inappropriate prescribing of antimicrobial drugs, thereby cause the emergence of resistant strains. According to CDC, 40% of vancomycin orders were inappropriate.[5] This suggests that a policy of administering limited duration, narrow spectrum antibiotics may reduce drug resistance.[6]
4. Failure to implement standard diagnostic and therapeutic guidelines prescribed by important bodies

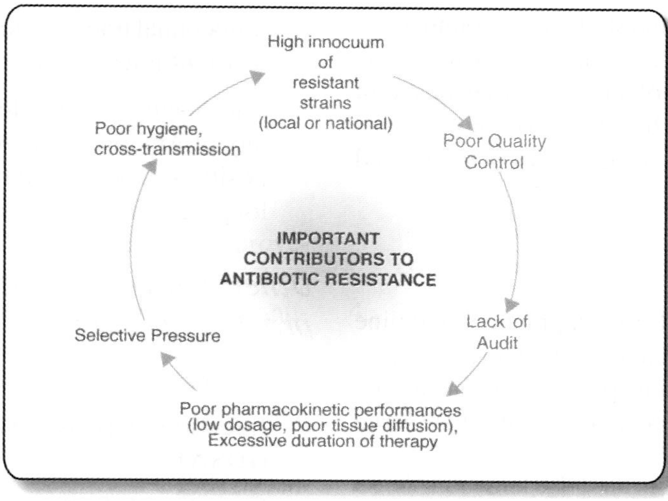

Figure 19.1: The activities which occur in a healthcare organization leading to antibiotic resistance

5. Leadership responsibilities not being taken up effectively at national, state and organizational levels

Antibiotic Resistance Is Directly Related to Several Factors Including

- physician behaviour/prescribing practices/ especially the misuse or inappropriate use of antibiotics
- the prescriber's understanding of the prevention and spread of resistant organisms
- the accuracy of clinical diagnosis

Therefore, it is important to optimize the use of antimicrobial agents to prevent development of resistant organisms by having strategic goals and practice guidelines.

Strategic goals for prevention of development of antimicrobial resistance includes optimizing the prophylactic, empiric and therapeutic use of antimicrobials in the hospital.[7]

1. Optimize antimicrobial prophylaxis for operative procedures.
2. Optimize choice and duration of empiric antimicrobial therapy.
3. Improve antimicrobial prescribing practices by educational and administrative means.
4. Establish a system to monitor and provide feedback on the occurrence and impact of antibiotic resistance.
5. Define and implement institutional or healthcare delivery system guidelines for important types of antimicrobial use.[8]

DEVELOP AND USE THE GUIDELINES AND TREATMENT ALGORITHMS GIVEN BY IMPORTANT BODIES[9,10]

Quality indicators to define and implement institutional and healthcare delivery system guidelines for antimicrobial use must be developed. This has been comprehensively

Hospital Acquired Infections

linked to resistance to other agents. Thus, excessive use of one antimicrobial may be the cause of a high incidence of resistance to several others.

4. To prevent the spillover of resistant strains from the hospital environment to the community at large
5. To improve education of doctors by providing guidelines for appropriate therapy
6. To make prescribers aware of the adverse effects of antimicrobials so that they can restrict their use. A study in France clearly shows that an antibiotic-use policy allowed a reduction not only in antibiotic-selective pressure, but also the costs linked to antibiotics and a selective reduction of nosocomial infections due to antimicrobial resistant microorganisms.[14]

Antibiotic Policy: Institutional and National

The setting up of an institutional antibiotic policy requires close cooperation between personnel from several disciplines including representatives from laboratory (microbiology), pharmacology, nursing, administration, practitioners with expertise in treatment, prevention and control of drug-resistant strains and representatives from local and state health departments. The antibiotic subcommittee can be formed within a Hospital Infection Control Committee (HICC). In hospitals where antibiotic policies are particularly successful, they are usually developed jointly by the infectious disease and pharmacy departments working in conjunction with the microbiology and clinical departments. The introduction of such a programme is often a difficult task and requires the existence of appropriate infrastructure. This infrastructure can be established with the collaborative efforts of members of the pharmacy, microbiology, infectious disease, nursing and administrative departments. Sometimes there is resistance to change on the part of medical staff either due to an imagined increase in workload or due to medical or legal concerns. That is why it is felt that education seems to have the greatest effect on influencing antibiotic prescribing behaviour.

It is recommended that each healthcare facility consider formulating its own institutional strategies, tailored to meet its own needs, for the control of drug-resistant strains on the basis of local considerations.

The Following Factors Are Essentially to Be Considered in Formulating a Policy

1. Prevalence of drug-resistant strains in the given facility
2. Prevalence of drug resistant strains in other facilities that refer patients for admission
3. The frequency of transmission
4. The risk factors in the patient population
5. Availability of resources
6. Level of compliance of the staff, with infection-control practices

National antibiotic policies are very vital, as can be seen from the Danish experience. This has prevented the emergence of resistant strains in a big way. But there are other reports that state that national policies have not been very successful.

Certain Key Persons to Be Included in the Antibiotic Policy Committee

As far as possible, it is advisable to include a pharmacist, a microbiologist, clinicians, nurses and administrators in the committee. It must be mentioned here that the clinical microbiologist plays a key role in implementing a restrictive antibiotic policy in the hospital. Experience has shown that a close personal contact with clinicians in the daily treatment of patients is the most efficient way to ensure a rational use of antibiotics and keep the consumption low. Other important measures include the elaboration of antibiotic usage guidelines and performance of audit. On the basis of periodic summaries of laboratory data and data on antibiotic consumption, the microbiologist can keep the clinicians informed about antibiotic resistance and compliance with the antibiotic guidelines.

ANTIBIOTIC PRESCRIBING AND APPROPRIATE USE OF ANTIMICROBIALS

One of the first points to bear in mind is that the aim of chemotherapy is principally to aid the natural defences of the body to eliminate the microbes from tissues by preventing their multiplication. A systematic approach for selection of antimicrobials in infections should consider the following:

a. Consider whether or not the patient actually requires an antibiotic. Many a time it is seen that physicians prescribe a drug when there is little need for one. One must not accede to patient demands for unnecessary antibiotics.[15]
b. Confirm the presence of infection conclusively (fever, symptoms and signs, predisposing factors), before prescribing antibiotics. Laboratory help must be sought for an accurate diagnosis. In the absence of laboratory confirmation that an infection would be responsive to antibiotics, prescriptions should be based on treatment guidelines that are updated regularly on the basis of local and national resistance surveillance.[16]
c. Consider local surveillance patterns if starting empirical treatment.
d. Identify the pathogen (by smears, culture, serology or other methods): Laboratory response time is important in preventing inappropriate usage.
e. Sample collection, transport, diagnostic criteria and diagnostic methods should all be fine-tuned to one's own institution.
f. Consider strategy for drug (guidelines and pathogen), dose (pharmacokinetics and dynamics, dose adjustments in different conditions), assays and duration of treatment.
g. Select presumptive treatment based on host factors, drug factors, etc. In order to have the desired effect, the blood and infected tissues must contain a concentration of the antibiotic, which is ideally 2–5 times higher than the Minimal Inhibitory Concentration (MIC) of the antibiotic for the infecting organism.[17]
h. Monitor therapeutic response (clinical assessment, laboratory tests, assessment of treatment failure).
i. In general, do not change treatment if clinical condition indicates improvement.

j. If there is no clinical response in 72 hrs, the clinical diagnosis, the choice of antibiotic and the presence of a secondary infection should be reconsidered.

k. Review the duration of antibiotic therapy (e.g. After 7 or 10 days).

l. Consider the site of infection.

m. For surgical prophylaxis start with the induction of anaesthesia and continue for a maximum of 24 hrs only.

n. Consider host factors.

o. Remove predisposing factors to infection.

p. Although it is tempting to use broad-spectrum antibiotics for the treatment of many infections and thus 'safely' cover a large range of less common pathogens, this has the distinct disadvantage of selecting out resistant organisms and hence the temptation must be curbed.[18]

q. Practice correct hand-washing and other Standard Precaution measures.

r. Avoid prescribing antibiotics over the phone as far as possible.

s. Isolate hospital patients infected with or colonized by resistant organisms.

t. Educate patients on taking the full course of antibiotics when prescribed.

u. Defer prescription of antibiotics when the infection is likely to be self-limited.

Selection of Strategies

(Figure 19.2)

Broad spectrum antimicrobial treatment

Antimicrobials given to cover everything (broad-spectrum treatment) is not very desirable because it is unsystematic, expensive, more toxic and leads to resistance and super infections which are difficult to treat. A study in a large teaching hospital in Israel reported that intravenous antibiotic consumption increased the incidence of candiduria.[19] The strongest correlation with candiduria was shown for the use of Meropenem and Ceftazidime, thus adding a new dimension to the strategy of restricting broad spectrum antibiotics.

Empiric antimicrobial therapy

This is begun in patients who have an illness and in whom there is an expectation of an infectious cause. The treatment is directed against organisms most likely to be the cause of illness. Quality indicators to optimize choice and duration of empiric anti-microbial therapy include:[7]

Outcome Measures

1. Number of infections due to isolates or number of patients infected and/or colonized with bacterial strains resistant to antimicrobial(s) used for empiric therapy/ total number of patients given this (these) drug(s)
2. Number of adverse effects of empiric therapy/total number of patients receiving empiric therapy
3. Cost or quantity of empiric antimicrobials administered in a specific period

Process Measures

1. Number of inappropriate empiric regimens/ total number of patients receiving empiric therapy

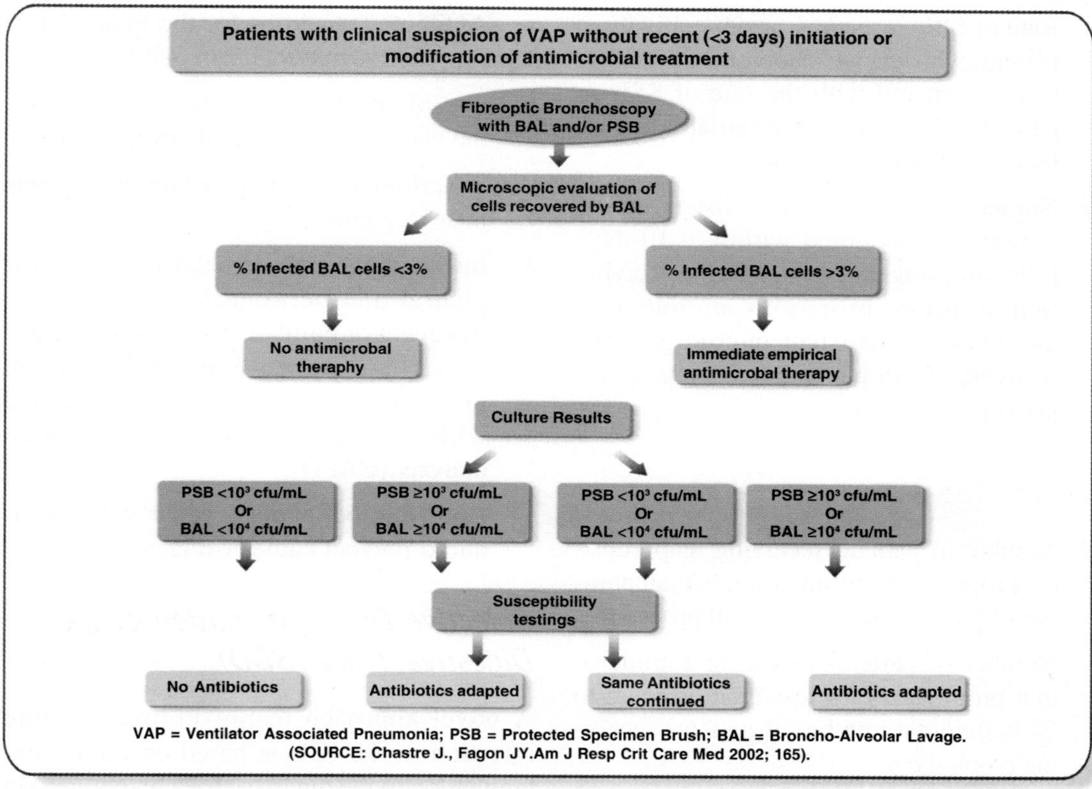

Figure 19.2: Specific antibiotic treatment in nosocomial pnuemonia

2. Number of patients given empiric therapy without having a culture obtained/total number of patients given empiric therapy
3. Mean and/or median time interval between the initiation of empiric therapy and arrival at a microbiological diagnosis in patients who eventually have a diagnosis
4. Number of patients with a microbiological diagnosis who are receiving inappropriate empiric therapy/total number of patients given empiric therapy
5. Mean and/or median duration of empiric therapy (may be stratified by antimicrobial type)

Prophylactic antimicrobial therapy

Antibiotic prophylaxis is administration of an antibiotic prior to the onset of symptoms in order to prevent clinical infection. For surgical procedures, the antibiotic should be started with the induction of anaesthesia and continued for a maximum of 24 hours only. Quality indicators to optimize antimicrobial prophylaxis for operative procedures include:

Outcome Measures

1. Surgical site infection (SSI) rates (Number of SSIs occurring postoperatively/total number of operative procedures)

2. Rate of SSIs occurring postoperatively in patients who receive inappropriate prophylaxis compared with the rate of SSIs in patients who receive appropriate prophylaxis, expressed as a ratio
3. Number of antimicrobial-resistant microorganisms recovered within 7–10 days following surgery from patients receiving inappropriate prophylaxis/number of antimicrobial-resistant microorganisms recovered from patients receiving appropriate prophylaxis

Process Measures

1. Number of patients receiving inappropriate prophylactic antimicrobials/total number of patients having surgical procedures
2. Number of patients receiving antimicrobial prophylaxis for less than or equal to 24 hours/total number of patients receiving prophylaxis
3. Number of patients receiving antimicrobials within 2 hours preceding a surgical incision or at the time of incision/total number of patients receiving prophylaxis

Specific Therapy or Antibiotic-Directed Therapy

Instituted when culture and sensitivity tests become available.

Local Antibiotic Therapy

There may be times when local application of antimicrobial agents may be indicated.

- Use of Chloramphenicol for the treatment of purulent conjunctivitis
- Antibiotic ear-drops for the treatment of suppurative external ear conditions
- Use of silver nitrate solution (0.5%) for the chemoprophylaxis of severe burns
- Silver sulphadiazine cream for prophylaxis in severe burns
- Instillation of antimicrobial agents into the pleural and peritoneal cavities in the treatment of purulent effusions or peritonitis. This route may be particularly useful in the treatment of peritonitis associated with continuous ambulatory peritoneal dialysis (CAPD).
- Antibiotic lock of minocycline and rifampicin to prevent catheter-related infections

Selective Decontamination of the Digestive Tract (SDD)

A novel approach to prevention of acute infection in the ICU is based on the decontamination of the digestive tract by polymyxin B, tobramycin, and amphotericin-B in patients requiring orotracheal intubation for more than five days. Oropharyngeal, tracheal and rectal colonizations with aerobic Gram-negative bacilli is markedly decreased in patients receiving SDD. This technique was first described by Stoutenbeek and co-workers. Infection rates are reportedly reduced by this technique. Other agents have also been used by other workers. The influence of SDD on mortality rates is still not established. There is also a decreased rate of development of resistant strains.[20]

Rotation of antibiotics

One of the strategies to prevent development of antimicrobial resistance is rotation of antibiotic. The combination of drugs is selected according to the organisms generally grown in the cultures and used for a fixed period. This is then changed to an equally effective combination. Three to four combinations are rotated and after a period of rotation (say 1–2 years) of the combinations, the initial combination is restarted.

Biocides rotation (collectively disinfectants, antiseptics and preservatives) in the healthcare setting plays an essential role in infection control and helps prevent the transmission of infectious organisms.[21, 22] Unlike antibiotics, which act on specific intracellular targets, biocides have a broad spectrum of antimicrobial activity and act on several targets on, or in, microbial cells. Presently, there are comparatively few reports of microbial resistance to in-use concentrations of biocides (except with intrinsically resistant microbes like Mycobacteria and spores). This is in stark contrast to antibiotics where reports of bacterial resistance to multiple antibiotics are common and increasing. More recently, however, concern has been expressed over biocide usage, that they could select for antibiotic resistant organisms such as MRSA or various GNB, and that these bacteria may have increased resistance to biocides. Therefore, alternating (rotating) biocides may help to prevent not only the development of biocide resistance, but also the selection of antibiotic-resistant bacteria.[23]

Unlike with antibiotics, MIC values should always be interpreted with caution for biocides, because they may precipitate or interact with the growth media, which could result in misleading data. In general, GNB are usually more resistant to biocidal action that GPB. This is due to the outer membrane found in GNB which impairs the uptake of biocides (intrinsic insusceptibility).[24]

Sequential antibiotic therapy/switch therapy/stepdown therapy

The cost saving policy of 'sequential antibiotic therapy', is the conversion of parenteral antibiotic treatment to oral with the same medication, ('switch therapy' is a similar term which generally refers to replacing parenteral therapy with oral therapy of the same therapeutic class).

Combination of Antimicrobial Agents

While most infections respond to single antimicrobial therapy, it may sometimes be necessary to provide more than one agent. These indications include:

- Tuberculosis infections: In order to prevent the development of bacterial resistance
- Polymicrobial sepsis (e.g. intra-abdominal sepsis): where more than one microbe is involved and hence necessary
- Septicaemia and endocarditis

Indications for clincial use of antimicrobial combinations

a. Prevention of emergence of resistant organisms: Justification for this is well documented only in the case of tuberculosis therapy (now for antiretro viral therapy too)

b. A carbapenem antimicrobial agent, if used, for anti pseudomonal activity, should be combined with either Ciprofloxacin or with an aminoglycoside

c. Polymicrobial Infection: If the polymicrobial flora has either an Enterococcus or

MRSA, or if the organisms are not covered adequately by a broad spectrum Cephalosporin (3rd or 4th generation) or a Carbapenem

d. Empirical therapy in neutropenic patients or in patients in whom the nature of infection is unclear only till the time culture and sensitivity reports are available. Two agents are generally sufficient. E.g. Ticarcillin-Clavulanate/Piperacillin-Taxzobactam + Gentamicin/Tobramycin. Once the culture reports are available, a switchover to single antimicrobial should be done as soon as possible

e. In a case of persistent fever with neutropenia after 5 days of empirical anti microbial therapy, it is advisable to add Amphotericin B, while waiting, to combat fungal infections

f. A combination of amphotericin B and 5 fluorocytosine is useful in treating cases of Cryptococcosis or Candidiasis

g. Synergism in Infection of Immunosuppressed or Immunocompetent patients:

   Even in cases of susceptible organism, two drugs shall have to be combined in cases of abnormal host defence systems. Generally, for Gram-negative bacilli, a combination of Cephalosporin or Ticarcillin or Piperacillin with an aminoglycoside is advocated.

   Caution: A combination of Beta Lactam–beta lactam antibiotic, e.g. Ceftazidime + Ceftriaxone or Cefuroxime or Amoxyclav will be antagonistic in nature. Their combination should be avoided except in situations like infections with *Burkholderia cepacia* and *Stenotrophomonas maltophilia* where Ceftazidime can be combined with Piperacillin + Tazobactam or Piperacillin or Ticarcillin + Clavulanate.

h. Synergism: This is used in cases of moderately resistant organisms showing such a resistant pattern for all or most of the drugs, which can be safely given in such a patient.

   Two drugs to which the organism shows moderate resistance or to which the MIC values are high (not in the sensitive zone) can be combined to have such an effect.

   Synergistic combinations have to be used in cases of bacterial endocarditis, especially with respect to *Enterococcus spp*. This will require Penicillin and Streptomycin/Kanamycin/Amikacin/Gentamicin combination.

   Many serious infections with *Pseudomonas aeruginosa* will respond to a combination therapy with Carbenicillin, Ticarcillin, Mezlocillin, Azlocillin, or Piperacillin with Gentamicin/Tobramicin/Amikacin or Ciprofloxacin.

   Cotrimoxazole as a fixed combination therapy can be used in selective situations or it can be combined with three or four other agents in infections with organisms like *Burkholderia cepacia* and *Stenotrophomonas maltophilia* where I/V Cotrimoxazole can be combined with Ceftazidime/Meropenem and Piperacillin + Tazobactam or Ticarcillin-clavulanate + Tobramycin/Amikacin.

De-escalation therapy

Start off with a broad spectrum antibiotic and then, as soon as the susceptibility reports are available, change to that specific drug.

RESTRICT USE OF CERTAIN ANTIMICROBIALS

These agents shall be called Restricted Usage Antimicrobials. Examples of drugs which are on the restricted list are given in Table 19.1.

Empiric Therapy with the following antimicrobial agents is generally avoided: Such drugs are to be used only under extraordinary life threatening conditons for empirical therapy. Infection-control team (ICT) shall be notified by the pharmacy within 48 hours of such drugs being dispensed.

EFFECTIVE PREVENTIVE MEASURES (PRACTICE GUIDELINES)

Quality indicators to increase adherence to policies and procedures, especially hand hygiene, barrier precautions and environmental control measures should include the following[7]:

Outcome Measures

1. Number of nosocomial infections due to pathogens known to be transmitted by indirect contact via contaminated hands or fomites (e.g. Respiratory Syncytial Virus or *C.difficile* infections)/Number of discharged patients hospitalized for at least 48 hours (or 100 or 1000 patient-days in patients hospitalized for at least 48 hours) trended over time

Process Measures

1. Number of contacts with patients or potentially contaminated objects during which healthcare workers wear gloves/ total number of contacts for which gloves should be worn
2. Number of contacts with patients or potentially contaminated objects after which care-givers remove gloves and wash hands immediately after caring for

Table 19.1: Examples of restricted antibiotics

1. Meropenem	2. Imipenem-Cilastatin
3. Teicoplanin	4. Rifampicin (other than for Mycobacteria)
5. Chloramphenicol	6. Polymyxin – B
7. Piperacillin – Tazobactam	8. Vancomycin
9. Ticarcillin + Clavulanate	10. Cefoperazone + sulbactam
11. Linezolid	12. Aztreonam
13. Amphotericin – B	14. Voriconazole
15. Caspofungin	16. Posaconazole

the patients/total number of contacts in which gloves are worn

3. Number of patient contacts that are followed by hand washing/total number of patient contacts.
4. Number of patients known to be carriers of specific antimicrobial resistant pathogens placed on appropriate isolation precautions/total number of patients requiring such precautions

Cost of purchasing or rate of consumption of gloves and hand-washing agents (may be unit specific) as a proxy for compliance with gloving and hand-washing policies.

PROMPT DIAGNOSIS (SEE PRACTICE GUIDELINES)

Quality indicators to develop a system to recognize and promptly report significant changes and trends in antimicrobial resistance include the following:[7]

Outcome Measures

1. Number of staff members who were sent an antimicrobial resistance trend report in a specified reporting period/total number of staff members
2. Number of staff members who recall receiving trend reports in a reporting period/total number of staff who sent reports
3. Number of staff members who can describe trends in resistance/total number receiving reports

Process Measures

1. Trend (over several reporting periods) of the time interval between the close of reporting periods and the availability of reports

Interval between the occurrence of an outbreak or other significant trend in resistance and recognition of the event's occurrence. Develop a system for rapid detection and reporting of resistant microorganisms in individual patients to appropriate personnel (care-givers and infection-control staff) and for rapid response by care-givers.

Process Measures

1. Number of bacterial strains tested for susceptibility within a specified threshold interval from the time of their isolation/ total number of bacterial strains tested
2. Mean or median time interval between bacterial isolation and susceptibility testing
3. Number of reports of antimicrobial resistant bacteria reaching the appropriate ward and/or infection-control staff within a specified threshold time from receipt of culture (or isolation of microorganism)/total number of resistant bacteria tested
4. Mean and/or median time interval from receipt of culture (or isolation of microorganism) in the laboratory until reporting of results
5. Number of patients placed on appropriate isolation precautions within a specified threshold time after receipt of the antimicrobial resistant report on the ward/total number of patients with antimicrobial resistant isolates

6. Mean and/or median time from receipt of report on the ward until patient is placed on isolation precautions
7. Number of patients for whom a change in antimicrobial therapy is ordered in response to a report of bacterial resistance/total number of patients receiving antimicrobials to which microorganisms are reported to be resistant

ADMINISTRATIVE AND MANAGERIAL INTERVENTIONS[25-27]

Quality indicators to incorporate the detection, prevention and control of antimicrobial resistance into institutional strategic goals and to provide required resources.

Outcome Measures

1. Number of team projects or quality improvement initiatives related to detection, prevention and control of antimicrobial resistance that are implemented and lead to demonstrable results

Process Measures

1. Frequency with which resistance issues are discussed at senior management meetings (or percentage of time devoted to this topic)
2. Whether resistance issues are included in institutional strategic goals and in goals of individual departments or services
3. Whether infection control and/or hospital epidemiology is represented on the facility's planning committee, product evaluation committee, or other relevant administrative committees
4. Whether antimicrobial resistance issues are included in hospital staff orientation, continuing education and the reappointment process. Hospital leaders can influence antibiotic control by the priority they give it.

System for Monitoring Antibiotic use and improvement strategies:

1. Antibiotic Utilization Review: Drug used per year, cost of drug per year, number of patients treated with each drug per year; these data are used to analyse patterns of use in different services.
2. Identify problems such as inappropriate choice of antimicrobial agents, incorrect timing, unnecessary use of prophylactic antibiotics, self-prescribing, erratic antibiotic supply, use of counterfeit or low-quality drugs, all of which contribute to the incidence of antibiotic resistance, especially in the developing world.
3. Improvement strategies: Physician education, pharmacy dispensing patterns
4. Clinical practice guidelines combined with clinical pathways for common infections.
5. Restriction of certain antibiotics
6. Linking antibiotic use with surveillance data for resistant pathogens
7. Long-term effectiveness of educational programmes and prescribing practices
8. Antibiotic utilization audits
9. Multidisciplinary antibiotic utilization team
10. Formulary control and restriction
11. Antibiotic approval system

12. Commitment from hospital administration
13. Computer-assisted antibiotic decision support using benchmarking and re-engineering
14. Wide consultation with all the hospital personnel concerned
15. Guidelines must be available in short, simple language so as to be understood even by the new doctors and nurses and educate them in the correct use of antimicrobials
16. Information on choice of antibiotics for empirical and targeted therapy of major infections.
17. Obtain information on use of antibiotic prophylaxis (e.g. in surgery—with details of timing, route, dosage and frequency).
18. Conduct an extensive review of all the available antimicrobials and formulate a basic formulary for the hospital.
19. Establish concrete guidelines for the use of antimicrobials in various settings viz. prophylactic, empirical, therapeutic.
20. If an antimicrobial agent has a narrow spectrum of activity or is known to be toxic, keep it in reserve and restrict its use.
21. As far as possible, enlist only those antimicrobials in the formulary which are capable of being tested for susceptibility patterns in the microbiology laboratory.
22. The policy makers should regularly monitor the susceptibility patterns of antimicrobials in use and provide a feedback to the user departments.
23. Specific antibiotics should be audited
24 Importantly, the policy makers should not give in to the pressures from pharmaceutical firms when they urge advocacy of their launches.

Quality indicators to develop a plan for identifying, transferring, discharging and readmitting patients colonized with specific antimicrobial-resistant microorganisms.

Outcome Measures

1. Number of patients who, on their discharge from the hospital, are not identified to be colonized with a specified resistant microorganism and are later discovered to be colonized on hospital readmission/ total number of patients with resistant microorganisms readmitted in a specified period
2. Number of hospitalized patients infected with a resistant microorganism who were not known previously to be colonized/ total number of patients admitted (or discharged) within a specified period (per 1000 patient-days)

Process Measures

1. Number of patients with antimicrobial resistance noted on discharge or transfer documents/total number of patients colonized with resistant microorganisms in a specified period

Quality indicators to improve antimicrobial prescribing practices by educational and administrative means include:[7]

Outcome Measures

1. See outcome measures for previous two goals. These measures should be physician specific when possible. If justified by the volume of antimicrobial use, these measures should be used to establish a physician's performance profiling system

2. Physician knowledge
3. Physician assessment of the hospitals educational and administrative interventions
4. Overall clinical indication: Specific (defined locally) trends in antimicrobial usage, costs and resistance
5. Physician knowledge of trends in antimicrobial usage, costs, and resistance

Process Measures

1. Number of educational or administrative activities in a specified period
2. Percentage of physicians attending educational sessions

PREVENT INAPPROPRIATE USE OF ANTIMICROBIALS IN ANIMAL HUSBANDRY

Use of antimicrobials in animal husbandry. *For example, Oxytetracycline is a drug that has been permitted and is used in beehives.

Similarly, Oxytetracyclines and sulfamerazine (a sulphonamide derivative) are used in commercially raised fish like salmon, catfish and trout to treat ulcers or furunculoses of skin, diarrhoea and blood-borne sepsis.[7, 8]

Note: Nearly 40% of antibiotics manufactured in the USA are given to animals. Although some are used to combat infections, most are mixed into feeds to promote growth. These antimicrobials include tetracyclines, penicillin G, neomycin, streptomycin and sulphur derivatives.

DEVELOPMENT OF NEWER AND NOVEL STRATEGIES

(TABLE 19.2)

Faced with this erosion in the efficacy of even the newest of antimicrobials, and with such unfailing regularity, clinicians have come to rely heavily on the ability of the pharmaceutical industry to develop novel agents. However, the costs of discovering, developing, testing and approving antimicrobials continue to escalate while the hazards of unexpected toxicity and clinical failure remain almost unchanged. Moreover, the projected useful lifespan of these newer agents diminishes with time. The bottom line is that the pharmaceutical industry is finding it increasingly difficult to keep pace with the development of antimicrobial resistance and the problems of the 'post antimicrobial era'.

Yet, in the words of R.E.O. Williams, the solution to control of antimicrobial resistance seems quite a simplified and encouraging prospect. He opined, 'The control of resistant bacteria is not different in principle from the control of sensitive bacteria. We need to discover, and if possible, eliminate the reservoir; and to discover, and if possible, control the routes and vehicles of spread.'

It is beyond the scope of this book to examine all medical subjects empowered by IT, yet it may be worthwhile taking a detailed look at the electronic drug formulary and prescription writing, commonest causes of medical errors resulting in avoidable morbidity and mortality.

The incorporation of digital drug formulary to the Electronic Patient Record, if used effectively, will not only enhance safety for the patients, but would be a great help to the physician as well. Following are but a few examples of what a ready access to drug formulary can possibly do:

1. The prescriptions will be legible and complete. Pharmacists/nurses would not have to 'guess' as to what the physicain

Table 19.2: Examples of "Specific Treatment" for microorganisms

Organism and type of disease	Drug order of choice	
	First-line drugs of choice	Alternative drugs
Infecting Gram-positive cocci		
Staphylococcus		
Methicillin-sensitive	Nafcillin or oxacillin	Clindamycin; macrolides; Trimethoprim Sulfamethoxazole + rifampin; Fluroquinoline + rifampin
Methicillin-resistant	Vancomycin	Quinupristin-dalfopristin; Linezolid
Vancomycin-intermediate	Quinupristin-dalfopristin Linezolid; Vancomycin + nafcillin or oxacillin	
Streptococcus pyogenes (group A)	Penicillin; Amoxicillin	A cephalosporin (Gen 1); Vancomycin; macrolide; Clindaycin
Streptococcus (viridans group)	Pencilllin G ± gentamicin	Ceftriaxone, Vancomycin
Streptococcus agalactiae (group B)	Ampicillin or penicillin G ± gentamicin	A cephalosporin (Gen 1); Vancomycin; Ceftriaxone or cefotaxime
Streptococcus bovis	See viridans streptococci	-
Streptococcus (anaerobic species)	Penicillin G	A cephalosorin (Gen 1); Clindamycin; Vancomycin
Streptococcus pneumoniae		
Pencillin-sensitive (MIC < 0.1 *mg*/mg) or intermediately resistant (MIC ³ 0.1 and < 1.0)	Penicillin; Amoxicillin	A Cephalosporin (Gen 1) ; Clindamycin; macrolide; Clindamycin Trimethoprim-sulfamethoxazole
Penicillin-resistant (MIC ³ 1.0)	Cefriaxone or cefotaxime; Vancomycin; Penicillin	Clindamycin; Fluroquinoline; Trimethoprim-sulfamethoxazole

Table 19.2: (Contd.)

Penicillin-sensitive (MIC < 0.1)	Penicillin	Ceftriaxone or cefotaxime; Vancomycin
Penicillin-intermediately resistant (MIC ^{3} 0.1 and < 1.0)	Cefotaxime or ceftriaxone	Vancomycin
Penicillin G-resistant (MIC ^{3} 1.0)	Vancomycin + rifampin or ceftriaxone or cefotaxime	Ceftriaxone or cefotaxime + rifampin
Enterococcus		
Vancomycin-susceptible	Penicillin G or ampicillin + gentamicin	Vancomycin + gentamicin
Vancomycin-resistant	Quinupristin-dalfopristin	Chloramphenicol; Doxycycline; Linezolid
Vancomycin-susceptible	Amoxicillin or ampicillin or penicillin	Vancomycin; Ciprofloxacin or Fluroquinoline
Vancomycin-resistant	Quinupristin-dalfopristin	Ampicillin or amoxycillin Fluroquinoline; Chloramphenicol; Doxycycline
Infecting Gram-Negative bacteria		
Acinetobacter spp	Imipenem; meropenem	Piperacillin; ciprofloxacin; trimethoprim-sulfamethoxazole
Bacteroides fragilis	Metronidazole; clindamycin	Imipenem; meropenem; cefoxitin
Bartonella henselae	Ciprofloxacin; Azithromycin	Trimethoprim-sulfamethoxazole; clarithromycin
Bordetella pertussis	Erythromycin	Trimethoprim-sulfamethoxazole
Burkholderia cepacia	Trimethoprim-sulfamethoxazole	Ceftazidime; chloramphenicol
Enterobacter spp.	Imipenem; meropenem	Third-generation cephalosporin; piperacillin-tazobactam; ciprofloxacin

Table 19.2: (Contd.)

Escherichia coli	Third-generation cehalosporin; fluoroquinolone	Trimethoprim sulfamethoxazole; aztreonam
Hemophilus influenzae	Cefotaxime; ceftriaxone	Cefuroxime; fluoroquinolone
Klebsiella pneumoniae	Third-generation cephalosporin	Imipenem; meropenem; Piperacillin tazobactam; aztreonam; ciprofloxacin
Legionella spp. ***Moraxella catarrhalis***	Azithromycin; fluoroquinolone Macrolide; trimethoprim – sulfamethoxazole; doxycycline	Erythromycin Fluoroquinolone; amoxicillin/ clavulanic acid; ceftriaxone; cefuroxime
Neisseria gonorrhoeae	Ceftriaxone; ciprofloxacin; ofloxacin; cefixime	Cefotaxime; spectinomycin
Neisseria meningitidis ***Proteus*** (indole+) Including ***Providentia rettgeri, Morganella morganii, and Proteus vulgaris***	Penicillin G Third-generation cephalosporin	Ceftriaxone; cefotaxime Imipenem; meropenem; piperacillin /tazobactam; ciprofloxacin; aztreonam
Proteus mirabilis	Ampicillin or amoxicillin (ß-lactamase (-) strains)	First-or second-generation cehalosporin; aztreonam; fluoroquinolone
Providencia stuartii	Third-generation cephalosporin	Imipenem; meropenem; piperacillin-tazobactam; aztreonam; ciprofloxacin
Pseudomonas aeruginosa	Piperacillin + an aminoglycoside (gentamicin; tobramycin; or amikacin)	Cefepime; ciprofloxacin; imipenem; or meropenem; + aminoglycoside
Serratia spp	Imipenem; meropenem	Third-generation cephalosporin; piperacillin aztreonam; ciprofloxacin
Stenotrophomonas maltophilia	Trimethoprim – sulfamethoxazole	Ticarcillin-clavulanic acid; ceftazidime; or minocycline; aztreonam + Ticarcillin-clavulanate
RSV—Respiratory Syncytial Virus		
Pneumonia and bronchiolitis of infancy	Ribavirin (aerosol)	-

Table 19.2: (Contd.)

Varicella zoster virus		
Herpes Zoster or varicella in Immunocompromised host, pregnancy	Acyclovir	Foscarnet (Trisodium phosphonosormate)
Varicella or herpes zoster in normal host	No therapy/Acyclovir/ Famciclovir/Valacyclovir	-

may have meant before administering a drug prescribed by the doctor in an illegible hand. The physician while writing the prescription will be forced to complete the details like strength, frequency and duration since all such fields will be marked mandatory.

2. It is humanly impossible for a physician to know all possible drug interactions while writing prescriptions. They do commit such mistakes, and society in general and the patient in particular does pay a price for such innumerable 'overlooks'. IT empowerment appears set to change all this. Whenever a physician is writing a prescription, if two or more drugs with known interactions appear together, the system will throw up a warning and thus avoid maybe a major mishap! It is imperative that physicians should not only accept their own limitations as against the power of the computer, but adopt computer-aided prescription writing even if it means deviation from age-old practice, some inconvenience and that little extra effort.
3. The physician may not be aware or may not remember each time he writes a prescription of special instructions that may have to be communicated to the nurse/ patient for executing the order. The application, by default, may give a printout of such instructions that must be followed, which not only enhances patient safety and improves outcomes, but also helps reduce costs.
4. A doctor, during history taking, may come across unfamiliar drug names that a patient may be taking. With the help of drug formulary, he can instantly find all that he needs to know about the drug and plan accordingly.
5. With an ever-increasing list of trade names, many physicians in the OPD do encounter medicines prescribed elsewhere that they may have never heard of. Empowered with ready reference to drugs and their trade names on his desktop, he doesn't have to feel embarrassed anymore trying to find out the composition.
6. A ready reference to drug dosage and in-built calculator can eliminate simple errors of arithemetic, not uncommon in clinical practice.
7. Checks can be built within the system, which do not allow over-dosage or wrong route of entry, as only the correct options would be available in the 'pull down menu' for the physician to select from.

8. Cross checks within the EPR and prescription module can help avoid many clinical errors. If a patient's EPR has entries like history of asthma and allergy to penicillin in relevant sections, whenever a physicain inadvertently prescribes a beta-blocker and penicillin, the system many not allow him to do so. It is believed that there are over 600 drugs that require adjustments of doses in the event of renal dysfunction.
9. Attempts have been made to build IT based 'intelligent systems' wherein site and method of injecting medications have been identified and standardized, and a specialized monitor placed at the drug delivery location with all this information digitized. The injection port is placed in a special mount reducing the risk of contamination or accidental needle sticks and standard syringes are held in a modified label causing automatic alignment with the injection port. This affords the opportunity to scan for an identifying bar-code and the plunger position. This data is thereby obtained for the digital record in a manner least disruptive to regular clinical practice and without the necessity of manual clinician input.

ANTIMICROBIAL ABUSE AND ITS IMPLICATIONS

1. Increase in antimicrobial resistance around the world suggests that more effective strategies are needed[28] to combat this problem.
2. This has led to increased mortality and morbidity with also an impact on increased duration of admissions, closure of wards due to outbreaks and increased waiting lists and bed shortages.[29]
3. Effective leadership can influence antibiotic control through the priority they give.[30]
4. Antibiotic intervention policies, efficient infection-control measures and an overall awareness of the serious public health implications can contribute to the management of antibiotic resistance.[26]
5. Physicians must understand that only using a clinical judgement for selection of antibiotics could be fallacious. This was shown in a study by Fagon et al where only 62% of the physicians arrived at a correct diagnosis and only 33% had a correct therapy based on this. They found the combination useful.[11]
6. Lack of preventive measures also contributes to development of resistance as this leads to cross-infection, which in turn leads to the development of resistance.
7. A prompt, correct and supportive diagnosis of specific infections must be carried out by adequate diagnostic criteria including sampling methods and laboratory methods. Rapid diagnostic tests help in avoiding antibiotics in patients who do not need them.[10]
8. Use or selection of a wrong antibiotic has shown increased mortality in serious infections. Therefore, empirical selection of antibiotics must be guided by guidelines such as the American Thoracic society for nosocomial pneumonias. These guidelines must be adequately modified by local bacterial flora.
9. The resistance gene pool is constantly multiplying, as are the numbers of microorganisms resistant to more than one antibiotic. If we ignore the problem, single drug therapy will simply become obsolete.

It is already so in the treatment of tuberculosis and HIV/AIDS infection. Thus, the aim is to maintain the efficacy of the antibiotics we have, by determining which diseases they can still eradicate and which microorganisms are still largely susceptible. We should develop newer antibiotics but use them appropriately.

The goal in the next decade is to make antibiotics more available in the areas where they are most needed and to discourage frivolous use in areas where they are currently being overused. Education must remove the false impressions and attitudes about these drugs in the minds of both the consumer and the prescriber.

REFERENCES

1) Ayliffe GAJ, Fraise AP, Geddes MS: Control of Hospital Infection- A Practical Handbook. Arnold Publications. 4th Edn. 2000; 263-280.

2) Paladino J, Holmes B, Schmitz FJ. Patient physician issues in appropriate use of Antimicrobials: A Practical Guide for Physicians. Science Press Ltd. 2002; 49-56.

3) Levy SB. In: The Antibiotic Paradox. How miracle drugs are destroying the Miracle. New York, London. Plenum Press 1992; 223-252.

4) Selwyn S. Hospital infection: The first 2500 years. J Hosp infect 1991; 18.

5) Thomas AR, Cieslak PR, Strausbaugh LJ, Fleming DW. Effectiveness of pharmacy policies designed to limit inappropriate van comycin use: population-based assessment. Infect Control Hosp Epidemiol. 2002 Nov; 23 (11): 683-8.

6) Franklin GA, Moore KB, Snyder JW, Polk HC Jr, Cheadle WG. Emergence of resistance microbes in critical care units is transient, despite an unrestricted formulary and multiple antibiotic trials. Surg Infect. 2002 3(2):135-44.

7) Levy SB. Antibiotic resistance. Microbial adaptation and evolution. In The Antibiotic Paradox. How miracle drugs are destroying the miracle. Plenum Press New York: London. 1992; 150-212.

8) Geissler A, Gerbeaux P and Granier IC. Rational use of antibiotics in the intensive care unit: impact on microbial resistance and costs. Intensive Care Med. 2003; 29(1): 49-54.

9) Bonten MJ and Mascini EM. The hidden faces of the epidemiology of antibiotic resistance. Intensive Care Med. 2003; 29(1): 1-2

10) Kolmos HJ. Interaction between the microbiology laboratory and clinician: what the microbiologist can provide. J Hosp Infect 1999; 43 (Suppl): S285-91.

11) Fagon JY, Chastre J, Hance AJ et al. Evaluation of clinical judgement. In: The identification and treatment of nosocomial pneumonia in ventilated patients. Chest 1993; 103: 547-553.

12) Evans RS, Pesotnik SL, Cassen DC, et al: A computer-assisted management programme for antibiotics and other anti-infective agents. N Eng J Med. 1998; 338(4): 232-238.

13) Pesotnik SL, Classen DC, Evan RS et al: Implementing antibiotic practice guidelines through computer-assisted decision support: Clinical and financial outcomes. Ann Intern Med. 1996; 124(10): 884-890

14) Fagon JY, Chastre J, Wolff M et al. Invasive and noninvasive strategies for management of suspected ventilator-associated pneumonia. Ann Intern Med 2000; 2: 621-630.

15) Rosamund J Williams, David L Heymann.Containment of Antibiotic Resistance. Science 1998:20; Vol.279: 1153

16) Koibuchi H, Shibuya Y, Kubo N and Itoh K. Selection of appropriate antimicrobial agents to test and report by clinical microbiology laboratories. Rinsho Byori. 2002; 50 (10): 992-9.

17) Paladino J, Holmes B and Schmitz FJ. Appropriate Use of Antimicrobials: A Practical Guide for Physicians. Science Press Ltd. 2002: 49-56.

18) Davis J. Inactivation of antibiotics and the dissemination of resistant genes. Science 1994: 264; 375-382

19) Weinberger M, Sweet S, Leibovici L et al. Cor relation between candiduria and departmental antibiotic use. J Hosp Infect. 2003; 53(3): 183-6

20) Wong A and Wenzel RP. Using Quality Improvement techniques for the prevention of Nosocomial Pneumonia. In: Jarvis WR, ed. Nosocomial Pneumonia. New York: Marcel Dekker Inc. 2000; 187-201.

21) Murtough SM, Hiom SJ, Palmer M et al. Biocide rotation in the healthcare: is there a case for policy implementation? J Hosp Infect 2001 48:1-6

22) Lelekis M and Gould IM. Sequential antibiotic therapy for cost containment in the hospital setting: why not? Journal of Hospital Infection 2001; 48: 249-257.

23) National Committee for Clinical Laboratory Standards. Performance standards for antimicrobial susceptibility testing. NCCLS, Wayne, Pa. Ninth informational supplement 1999; MS100.

24) Jardine MA, Kumar Y, Kausalya S et al. Reducing antibiotic use on the neonatal unit by improving communication of blood culture results: a completed audit cycle. Arch Dis Child Fetal Neonatal Ed 2003; 88: F255-F258.

25) Goldman D A; Weinstein R.A; Wenzel R.P et al. Strategies to prevent and control the emergence and spread of antimicrobial-resistant microorganisms in hospitals-a challange to hospital leadership. J AmMed Assoc 1996 ; 275 (3): 234-240.

26) Struelens MJ, Mertens R. National Survey of methicillin-resistant *Staphylococcus aureus* in Belgian hospitals: detection methods, prevalence trends and infection control measures. The groupment pour le Depistage L'Etude et la prevention des infections Hospitalieres. Eur J Clin Microbiol Infect Dis. 1994; 13 (1): 56-63.

27) Laboratory capacity to detect antimicrobial resistance, 1998. MMWR 2000; 48:1167-71

28) Hosein IK, Hill DW, Jenkins LE et al. Clinical significance of the emergence of bacterial resistance in the hospital environment. J Appl Microbiol. 2002; 92 Suppl 90S-97S

29) Hamberger H, Diekema D, Fluit A, Jones R, Struelens M, Spencer R, Wolff M. Surveillance of antibiotic resistance in European ICUs. J Hosp Infect. 2001; 48 (3): 161-76

30) Masterson RG. Antibiotic policies and the role of strategic hospital leadership. J Hosp Infect 1999. 43 (Suppl): S261-4.

Chapter 20

Blood Transfusion, Solid Organ Transplantation and Implants

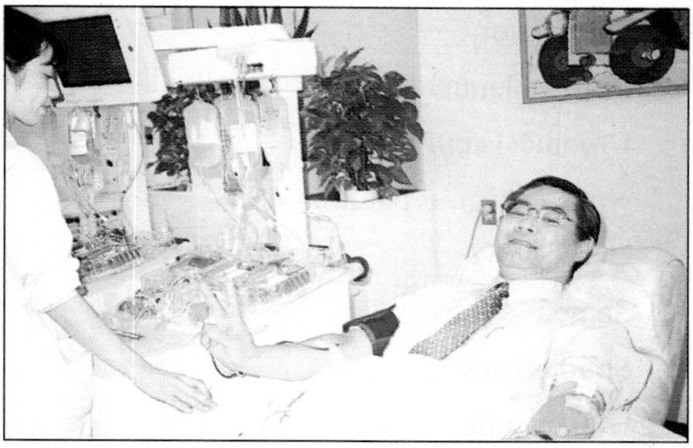

Today knowledge has power. It controls access to opportunity and advancement.

—Peter F. Drucker

Highlights

Transfusion-Related Infections

Reducing Infectious Risks of Blood Transfusion

Solid Organ Transplantation Related HAI

Infections Associated with Indwelling Medical Devices and the Concept of Biofilms

INTRODUCTION

Blood transfusion is one of the oldest forms of tissue transplant after which different kinds of tissues and organs for transplantation have been increasing over the years. Specific tissues listed as biological products which can transmit infections include:

- Blood
- Duramater
- Corneal lenticules
- Umbilical veins
- Nonautologous cultured skin
- Heart valves
- Semen
- Solid organs
- Human milk
- Bone marrow and
- Bone (solid)

This has led to the design of detailed protocols in retrieval, storage, processing and transplantation of these tissues keeping in mind the various infections that can be transmitted. With the evolution of technology, novel methods, such as tissue culturing and cloning, are evolving and may need to be regulated to prevent HAI transmission. Infections in transplant recipients are a serious problem due to the transmission through transplanted tissues, immunosuppressive treatment and the highly invasive nature of the surgeries. In fact, the success of surgery depends on how successfully one is able to prevent infections. Therefore, bone marrow units and liver transplant units need a lot of planning in construction (engineering controls) and design, recruiting highly trained and motivated staff, designing barrier precautions, an efficient and advanced laboratory, efficient surveillance systems, early detection of outbreaks, antibiotic and prescribing protocols, vaccinations, etc., and multiple strategies which have been discussed in this book.

In recent years, there has also been an increasing trend of replacing parts of the body by prosthetics and artificial implants, e.g. joint replacement, valves, vessels, CAPD (continous ambulatory peritoneal dialysis), mesh repairs for hernias, etc. This chapter also discusses HAI associated with implants and indwelling medical devices (Photo 20.1).

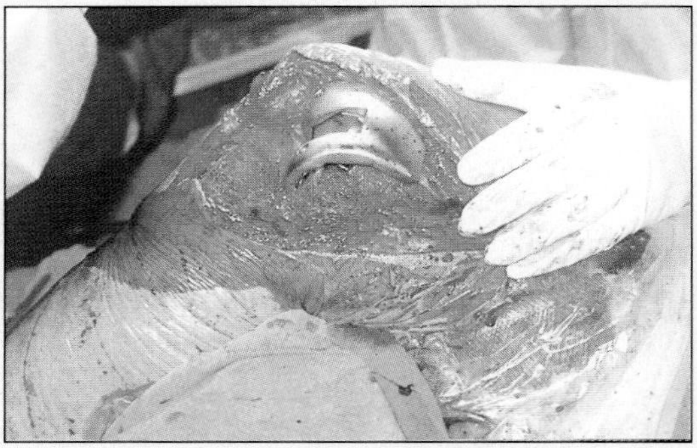

Photo 20.1: A knee replacement in progress

TRANSFUSION-RELATED INFECTIONS[1-4]

Strategies which can decrease blood transfusion and therefore reduce infective complications include autologous transfusion, changing indications of transfusion and use of artificial blood. However, till alternative strategies evolve, the infective dangers remain. These can be countered by donor and recipient testing, having strict guidelines, regulations and laws related to blood transfusion.

There are a number of infections (bacterial, viral, protozoal, fungal) that are transmitted by blood transfusion. But the commonest are the viral, followed by bacterial infections. Infections are also dependant on endemic infections prevalent in a particular country or state.

Common Blood-Borne Infections

Bacterial

- *Pseudomonas spp*
- *Yersinia spp*[5]
- *Brucella spp*
- *Salmonella spp*
- *Enterobacter agglomerans*
- *Enterobacter cloacae*
- *T. pallidum*

Fungal

- Candida spp

Viral

- Hepatitis B
- Hepatitis C
- Other types of Hepatitis viruses
- CMV
- EBV
- HIV-1 & 2

Parasitic

- *Plasmodium spp*
- *Toxoplasma gondii*
- *Babesia spp*
- *Trypanasoma cruzi*

REDUCING INFECTIOUS RISKS OF BLOOD TRANSFUSION

Risk of blood transfusion is expressed per unit of blood transfused rather than per patient as this allows a more accurate computation of risk for a given patient (multiply per unit risk times the number of units transfused). The risk calculation is difficult to accurately measure and is usually by mathematical modelling of data from infectious disease testing in donors or follow-up results from recipients. The risk also varies with the location of the pathogen. Intracellular or leucocyte-associated viruses (Human T cell Lymphotrophic Virus Types I and II (HTLV-I/II) are not transmitted through acellular blood products (FFP or cryoprecipitate), whereas the risk of transmission is the same for each type of blood component used in the case of other viruses (HIV, HCV, HBV). For the most important transfusion transmissible agents like HIV, HCV, HBV, etc., the per unit risk is the same for each type of blood component received (i.e, red cells, platelet, FFP, Cryoprecipitate).[6]

Per unit risk of transmitting infectious agents through blood transfusion reported in some centres:[7]

Agent	**Per unit risk**
HIV	1 in 450,000
HTLV-I/II	1 in 50,000
HBV	1 in 200,000
HCV	1 in 5000
Others	less than 1 in 10,00,000

Donor Testing

A clinical examination must be carried out to

rule out any signs of infection in the donor. Signs of infection, inflammation, fever, history of hepatitis and high risk activities and signs of drug abuse are noted. A number of tests are carried out in the donor or the blood donated. These tests include:

- Serological tests for syphilis
- Hepatitis B surface antigen (HBsAg)
- HIV-1, HIV-2 tests for antibody
- Antibody to hepatitis B core antigen (Anti-HBc Ag)
- Antibody to Human T-cell Lymphotrophic virus Type I, II
- Antibody to Hepatitis C virus
- HIV – p24 antigen
- NAT (nuclear antibody testing) for HCV, HBV, HIV has reduced the window period for various important infections. It is however costlier than the routine tests but in the longer run may be more cost effective.

The choice of tests depends on the incidence, prevalence of specific infections in a country/ state. Changing technology (e.g. NAT testing) may replace traditional tests and also decrease risks associated with blood transfusion.

Leucocyte reduction[8]

CMV sero negative blood is used to prevent transmission of cytomegalovirus.

This is indicated in specially susceptible patients. Leucocyte reduced blood may be used instead of CMV seronegative products in some situations (e.g. Auto-BMT or lack of CMV seronegative blood). Leucocyte reduction is carried out by leucocyte reduction filters.

Irradiated blood

This is not used for leucocyte reduction but is used for reduction of transfusion associated graft versus host disease in susceptible patients.

Alternative Strategies

Alternative strategies prevent infections by decreasing the need for allogenic blood (by questioning the traditional indications for blood products) and promoting use of autologous blood and artificial blood.

Blood Salvage and Containment of Loss

Better surgical techniques and equipment, e.g. argon laser, laser resections, have reduced the blood loss which in turn has reduced the need for transfusions. Other methods include management of:

1. Hypotensive techniques: Generalized bleeding which cannot be controlled with surgical sutures or cautery
2. Correction of coagulation problems perioperatively, e.g. partial thromboplastin time within 1.5 times normal
3. Correction of bleeding problems, e.g. a platelet count greater than 70,000/mm^3 (to ensure that thrombocytopenia is not the cause of the bleeding)

Autologous versus Allogenic[9-12] Blood

(Photo 20.2)

Autologous transfusions could be preoperative, intraoperative or postoperative.

Preoperative techniques include preoperative collections from the patient in the period preceding the surgery. Once the blood is collected, the blood is reserved for the patients' own use. This theoretically reduces the need for allogenic blood and the need for testing

The other method is the intraoperative collection of blood target (haematocrit 30%). Acute normovolemic haemodilution can be used to dilute blood reducing the number of cells per unit volume and hence reducing the loss of cells per unit volume lost. The targeted haematocrit could also be < 20% (profound) but needs a higher level of monitoring. Autologous techniques need to be popularised .

Autologous blood is also retrieved with equipment such as the cell saver (Photo 20.3).

Post operative autologous transfusions include the use of blood left over in the circuits and cardiotomy reservoirs.

Autologous transfusions at this point of time need to be promoted and hold a promise of decreasing blood requirements and decreasing infective complications of transfusion. But, autologous blood does have risks. One out of 16,000 autologous blood donations results in a reaction severe enough to require hospitalization. In fact, some complications associated with autologuos blood transfusion are listed below.

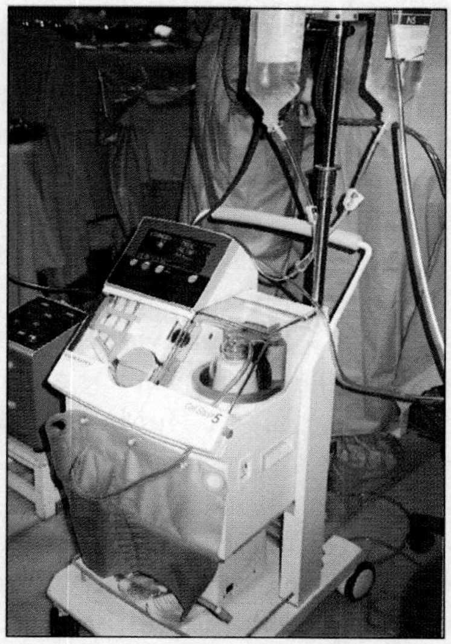

Photo 20.3: A cell seperator for intraoperative autologous transfusion

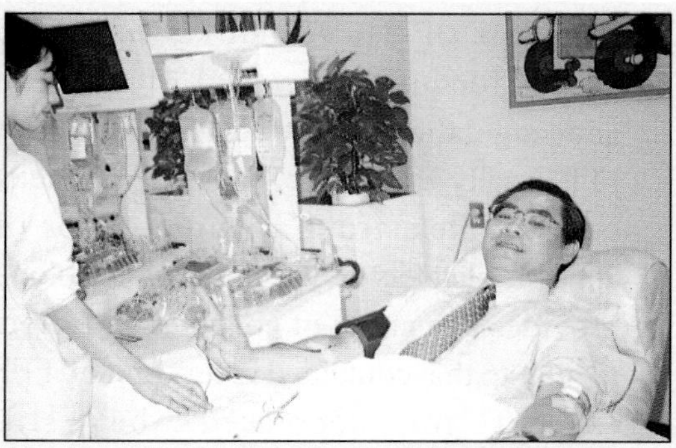

Photo 20.2: Preoperative autologous transfusion involves preoperative blood donations

Perils of autologous transfusions

1. Anemia
2. Preoperative myocardial ischemia from anemia
3. Wrong unit (1:100,000)
4. More frequent blood transfusions
5. Infections

Redefining Indications for Blood and Blood Product Transfusions[13-17]

Reducing transfusions of blood and blood products indirectly reduces the risk of transmission of infections. Many studies and audits have noted that patients were often transfused blood even when the haematocrit exceeded 33–34%. This means that many of the transfusions performed are actually unnecessary.

The indications for blood transfusion are increasingly being questioned. Blood transfusions usually are given to increase oxygen carrying capacity and intravascular volume. Since intravascular volume can be augmented with administration of fluids that do not transmit infections (e.g. crystalloids or some colloids) blood and blood products need not be transfused without specific indications. Therfore, increasing oxygen-carrying capacity is the only real indication for blood transfusions.

RBC (red blood cell) and plasma transfusions

According to the ASA 1996[18], recommendations for transfusing RBCs, transfusion is rarely indicated when the haemoglobin concentration is greater than 10g/dL and is almost always indicated when it is less than 6g/dl, especially when the anemia is acute. Less complicated guidelines would be helpful. For example, with the help of Habibi[19] et al, the following guidelines are recommended with the rule of thumb that administration of one unit of packed red cells will increase hematocrit by 3–5%. Indications are:

- Blood loss > 20% of blood volume or more than 1000 ml
- Haemoglobin < 8 gm/dL (Normal patient with no other co-existing disease)
- Haemoglobin < 10 gm/dL with major disease (e.g. emphysema, ischaemic heart disease)
- Haemoglobin < 10gm/dL with autologous blood
- Haemoglobin < 12 gm/dL and ventilator dependent

The ASA task[18] force guideline recommends the administration of fresh frozen plasma only in the following situations:

1. For urgent reversal warfarin therapy
2. For correction of known coagulation factor deficiencies, for specific concentrates which are unavailable
3. For correction of microvascular bleeding in the presence of elevated (>1.5 times normal) prothrombin time (PT) or Partial Thrombo plastin time (PTT)
4. For correction of microvascular bleeding secondary to coagulation factor deficiency in patients transfused with more than one blood volume and when PT and PTT cannot be obtained in a timely fashion.
5. Fresh Frozen Plasma (FFP) should be given in doses calculated to achieve a minimum of 30% of plasma factor concentration (usually achieved with administration of 10–15 ml/kg of FFP), except for urgent reversal of warfarin anticoagulation, for which 5–8 ml/kg of FFP usually will suffice. Four to five platelet concentrates, from a single donor of aphersis platelets or one unit of whole blood provides a quantity of coagulation factors similar to that contained in one unit of FFP (except for decreased, but still haemostatic, concentrations of factors V and VIII in whole blood).

Fresh frozen plasma[20] contraindications

Recent guidelines also direct that fresh frozen plasma should not be given:

1. For volume expansion and as a nutritional supplement
2. Prophylactically with massive blood transfusion
3. Prophylactically following cardiopulmonary bypass

Cryoprecipitate[21-24]

Cryoprecipitate contains Factor VIII: C (the procoagulant activity), Factor VIII:vWF (von Willebrand factor), fibrinogen, Factor XIII and fibronectin, which is a glycoprotein that may play a role in reticuloendothelial clearance of foreign particles and bacteria from the blood.

With low fibrinogen levels being more common with packed red blood cells, the ASA task force recommends considering the administration of cryoprecipitate for:

1. Prophylaxis in nonbleeding perioperative or peripartum patients with congential fibrinogen deficiencies or von Willebrand's disease unresponsive to DDAVP. (Whenever possible, these decisions should be made in consultation with the patient's haematologist)
2. Bleeding patients with von Willebrand's disease
3. Correction of microvascular bleeding in massively transfused patients with fibrinogen concentrations less than 80–100mg/dl or when fibrinogen concentrations cannot be measured in a timely fashion

A new approach has been described–administration of recombinant activated coagulation in coagulation defects even after above mentioned therapies-Factor VII (rVIIa) (Novonordisk) which has been successful. This exciting product should be a 'rescue' therapy until FDA approval is given.

Platelets[25-26]

Bacterial infection is more common with platelet transfusions than with red cells as they are stored at room temperature. This may be as high as 0.3% of platelet concentrates transfused. There is no accurate data on the morbidity and mortality implications of bacterial contamination. Because of storage at room temperature, bacteria can grow rapidly. A fever six hours after platelet transfusion should be considered as platelet sepsis. Symptoms may vary from fever, chills, hypotension, abdominal pain, vomitting, to DIC, renal failure and circulatory collapse. A warm shock picture can occur within minutes of starting transfusion. This reaction is potentially fatal.

Treatment: Treatment consists of administering antibiotics, corticosteroids, maintaining volume and vasopressors. Prevention consists of carefully adhering to collection, handling, and storage procedures, inspecting all blood components before transfusion, infusing components quickly (less than four hours preferred), promptly returning the blood to blood bank (within 20 min) if transfusion cannot be started.

As with red blood cells and fresh frozen plasma, the July 1989 FDA Drug Bulletin has tried to provide specific guidelines and has stated that platelets should not be given prophylactically to patients with immune thrombocytopenic purpura (unless there is life-threatening bleeding), or patients with massive blood transfusion, following cardiopulmonary bypass. Indications in the perioperative period has also changed, and if the quality of platelets is normal, then even a value of 50,000/ml is all right. Invasive techniques such as epidural anaesthesia may be avoided in such situations.

Transfusion-related immunomodulation[27-33]

Many authors have presented data to indicate that blood transfusion increases susceptibility to infection and enhances progression of malignant tumours.This may be because homologous blood transfusion exerts a nonspecific immunosuppressive action on the recipient. This effect is therapeutic for kidney transplant recipients.

Synthetic Blood

There are a number of trials with different products to replace natural blood, and these were summarized by Dietz et al.[34] Basically these products are:

1. Stroma-free human or bovine haemoglobin solutions containing some modifications of the haemoglobin molecule
2. Genetically-engineered haemoglobin (e.g. having *E. coli* produce human red cells)
3. Liposome-encapsulated haemoglobin solutions containing haemoglobin with a synthetic membrane
4. Perfluorocarbons, which are organic solutions with high oxygen solubility
5. Attachment of nonimmunogenic material (ethyl glycol) to the cell to prevent reactions in multiply transfused patients[35]

Various Phase II and III studies[36] have been, and are being, conducted. So far, most products cause slight hypertension and increases in amylase and lipase concentrations, the significance of which has yet to be determined. In the late 1980s, companies were stimulated to produce synthetic red cells because of the infectivity threat of blood (i.e. Hepatitis and AIDS). Haemopure will probably be approved by the FDA in the near future.

SOLID ORGAN TRANSPLANTATION RELATED HAI[37]

Infections are also related to intervention-related activities, for example, infections in transplant recipients, depending on the time elapsed after the event (operation, diagnostic test). A patient with a transplant is susceptible to a number of infections by various pathogens, after varying time intervals from the date of surgery.

Early

The early infections are those which occur within 1–4 weeks and are mainly caused by bacteria (Gram positive and negative), which are related to the various invasive procedures such as, intubation and ventilation, catheterization and venous cannulation. After this period is over the patient shows an increased susceptibility to pathogens due to immune suppression or pathogens which have a longer period of latency. Early infections associated with specific transplants are:

Liver transplant

Cholangitis, peritonitis (polymicrobial), *fungal* infections, *CMV, EBV* infections

Lung transplant

Pneumonia due to Gram-negative bacteria *(Enterobacter, Pseudomonas), Candida, Aspergillus, Cryptococcus.* Mediastinitis *(Staphylococcus, Candida, CMV).*

Heart transplant

Mediastinitis (*S.aureus, Pseudomonas, Candida, Mycoplasma hominis)*

Renal transplant

Urinary tract infections *(E. coli, Klebsiella, Enterobacter, Candida)*

Bone marrow transplant

Staphylococcus, Streptococcus, Pseudomonas, Enterobacteriaceae, Candida, Aspergillus, HSV-1

Intermediate

These infections occur between 1–4 months (middle group), the infections mainly seen are *CMV infections, EpsteinBarr virus infections, Legionellosis, Tuberculosis, Nocardiosis, Aspergillosis, PC pneumonia, Candidiasis, RSV infections, Influenza, Parainfluenza* and transfusion related infections.

Late

These infections occur more than six months after transplant. They include infections such as *P. carinii pneumonia, Cryptococcosis, Herpes zoster virus infections,* CMV retinitis and infections by community acquired pathogens such as *Streptococcus pneumoniae*

Preventing Infections related to Solid Organ Transplantation

Standards (guidelines, regulations, laws) related to transplant of tissues are dependant on the tissue or organ (tissue specific) itself, as well as the countries and states (country specific). They apply to retrieval, processing, storage and transplantation of each tissue. However, some common strategies for prevention include the following:

a) Donor testing

Donors need to be screened for various diseases as per checklist. These are specific for type of organ, place, organization and country. Tests also vary with time and technology.

b) Recipient screening

Recipients are also screened as per a check list. The indications and contraindications of transplantation have been changing. For example: patients with HIV, HBV, HCV can receive transplants. They were contraindicated in the past.

c) Behaviour/History/exclusion criteria

History of risky behaviour is checked for, as this can lead to a greater risk of infection after transplantation. Such patients should also test negative for infections, if present, in the window period. Donors with risky behaviour must wait beyond the incubation period or have to undergo repeated testing after the period of incubation or window period before they are cleared for donation.

d) Laboratory exclusion criteria

Tissues may be tested in some cases for presence of specific infections if donor testing has not been possible.

e) Quarantine (for semen)

Keep sample at low temperatures for beyond incubation period of the relevant diseases and test for antibodies, e.g. HIV testing for semen donations.

f) Record keeping and tracking of recipients and tissues

Registers maintained by hospitals, physicians or bodies such as UNOS, NHLBI must be complete and confidential. Further testing and reporting of recipients is also carried out as and when necessary.

Recall of stored tissue and tracking of recipients of organs/tissue from infected donors is carried out in countries that have an organized system of tracking recipients.

g) Inactivation of disease in tissues

There are some reports of inactivation of HIV in bone tissue after treating with chemicals by recommended methods. However, it is not clear whether it is due to avascularity or processing.

h) Other methods of prevention include vaccination against

1. Pneumococci
2. *H. influenzae*
3. Meningococci
4. Influenza virus
5. Polio virus
6. *C.diphtheriae*
7. Measles, Mumps and Rubella viruses

i) Isolation

Strict clinical protocols are to be followed in handling patients and isolation precautions should be undertaken wherever necessary.

INFECTIONS ASSOCIATED WITH INDWELLING MEDICAL DEVICES AND THE CONCEPT OF BIOFILMS[38,39]

(TABLE 20.1)

Many HAI are associated with invasive devices. Tubings or catheters inserted into intravascular system body cavities, e.g. in CAPD, CNS shunts, urinary catheters and endotracheal tubes, etc. may become colonized with bacteria and lead to clinical infection. Bacteria initially adhere to the surface of the device and form microcolonies which generate a matrix of slime (exopolysaccharide). This is termed a biofilm. Infection of indwelling medical devices depends on a number of factors:

a. The type and properties of the organisms: This, in turn, depends on the site and location of the medical device and the bacterial adhesin characteristics.
b. The predeliction of various organisms to various devices is well known. This helps in understanding the treatment and preventive modalities of infection.
c. The type of surface (prosthetic joints, endotracheal intubation, tracheostomy tube, intravascular device used for

infusion therapy, pacemakers, prosthetic valves, vascular grafts, shunts, urinary catheters, intrauterine loops) influences the adsorption of the most active host proteins, thus promoting bacterial adhesion. The presence of extracellular matrix protein, fibronectin, is shown to play an important role in promoting initial Staphylococcal attachment to subcutaneously located polymer and metallic surfaces, thus leading to bacterial colonization and infection of indwelling devices.

d. The environment of the indwelling device may decrease the susceptibility to bactericidal antibiotics.

e. Coagulase negative Staphylococcus and Gram-negative bacteria are commonly associated with biofilm formation on medical devices. Although colonization of a catheter is not in itself harmful, local infection can occur and small pieces of biofilm released into the blood stream may be responsible for bacteremia and less frequently septicemia or endocarditis. Gram-negative bacterial and fungal infections have also been reported.

f. Since the devices are very expensive, the treatment of these infections is not always removal of the device. There are specific guidelines for various problems and this may vary from antibiotic treatment to surgery. The readers are advised to refer to books for specific device-related problems.

Table 20.1: Guidelines for prevention of infections related to implants

Prosthetics, implants and equipment	a. Follow manufacturers orders, e.g. do not use after date of expiry
	b. Do not use in case of damaged packaging
	c. Ensure proper storage
	d. Do not re-sterilize if it is a single use item
	e. Guarantee and warranty period must be checked

REFERENCES

1) Busch MP, Kleinman SH and Nemo GJ: Current and emerging infectious risks of blood transfusions J Am Med Assoc 2003; 289: 959.

2) Purdy RF, Tweeddale MG and Merrick PM: Association of mortality with age of blood transfused in septic ICU patients Canad J Anaesth 1997; 44: 1256.

3) Kim DM, Brecher ME, Estes TJ et al. Relationship of hemoglobin level and duration of hospitalization after total hip arthroplasty: implications for the transfusion target. Mayo Clin Proc. 1993; 68: 37.

4) Williams AE, Thompson RA, Schreiber GB et al: Estimates of infectious disease risk factors in US blood donors. JAMA 1997; 277: 967

5) Centers for Disease Control (CDC): Red blood cell transfusions contaminated with Yersinia enterocolitica. J Am Med Assoc. 1997; 278:553.

6) Practice recommendation for Healthcare Facilities Implementing the US Public Health Service Guidelines for Management of Occupational Exposures to Blood-borne Pathogens. Morbidity and Mortality Weekly Report (MMWR) Recommendations and Reports. 2001: RR-11

7) Informed consent, infectious complications of transfusion, and transfusion alternatives. In: Transfusion Therapy Manual. UCLA Medical Center, Division of transfusion medicine. 1996: 30-35.

8) Corwin HL, Buchon Au JP: Is leuko-reduction of blood components for everyone? J Am Med Assoc. 2003; 289: 1993.

9) Etchason J, Petz L, Keeler E et al: The cost effectiveness of Preoperative autologous blood donations. N Engl J Med 1995; 332: 719-724.

10) Kanter MH, Maanen VD, Anders K et al: Preoperative autologous blood donations before elective hysterectomy. J Am Med Assoc1996; 276: 798.

11) Popovsky MA, Whitaker B and Arnold NL: Severe outcomes of allogenic and autologous blood donations: frequency and characterization. Transfusion 1995; 35: 734-737.

12) Miller RD, Ehrenberg VW. Should the same indication be used for both autologous and homologous transfusions. Transfusion 1995; 35: 703.

13) Thurer RL. Evaluating transfusion triggers. J Am Med Assoc 1998; 279: 238.

14) Ely EW and Bernanrd GR. Transfusion in critically ill patients. N Engl J. Med 1999; 340: 467.

15) Centers for biologics evaluation and research: Points to consider in the safety evaluation of hemoglobin-based oxygen carriers.Tranfusion 1991; 31: 369.

16) Hughes GS, Yancey EL, Albrecht R et al: Hemogloin-based oxygen carriers preserves sumaximal exercise capacity in humas. Clin Pharmacol Ther 1995; 58: 434.

17) Madjpour C, Spahn DR. Allogenic red blood cell transfusions: Efficacy, risks, alternatives and indications. Br J Anaes 2005; 95(1): 33-42.

18) ASA Task Force: Practice guidelines for blood component therapy, Anesthesiology. 1996; 84:32.

19) Habibi S, Coursin DB, McDermott JC et al: trauma and massive hemorrhage. In: Muravchick S, Miller RD, eds. Churchill. Atlas of Anesthesis subspeciality care. Livinigstone 1997; 6.2-6.17.

20) NIH Consensus Conference: Fresh Frozen plasma: Indications and risks. JAMA 1985; 253: 551.

21) Murray DJ, Pennell BJ, Weinstein SL et al : Packed red cells in acute blood loss: dilutional coagulaopathy as a cause of surgical bleeding. Anesth Anlg 1995; 80: 336.

22) Miller RD: coagulation and packed red blood cell transfusions Anesth Analg 1995; 80:263

23) Weiskopf RB: Intraoperative use of recombinant activated coagulation Factor VII. Anesthesiology 2002; 96: 1287.

24) White GC, McMillan CW, Kingdon HS, Shoemaker CB: Use of recombinant anti-hemophiliac factor in the treatment of two patients with classic hemophilia. New Engl J Med 1989; 320:164.

25) Reed RD. Heimback DM, Counts RB, et al: Prophylacic platelet administration during massive transfusion. An Surg 1986; 203:40.

26) Kruskalll MS: The perils of platelet transfusions. N Engl J Med 1997; 337:650.

27) Weiskopf RB, Viele MK, Feiner et al: Human cardiovascular and metabolic responses to acute, severe isovolemic anemia. J Am Med Assoc.1998; 279; 217

28) Collins JA. Recent developments in the area of massive transfusions. World J Surg 1987; 11: 75.

29) Counts RD, Haisch C, Simon TL et al: Massive blood transfusion: Is there a limit? Critical Care Med 1989; 17:699.

30) Waymack JP, Warden GD, Alexander JW et al: Effect of blood transfusion and anesthesia on resistance to bacterial peritonitis. J Surg Res 1987; 42: 528.

31) Heal JM, Chuang C and Blumberg N: Perioperative blood transfusions and prostate cancer recurrence and survival. Am Surg 1988; 156: 374.

32) Schriemer PA, Longnecker DE and Miniz PD: The possible immunosuppressive effects of perioperative blood transfusion in cancer patients. Anesthesiology. 1988; 68: 422.

33) Murray DJ, Olson J and Strauss R: Coagulation changes during packed red cell replacement of major blood loss. Anesthesiology. 1988; 69: 838.

34) Dietz NM. Al: Blood substitutes: fluids, drugs, or miracle solutions? Anesth Analg 1996; 82: 390.

35) Murad KL, Mahany KL, Brugnara C et al: Structural and functional consequences of antigenic modulations of red blood cells with methoxypoly ethylene glycol. Blood. 1999; 93: 2121.

36) Viele MK,Weiskopf RB and Fisher DM: Recombinant human hemoglobin does not affect renal function in humans: Analysis of safety and pharacokinetics. Anesthesiology. 1997; 86: 848.

37) Finberg R, Fingeroth J. Infections in the transplant recipients. Harrison's Principles of Internal Medicine Vol. 1 15th edn. Mc Graw Hill Publishers 2000; 860-867

38) Aylifte GAJ, Babb JR and Taylor LJ. Hospital Acquired Infecion – Principles and prevention. 3rd edn. Arnold Publishers. 2001; 21-23.

39) Vaudaux PE, Lew DP, Waldvogel FA. Host factors predisposing to and influencing therapy of foreign body infections. In: Bisno AL, Waldvogel FA, eds. Infections associated with Indwelling Medical Devices. Washington DC: 2nd edn. ASM Press.1994; 1-29.

Chapter 21

Occupational Hazards and Hierarchy of Controls

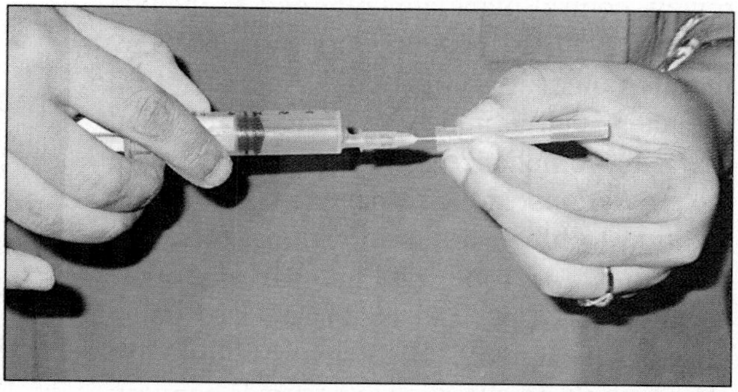

All our goods must be of proven value and they must provide means of curing, better still of preventing, sickness and disease.

—Harry Jephcott

Highlights

Infectious or Biological Hazards

Chemical Hazards due to Disinfectants and Sterilants

Strategies of Control

Administrative Controls and Policies

Engineering Controls

Work Practice Controls

Personal Protective Equipment (PPE)

INTRODUCTION

Countries around the world have started taking steps to curb occupational hazards. A code of practice standards has been introduced in UK and Australia (similar to standards of practice in infection control, US). There is also a strong recommendation by regulatory bodies such as the OSHA (US) to shift to safer medical devices (engineering controls), to review control plans annually and to include reporting of needle-stick injuries to HCWs by maintenance of a log book. Accreditation agencies such as the JCAHO have included assessing compliance of the organizations with the regulations in the respective countries. In addition to blood-borne infections, there are strategies and tools against various other hazards, e.g. tuberculosis. The rate of transmission of Hepatitis B to susceptible HCW after a single needle-stick exposure is between 6% and 30% (for nonimmunized HCW), 1.8% for Hepatitis-C, and 0.3% for HIV. Other routes of exposure also carry a risk, although lower, e.g. exposure through conjunctiva. These are the most commonly researched pathogens. The average combined cost of employee time, laboratory testing, case investigation and initial treatment is high, in the US, $ 3000 per injury. Many countries have a plan worked out for the cost consideration of worker's compensation benefits and litigation by the employee.

Five categories of hazards have been identified and these include:

1. Infectious or biological hazards
2. Chemical hazards
3. Environmental hazards
4. Physical hazards
5. Psychological hazards

Only the first two are within the scope of this book and are thereby discussed. An unsafe environment can lead to various problems in a healthcare worker. First of all, every HCW should be aware of methods to prevent exposing themselves to hazards. Also, 'the system' or 'the organization' has a responsibility towards its employees. This is regulated in some countries and not so organized in others. An attempt is made here to improve awareness of existing systems and protocols.[1-4]

Examples

Case 1: A healthcare worker develops Hepatitis C infection. He is worried about cost of treatment, loss of working hours, loss of a job, morbidity, death.

Case 2: A doctor develops allergy to latex gloves.

Case 3: A clinician delivers a baby with birth defects—could it be due to the disinfectants she has been exposed to?

INFECTIOUS OR BIOLOGICAL HAZARDS[5]

(PHOTO 21.1)

Infectious risks (occupational hazards) have been changing over a period of time and newer and emerging infections are being added to the already existing ones. The range of infectivity and the virulence of the organisms also vary. Newer infections such as the Severe Acute Respiratory Syndrome (SARS), which are emerging in the community, are a serious threat to healthcare workers. Victims of bioterrorist attacks also are a source of infection about which not much information is available. Common infectious hazards can be grouped into:

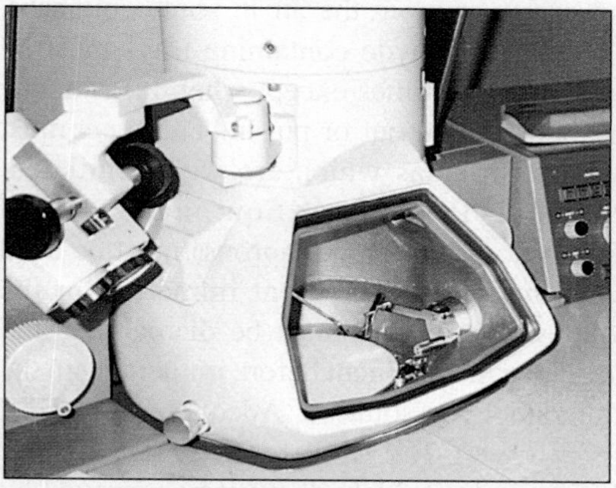

Photo 21.1: An electron microscope. Newer technologies and diagnostic methods are required to diagnose the whole spectrum of hazards.

I. Infections Transmitted by Patients to HCWs

Blood-borne infections like HIV infection, Hepatitis B, Hepatitis C, Cytomegalovirus infections, Ebola virus infection.

Airborne infections like Tuberculosis, Chickenpox, Measles, Rubella, Parvovirus B19 infection, RSV infection, Adenovirus infection, Pertussis.[6, 7]

Enteric infections like Hepatitis A, Salmonella Gastroenteritis, Diarrhoeas due to Cryptosporidium, Norwalk virus or *Clostridium difficile.*

II. Infections Commonly Transmitted from HCW to Others

There are a number of infections which can be transmitted from a HCW to others. Some of the common infections are Hepatitis B, Hepatitis C, infections due to MRSA and Group A Streptococci, *Salmonella Gastroenteritis,* Tuberculosis and Measles.

Staff with infections

Consider removing such HCWs from patient contact e.g. conjunctivitis, diarrhoea, acute respiratory tract infections, Group A Streptococcal infections, pyogenic skin infections, MRSA, scabies, rubella, measles, mumps, chickenpox.

III. Infections in Laboratory Workers

Laboratory workers are prone to a separate set of infections.

The commonly reported infections include those due to HIV, Hepatitis B and C viruses, Rickettsia, *Francisella tularensis, Salmonella typhii, S. paratyphi A & B*, Shigella, non-typhoidal Salmonella, Campylobacter, *Vibrio cholerae, Neisseria meningitidis, Mycobacterium tuberculosis, Coccidioides immitis, Blastomyces dermatitidis, etc.*

CHEMICAL HAZARDS DUE TO DISINFECTANTS AND STERILANTS

(PHOTO 21.2)

Chemical exposure can occur under various circumstances and due to various commonly used disinfectants and sterilants:

Chlorhexidine

The use of chlorhexidine in hand-washing preparations has been reported to cause birth defects in children when used by pregnant mothers (especially with non-intact skin). There are still no clear guidelines on the use of chlorhexidine for skin preparation in very small children and are therefore not being used.

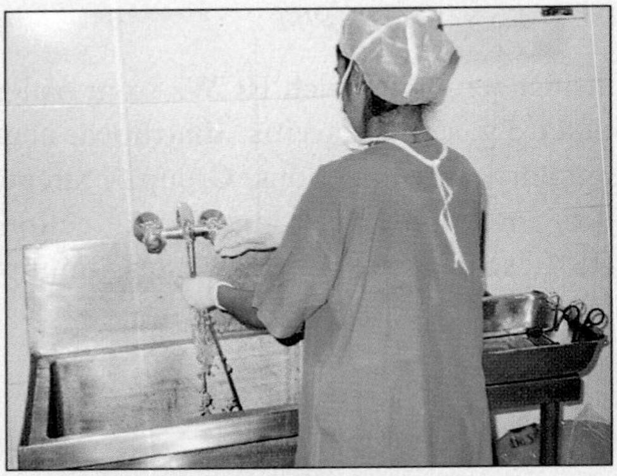

Photo 21.2: A nurse cleaning equipment after a surgery is prone to chemical hazards posed by sterilants and disinfectants.

Phenols and Phenol Derivatives

These are rapidly absorbed by the skin to act systemically, leading to side effects, which include sinus congestion, phenol burns, skin ulceration, gangrene and dermatitis.

Gluteraldehyde Vapours

Source of guideline: Occupational Safety and Health Organization (OSHA) has adopted 0.2 ppm of gluteraldehyde air vapour as the permissible exposure limit (PEL) in the workplace (1989). Routine monitoring of theatre environment is not recommended. The PEL may be achieved by a combination of engineering controls, work practices, and personal protective equipment. This ceiling limit is based on an uncomfortable irritation to the nose, eyes and throat. It is not a toxicity level. The PEL is far below the toxicity level for glutaraldehyde, thus allowing a safety margin for healthcare workers. Routine air monitoring for any chemical is still not recommended. But, there are air monitoring devices and badges available that monitor the level of glutaraldehyde vapours in the air in some countries. The gluteraldehyde containing trays must be covered at all times except when instruments are being taken out or put in. The trays must be kept in areas which are well ventilated. Personal Protective Equipment (PPE) (impervious gloves and aprons) must be used when handling equipment immersed in the solution.Equipment must be dismantled and cleaned with detergent before immersing in the gluteraldehyde solution. Adequate time must be allowed for disinfecting/sterilizing. Residual gluteraldehyde must be removed by adequate washing—manually or by using an automatic washer. The residuals have a number of effects on the body depending on the region with which they come in contact—allergic contact eczema, proctitis, etc. are known to occur. Engineering and work practice controls to ensure the proper ventilation of glutaraldehyde air vapours for routine handling and for spills should be in place. These recommendations are also given by the manufacturers of gluteraldehyde, e.g. Johnson and Johnson.

Precautions: Use a large, well- ventilated area to ensure that not more than 2 ppm glutaraldehyde vapours is exceeded. Keep lids on the disinfecting trays at all times except when transferring instruments in or out of the solution. Dispose of any glutaraldehyde-soiled rags or towels by rinsing with water and disposing in a closed plastic bag. While building or remodelling areas where disinfectants are used, strive to achieve ten air exchanges per hour and place vents at floor level. Glutaraldehyde vapours are heavier than air and this pulls the vapours down away from the face. For spills, use ammonia solution to neutralize, and for large spills use ammonium carbonate 500 gms per gallon of gluteraldehyde estimated to be spilled. And then clean after five minutes using safety precautions and personal protective equipment. In case of spills, use safety glasses, latex gloves for mopping or sponging and a plastic trash bag for collection and disposal. For large spills, breathing equipment with an organic vapour filter is recommended by the company in addition to rubber boots and use of plastic scoop. These guidelines can be further specified into hospital protocols or standard operating procedures (SOPs).

Formaldehyde

Formaldehyde is highly irritating to eyes and respiratory tract (<3–4 ppm). The chronic effects include pneumonitis, pulmonary oedema, residual cardiac impairment and ocular damage. It is also known to be potentially carcinogenic. Another form of formaldehyde (1, 6 dioxhexane which is chemically bound formaldehyde, gluteraldehyde, benzalkonium chloride and alkyl urea derivatives), marketed as Bacillocid, is not cleared by the EPA (USA) because of stringent standards, but is accepted by the CEN and is used in European hospitals. Glutaradehyde and Formaldehyde (1, 6-Dihydroxy-2, 5 dioxahexane is a releaser of formaldehyde) are well-known sensitizers (R43 classification in the European council EC). That is why at higher concentrations a solution of Bacillocid may cause an allergic contact eczema after direct contact with the skin. Several epidemiologic and occupational health studies (e.g. Pickering et. al., England, 1997) as well as several expert evaluations (e.g German MAK commission for occupational health, 1998) could not conclusively prove the suspicion. The debate on the use of formaldehyde containing preparation and their ill effects [Carcinogenicity, Mutagenicity, Teratogenicity (CMT)] is still not resolved and it is commonly used for disinfection and fumigation. The usage of these chemicals have been banned by the FDA (USA) on the fears that they are carcinogenic and mutagenic. However, it is still used in Europe. 1,6 Dihydroxy-2, 5 dioxahexane as a formaldehyde-releaser showed results comparable to that of formaldehyde. It was positive in some in-vitro-mutagencity tests, but not in all. It failed to be mutagenic in in-vivo tests, according to an official document by BODE, Germany (manufacturers of Bacillocid). Although formaldehyde is classified as a mutagenic/carcinogenic, worldwide epidemiologic investigations by the World Health Organisation (Geneva) did not find any conclusive evidence for concern in human use.

STRATEGIES OF CONTROL

Whatever may be the type of occupational hazard, Castillo, Pizatella and Stout (2000) have recognized a framework to evaluate risks and identify the most appropriate intervention to be used. This is called the 'hierarchy of controls'.[3] This framework prioritizes intervention strategies. There are a number of controls which can be applied in the workplace to reduce the risks. But which one is better? The list given below gives the most effective to least effective control measures:

a. Elimination/substitution controls (see chapter on risk management)

b. Engineering controls (see chapter on engineering controls)

c. Administrative controls (policy and management controls: e.g. Policy on active training, resource allocation, adoption of exposure control programmes)

d. Work practice controls (changes in behaviour with support from the management—ban on certain types of risky behaviour, mandates to follow certain practices)

e. Personal protective equipment controls. This is the least effective. The devices must be appropriate and must not impede patient care

The hierarchy of controls can be applied to a variety of safety hazards. For example, the incidence of needle-stick injuries has started to decline because of the application of engineering controls (safer designs) rather than work practice controls (e.g. recommendations not to recap needles was practical and logical but it did not change the workers' behaviour). A combination of controls can also be used and may be more effective than a single control tool. Controls are only end of spectrum of tools which can be used. The other tools available can be seen in the performance management map (Fig. 7.1)

ADMINISTRATIVE CONTROLS AND POLICIES

Workers are more likely to comply with hazard reduction protocols if there is senior management support for programmes (e.g. appropriate work sites, clean units, less barriers).[1-3, 8, 9] Every hospital must have written guidelines for:

1. Pre-employment screening for Hepatitis B
2. Vaccination and seroconversion testing
3. Protocols for low and non-responders to vaccination
4. Management of occupational exposures
5. Monitoring of sharp injuries
6. Training in standard precautions

Examples of Important Policies

A well made out administrative policy can help hospital personnel administer a planned treatment–

The Blood-borne pathogen policy

(Table 21.1)

In the US regulations and policies, such as the blood-borne pathogen policy, are used as a tool to ensure a system that takes care of occupational exposure of employees to blood (needlestick exposures).[1-3] However, such regulations may not be present in other countries. A blood-borne pathogen policy gives us the steps individuals and organizations should take after an exposure occurs. It places a large responsibility on the healthcare organization to prevent, diagnose, monitor or treat exposure to blood in the form of needlepricks, splashes, etc. Regulations by OSHA also enforces teaching and training of standard precautions to all employees by the 'Blood-borne Pathogen Standard'. This also makes the availability of personal protective equipment mandatory. This however, is not directly applicable in other countries, but it serves as a model and appropriate changes may be made when adopted by other countries or organizations.

Blood-Borne Pathogen Standard

Management of occupational blood exposures

There must be written-down guidelines and protocols for the management of exposure.

Provide immediate care to the exposure site

- Wash wounds and skin with soap and water.
- Flush mucous membranes with soap and water.

Determine risk associated with exposure by noting:

- Type of fluid (blood, visibly bloody fluid, other potentially infectious fluid or tissue, and concentrated virus)
- Type of exposure (i.e. percutaneous injury, mucous membrane or non-intact skin exposure and bites resulting in exposure)

  Healthcare workers must promptly report blood/body fluid exposures to infection control, occupational health, or a supervisor in accordance with the exposure control plan at their hospital, clinic or office practice.
- Evaluation of the exposure includes documentation of date, time, and location of exposure; route of exposure and type of potentially infectious material; detail of exposure incident, task being perfomed, etc.

Identification of the source person, if known

If a person is a suspected source of infection to a healthcare worker (HIV, Hepatitis B and Hepatitis C testing), testing of the source is performed after appropriate consent is obtained. Informed written consent after counselling is required for HIV testing. The rapid HIV test may be available to screen patients. Persons already known to be HIV, HBV and/or HCV infected need not be retested.

Medical evaluation, treatment and follow-up of the exposed healthcare worker includes

- Review of HBV vaccination status
- Baseline serologic testing for HBV, (if necessary) and HIV (after counselling and written consent)
- When a source is found to be Hepatitis C antibody positive, additional follow-up testing is recommended (such as LFTs and Hepatitis C viral studies)
- Counselling about the risk of infection resulting from the exposure, recommended post-exposure treatment and follow-up, and precautions to prevent possible HIV transmission to others, must be given.

Evaluate exposure source by the following:

- Test known sources for HBsAg, anti-HCV, and HIV antibody (consider using rapid testing).
- For unknown sources, assess risk of exposure to HBV, HCV, or HIV infection.
- Do not test discarded needles or syringes for virus contamination.
- Evaluate the exposed person.
- Assess immune status for HBV (i.e., by history of hepatitis B vaccination and vaccine response).

Table 21.1: Blood-borne pathogen policy: An example of administrative control policy. Guidelines by Occupational Safety and Health Agency (OSHA). Asbstracted and modified from MMWR recommendations and reports (June 29, 2001/vol50/ RR-11)

Practice recommendation	Implementation checklist
Establish a blood-borne pathogen policy	All institutions where healthcare personnel (HCP) might experience exposures should have a written policy for management of exposures.
	The policy should be based on the US Public Health Service (PHS) guidelines. The policy should be reviewed periodically to ensure that it is consistent with PHS recommendations.
	Healthcare facilities (HCF) should provide appropriate training to all personnel on the prevention of and response to occupational exposures.
Implement management policies	HCF should establish hepatitis B vaccination programme.
	HCF should establish exposure-reporting systems. They should have readily available personnel who can manage an exposure at all hours of the day.
	HCF should provide ready access to post-exposure prophylaxis (PEP) for use by exposed personnel as necessary.
	HCF should provide prompt processing of exposed person and source person specimens to guide management of occupational exposures.
	Testing should be performed with appropriate counselling and consent.
Establish laboratory capacity for blood-borne pathogen testing.	HCF should develop a policy for the selection and use of PEP antiretroviral regimens for HIV exposures wihin their institution.
	Hepatitis B vaccine and HBIG should be available for timely administration.

Table 21.1: (Contd.)

Select and use appropriate PEP regimens.	HCF should have access to resources with expertise in the selection and use of PEP.
	HCF should provide counselling for HCP who might need help dealing with the emotional effect of an exposure.
	HCF should provide medication adherence counselling to assist HCP in completing HIV PEP as necessary.
Provide access to counselling for exposed HCP.	HCP taking antiretroviral PEP should be monitored periodically for adverse effects of PEP through baseline and routine testing (every 2 weeks) and clinical evaluation.
Monitor for adverse effects of PEP.	HCF should develop a system to encourage exposed HCP to return for follow-up testing.
	Exposed HCP should be tested for HCV and HIV.
	HCF should develop a system to monitor reporting and management of occupational exposures to ensure timely and appropriate response.
Monitor for seroconversion.	
Monitor exposure management programmes.	

Recommendations for evaluation for specific diseases

Advise exposed persons to seek medical evaluation for any acute illness occurring during follow-up.

HBV Exposures

- Perform follow-up anti-HBs testing in persons who receive Hepatitis B vaccine
- Test for anti-HBs antibodies 1–2 months after the last dose of vaccine.
- Anti-HBs response to vaccine cannot be ascertained if HBIG was received in the previous 3–4 months.

HCV Exposures

- Perform baseline and follow-up testing for anti-HCV and alanine amino transferase (ALT) 4–6 months after exposure.

- Perform HCV RNA at 4–6 weeks if earlier diagnosis of HCV infection desired.
- Confirm repeatedly reactive anti-HCV enzyme immunoassays (EIAs) with supplemental tests.

HIV Exposures

- Perform HIV-antibody testing for at least six months post exposure (e.g. at baseline, six weeks, three months, and six months).
- Perform HIV antibody testing if illness compatible with an acute retroviral syndrome occurs.
- Advise exposed persons to use precautions to prevent secondary transmission during the follow-up period.
- Evaluate exposed persons taking PEP within 72 hours after exposure and monitor for drug toxicity for at least two weeks.

PEP for exposures posing risk of infection (e.g. HBV, HCV, HIV) transmission should include the following

- Initiate PEP as soon as possible, preferably within one to six hours of exposure.
- Offer pregnancy testing to all women of childbearing age not known to be pregnant.
- Seek expert consultation if viral resistance is suspected.
- Administer PEP for 4 weeks if tolerated.

Post exposure prophylaxis (PEP)

(Figures 21.1 and 21.2)

Commonly occurring infectious exposures must have standard protocols and regimen for prophylaxis, e.g. HIV, HBV, HCV. These are generally called PEP programmes. Counselling must be available immediately after exposure. There must be management support for investigations, prophylaxis, prevention and follow-up.

Examples

1. **HBV exposure** (Table 21.2)**:** HBV vaccination and HBV immune globulin (HBIG) are recommended for unvaccinated healthcare workers and known non-immune individuals. Previously vaccinated healthcare workers may require HBV vaccine booster.
2. **HIV exposure:** combination antiretroviral prophylaxis should be recommended.
3. **HCV exposure:** No effective prophylaxis for HCV is available.

Vaccination for hospital staff and immunization of laboratory staff [10-12]

Several categories of healthcare workers, in the course of their routine work, are exposed to a variety of pathogens. The Control of Substances Hazardous to Health (COSHH) (USA), Regulations 1994 dictates that an assessment be made of the workers exposed to biological agents. An approved Code of Practice entitled 'Control of Biological Agents' advises the control measures required to prevent or control such exposure to infection. Wherever it is possible to recognize the risk of infection and when effective vaccines are available, exposure reports have to be evaluated for completeness and accuracy, access to care (i.e., the time of exposure to the time of evaluation), and laboratory result reporting time.

Immunization of hospital staff must be a high priority. Healthcare workers' education with dissemination of information and the recent guidelines is crucial to the success of the immunization programme. In addition to the immunizations in hospitals, a programme to vaccinate the public is also essential. Immunization of staff is carried out for two reasons:

1. Protection of self
2. Prevention of transmission to patients

Immunization recommended for HCWs

- Hepatitis A
- Hepatitis B
- Influenza
- Measles
- Mumps

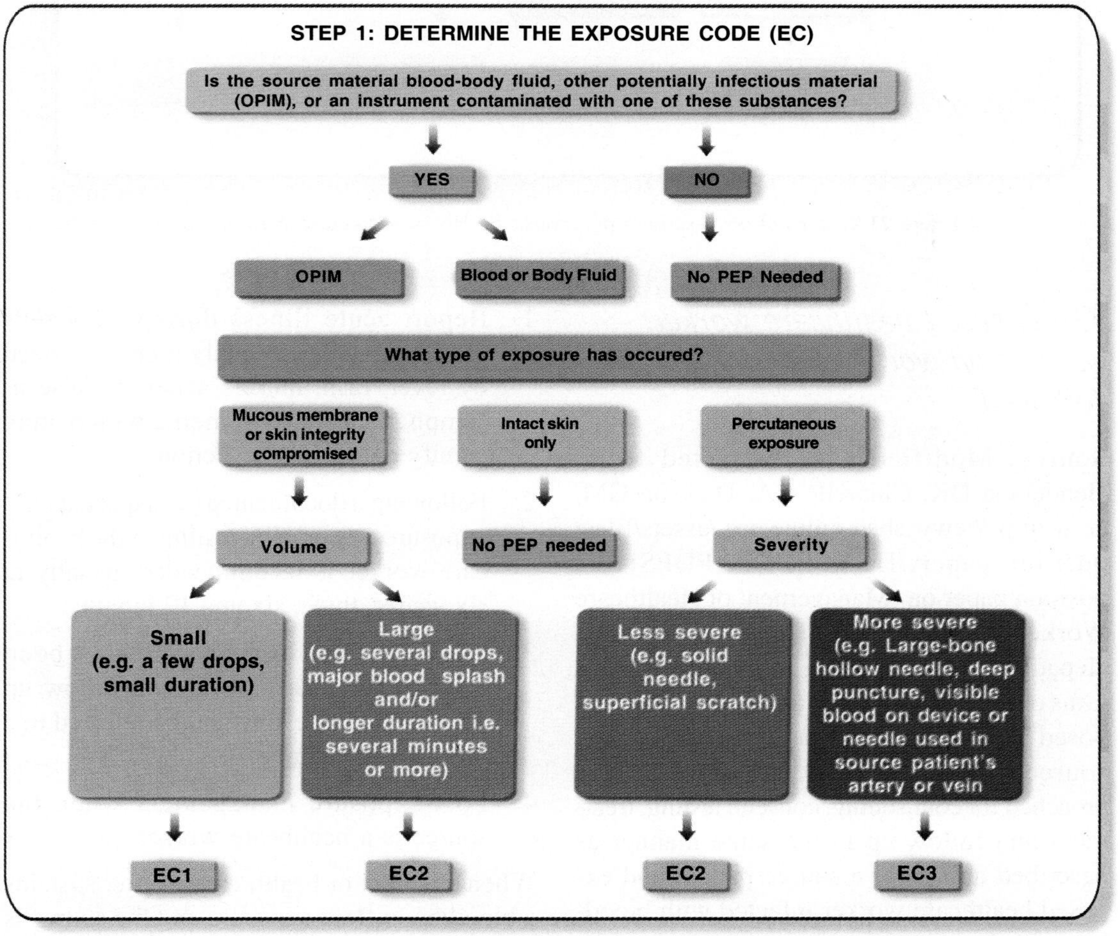

Figure 21.1: Steps of post-exposure prophylaxis for HIV now accepted the world over

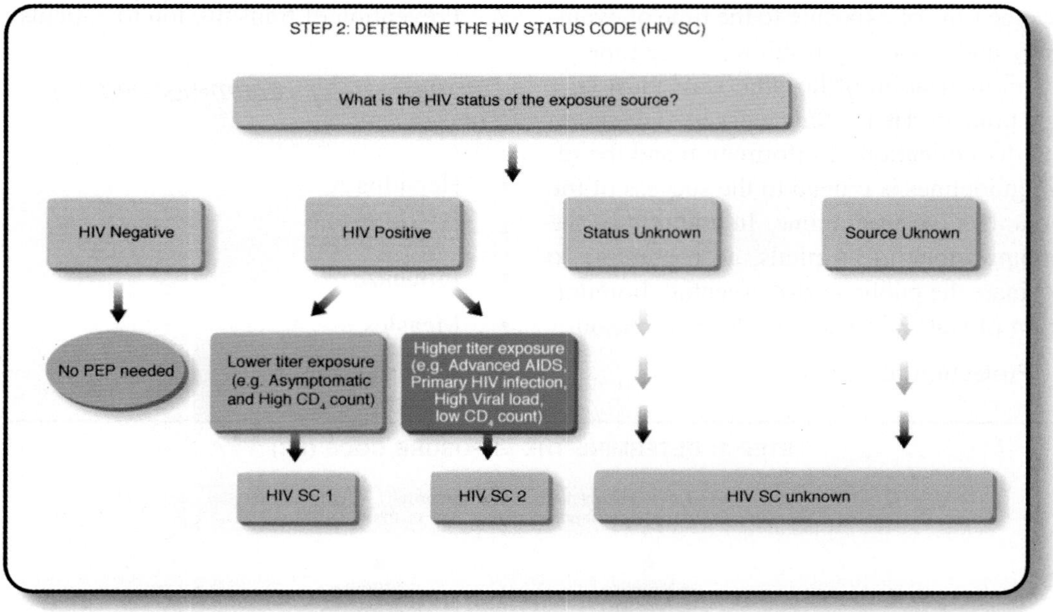

Figure 21.2: Steps of post-exposure prophylaxis for HIV now accepted the world over

The exposed healthcare worker: policies on work restriction and follow-up

Source: Modified and abstracted from, Henderson DK, Chiarello LA, Dickson GM, et al http://www.shea-online.org./assets/files/position-papers/HCW-BBP97.PDFSHEA position paper on 'Management of Healthcare Workers Infected with Hepatitis B Virus, Hepatitis C virus, Human Immunodeficiency virus or other blood-borne pathogens.' The exposed patient or healthcare worker and the source healthcare worker should be approached for counselling, consent, testing, treatment and follow-up in the same manner as described above for a source patient and exposed healthcare worker infected with blood-borne pathogens.

1. Report acute illness during 12 weeks after exposure, especially if characterized by fever, rash, muscle aches, malaise or lymph node enlargement, which may signify recent HIV infection.
2. Following a documented or suspected HIV exposure, repeat HIV testing of the healthcare worker is recommended, usually at six weeks, three, six and 12 months.
3. A healthcare worker who has been exposed to hepatitis C should follow up with serologic testing and be referred to a physician if positive.
4. Post-exposure management when the source is a healthcare worker–

When a patient or health care worker sustains a blood/body fluid exposure and the source is a healthcare worker, the hospital/clinic has an ethical obligation to notify the exposed patient or healthcare worker.

Mandatory HIV screening of healthcare workers is discouraged by OSHA; Voluntary HIV, HBV and HCV screening of healthcare workers for infection is encouraged so they may benefit from medical intervention; all healthcare workers who have been potentially exposed to HIV, HBV or HCV through personal risk behaviour, blood products or occupational accidents should be strongly advised to seek testing.

In USA, healthcare workers are not required to inform patients or employers if they are HIV, HBV or HCV positve. Employers should be infomed if infection results in impairment affecting job performance. A patient should be informed if that patient has sustained a significant exposure to the healthcare worker's blood.

Evaluation of infected healthcare workers for risk of transmission

There is a dearth of established laws, regulations and guidelines in most countries to evaluate risk of transmission in infected healthcare workers. OSHA recommends that each hospital or institution establish an expert panel to confidentially evaluate cases of blood-borne disease infected healthcare workers with respect to work-related issues. A panel can recommend practice limitations (the kind of practice a healthcare worker is allowed to continue), modifications or restrictions where the evidence suggests there is a significant risk

Table 21.2: Post-exposure prophylaxis for Hepatitis-B

ALGORITHM FOR HBV TREATMENT AFTER EXPOSURE

Exposed person is / Source	HBsAg +ve	HBsAg -ve	Unknown
Not HBV vaccinated	Test exposure for HBsAg. If +, no treatment	Vaccinate	In correctional setting, treat as if source were HBsAg +
HBV vaccinated; Unknown response	HBIG x 1 and vaccinate	No treatment	Test exposed for HBsAg. If -, revaccinate
HBV vaccinated; known Non-responder	HBIG x 1 and vaccinate	No treatment	In correctional setting, treat as if source were HBsAg +
HBV vaccinated; known Responder	No treatment	No treatment	No treatment

HBIG = Hepatitis B Immunoglobulin

to patients. Any modification of work practice must seek to impose the least restrictive alternative in accordance with disability laws. HIV, HBV or HCV infection alone does not justify limiting healthcare workers' professional duties. Limitations, if any, should be determined on a case-by-case basis considering the factors that influence transmission risk, including:

1. Nature and scope of professional practice
2. Techniques used in invasive procedures which may pose a risk to patients
3. Compliance with infection-control standards.
4. Presence of weeping dermatitis or skin lesions
5. Overall health status: physical and cognitive functions

Viral load testing

Can a HCW with Hepatitis B continue to work? Healthcare workers with positive results should be restricted from performing 'exposure-prone procedures' or be reviewed by an expert panel to determine which procedures they may safely perform. In some countries, guidelines are being laid for permission to work, based on viral load assays, e.g. Scandinavian countries, the UK, etc.

The upper limits of viral load are:

UK HBV viral load $>10^3$ DNA copies/ml

Netherlands viral load $> 10^5$ DNA copies/ml

Position statements on HIV

The CDC guidelines have stimulated enormous controversy, therefore, position statements from a variety of professional organizations and interest groups are given from time to time. In 1991, the American Medical Association Source (AMA) issued the following statement: 'Physicians who are HIV positive have an ethical obligation not to engage in any professional activity, which has an identifiable risk of transmission of the infection to the patient. Physicians must abstain from performing invasive procedures which pose an 'identifiable risk of transmission', or disclose their seropositive status prior to performing a procedure and proceed only if there is informed consent.' In the midst of this controversy are some points of agreement. There is a consensus that implementation of universal precautions and prevention of provider injuries are likely to produce the greatest overall public health benefit. An employee's HIV status must be protected as private and confidential medical information. To ensure care of HIV-infected patients, hospital authorities, clinicians or supervisors should educate and inform all healthcare workers, of the mechanisms of HIV transmission and reassure them that casual contact (touching, holding, kissing on the cheek) and protected handling of patients with PPE does not transmit HIV.

ENGINEERING CONTROLS

(PHOTO 21.3)

Replacement of equipment with safer devices is discussed in chapter on engineering controls. This must be combined with appropriate use of safety protocols, devices with special training and education. Institutions must organize classes for the benefit of the employees. Employees also need adequate motivation to change from older to newer methods. They

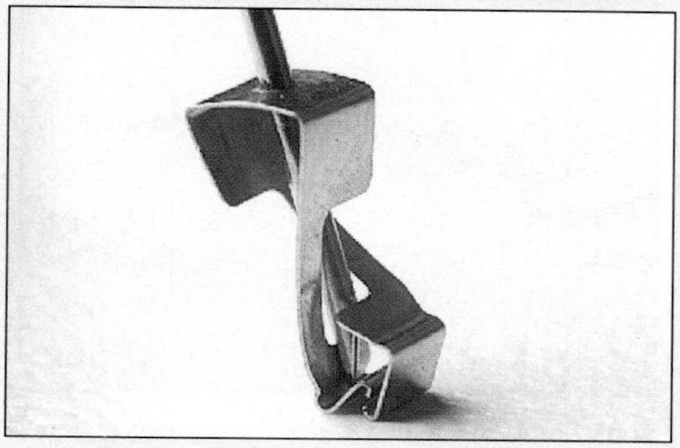

Photo 21.3: Engineering controls: development of a protected stylet tip (Courtsey B Braun India): This opens up when the stylet is withdrawn after intravenous cannulation.

must learn how new safety devices operate and practice with them.

1. Always deactivate the safety mechanism.
2. Do not bypass the safety mechanism.
3. Training sessions are also the responsibility of the manufacturers—involve them in training.

1. Hazards of Particular Equipment and Materials[13]

a. Centrifuges

The biggest threat from centrifuges comes from the rotation assembly. This is a threat both to the user and to others in the vicinity. The International Federation of Clinical chemistry (IFCC) guidelines for selection and use of centrifuges is recommended to prevent hazards arising out of centrifuges.

b. Autoclaves and pressure vessels

These may fail in their function and the reasons for this could be inadequate venting of a pressure-controlled autoclave, improper temperature monitoring or inadequate time. The effectiveness of the sterilization process is determined by the 'holding time at temperature' (HTAT), i.e. taken from the time when the temperature of the load reaches the required levels.

User errors are an important factor in the safe operation of small autoclaves. The precautions which need to be taken are as follows:

- Manufacturer's instructions to be followed
- Vessel inspected daily for corrosion and vent for evidence of blockage

c. Avoiding needles[14]

Bionectors (vygon): This is a closed IV connection system with standard Luer fittings and a self-sealing membrane for IV injections without a needle. The same connection can be used for sampling, infusions and injections. Staff have to be trained adequately in their usage and care, because, often it is seen that they appear unconcerned and rarely, if ever, document their practice.

There are a number of needleless devices which are available, and more are being developed. The cost of incorporating newer devices must be weighed against the benefit.

WORK PRACTICE CONTROLS

Work practice controls are aimed at reducing exposure to an infectious agent by removing the hazard or isolating the staff from the hazard.

Improper practices /procedures in the healthcare setting pose a high risk of infection to all concerned, many of whom are, more often than not, unsuspecting victims of the carelessness of others. These hazards can be minimized to a great extent by the simple policy of specifying how a particular procedure is to be performed and by whom. In some settings, these are laid down as Work Practice Controls, which are policies relating to patient and HCW safety. By definition, work practice controls are policies intended to ensure compliance in carrying out preventive strategies, and need managerial commitment for a consistent pursuit of safety. It is a strategy in which there is an attempt to control the manner in which various tasks are carried out, ensuring a safer and protected methodology. Generally, guidelines are laid down in order to alter unsafe behaviour or practices and in some settings, these are printed out as Work Practice Controls. It is mandatory for the healthcare workers to follow a particular standard of care, failing which action could be taken against them.

Work practice controls are modifications in technique that reduce or eliminate the likelihood of risk exposure by altering the manner in which the task is performed.

Behavior management + Administrative mandates = workpractice controls.

In many places, if the administrative support, in the form of policies, regulations or laws, is not present, the healthcare workers may be educated only about the changes in behaviour required to reduce risks.

Examples of Work Practice Controls for Prevention of Percutaneous (Needle-Stick) Exposures[15-18]

(Photo 21.4)

1. Avoid unnecessary use of needles and other sharps

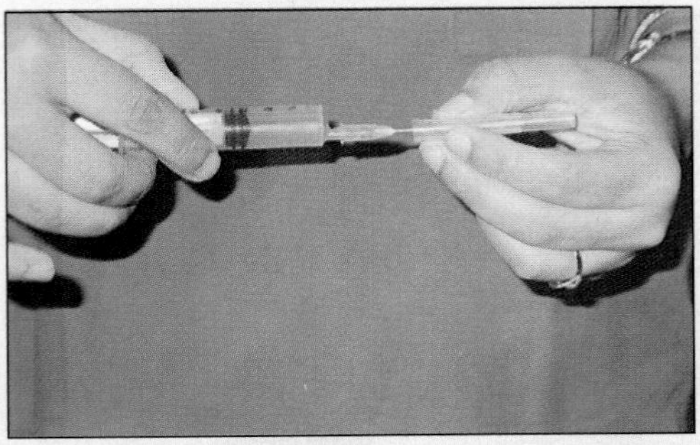

Photo 21.4: Recapping a needle—an occupational hazard

2. Take special care in handling and disposal of sharps
3. Do not recap needles or, if absolutely necessary, use a 'one-handed recapping technique'. Recommended method of recapping is as follows:
   - Place one hand behind your back.
   - Place needle cap on a flat surface.
   - Take hand away from cap and away from needle.
   - Holding only the syringe, guide needle into cap and scoop up the cap.
   - Lift up syringe so cap is sitting on needle hub.
   - Secure needle-cap into place.
4. In surgery, dentistry or emergencies, pass sharps using a basin or tray designated as a 'safe zone' (not hand-to-hand).
5. Disassemble sharp equipment only by using forceps or other devices
6. Always dispose of sharps you have used. Never leave sharps behind on trays, counters or beds for someone to pick up.

7. Watch out for over-filled sharps containers when disposing of sharps.

Avoiding Needle-Stick Injury During Surgery (Guidelines by CDC)

1. Use forceps, suture holders or other instruments for holding needles and suturing.
2. Do not use fingers to hold tissue when suturing.
3. Never leave sharps in a surgical field.
4. Do not blindly reach into a sink or basin of water to retrieve contaminated sharp instruments.
5. Seek help prior to any procedure when dealing with aggressive, violent patients.
6. Destroy trays and other instruments with jagged, broken edges.
7. Do nor remove or insert scalpel blades with bare fingers; use forceps, etc.

Behaviour ⟶	**Changed Behaviour**
Dangerous ⟶	**Less dangerous**
Recaping needles	Do not recap needles
Handling patients without protection	Handle with standard precautions
Mouth pipetting	Automated/safer pipetting
Handling sterilants	Protected handling

Develop SOPs for Specific Tasks

E.g. venepuncture

- The patient must be positively identified.
- The patient must give verbal consent. If the patient withdraws consent during the procedure, the procedure must stop.
- Before starting the procedure, the operator must wash her/his hands and wear gloves.
- Gloves must always be worn in the following situations:
  a. When the operator has any cut, scratch or abrasion on her/his skin
  b. When the operator judges that hand contamination with blood may occur, e.g. a semi-conscious patient
  c. When performing finger or heel pricks
  d. When learning or training how to do venepunctures
- Clean the venepuncture site with an alcohol wipe or other approved antiseptic
- Following the venepuncture, put the uncapped needle into a designated sharps box
- Put all bloodstained cotton wool or other materials into a designated impervious, labelled bag for incineration. The bag should be labelled either with a biohazard sign or 'medical waste', or both.

Recommended Behaviour in the Areas of Potential Exposure -

(Photo 21.5)

Do not

- Eat or drink in the area
- Apply cosmetics or lip balm
- Handle contact lenses
- Store food or drink
- Bend, break, or remove needles from disposable syringes
- Recap needles with two hands

Use of gloves

- Avoid touching phones, door knobs and light switches when wearing gloves, to prevent contamination
- Do not snap gloves while removing them, as it aerosolizes leading to contamination

Handling sharps

Source: Reproduced with permission from 'Element III: use of engineering and work practice controls to reduce opportunity for patient and healthcare worker exposure to potentially infectious material.' www. laboratoryconsultationservices.com LCS%infectioncontrolcourse.htm (02.06.2006)

- Do not try recapping needles.
- Do not bend contaminated needles.
- Use forceps or any other device to remove contaminated needles.
- Immediately or as soon as possible place sharps in a puncture-proof container which is leak proof and labelled with a biohazard symbol.

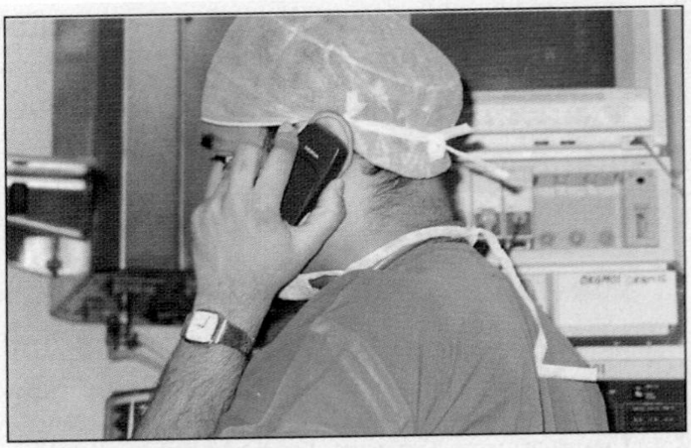

Photo 21.5: Work practice controls aim at changing high risk behaviour. E.g. use of phones with contaminated hands can lead to increased transmission.

- Suture needles should be placed in the sharps bin with forceps.
- Scalpel blades should be removed from a handle using needle holder with sharp edge facing away.
- Do not put a syringe in your pocket.

Eating and drinking habits

- Eating, drinking, smoking, application of cosmetics or handling of contact lenses should not be done in the work areas where there is reasonable likelihood of exposure.
- Food and drink must not be stored in refrigerators, cabinets or counters where blood and other potentially infectious materials are present.
- Disposable cups must be provided for patients.

Transport of specimens

- Specimens of blood or other tissue should

be placed in a container that is leak-proof during collection, handling and transport.

- It should preferably be a double container with a biohazard label.

Special precautions in potentially infected patients

- Patients with rashes and/or fever should be kept in a room to wait rather than in a common area.

Exposure to eyes

- If eyes are exposed, wash the area with water.
- Flush eyes in an eyewash.
- Report the exposure to a supervisor immediately.

Decontamination

- Anything that comes in contact with blood or potentially infectious material must be cleaned and decontaminated before reuse.
- Use an employee-friendly tuberculocide. E.g. a solution of 1:10 and 1:100 sodium hypochlorite.
- Soak in disinfectant for at least twenty minutes before continuing.

PERSONAL PROTECTIVE EQUIPMENT (PPE)

PPE against infectious pathogens have already been discussed in the chapter on barrier precautions and PPE. Appropriate transmission based precautions must be followed with different conditions or infections. Gloves must be worn when there is direct contact with contaminated instruments. Use high-quality impervious gloves when working with chemical disinfectants such as glutaraldehyde. Studies show natural rubber latex gloves meet these requirements. Masks and/or protective eyewear must be used during manual cleaning of instruments prior to immersion in glutaraldehyde solution. Impervious gowns/aprons must also be worn when engaged in cleaning of instruments. Preclean instruments with a neutral pH, protein dissolving detergent solution prior to disinfection. Proper pre-cleaning can reduce the bioburden by as much as 99% and make the instruments safer for healthcare workers to handle. Avoid direct skin contact.

Guidelines for Glutaraldehye Spills

PPE should also be used against chemical hazards. Glutaraldehye, as well as any chemical agent, should be handled with caution. If a glutaraldehyde spill should occur, follow the procedures below to ensure safety to healthcare workers:

1. Safety glasses
2. Latex gloves
3. Mop and bucket
4. Sponge, towels
5. Plastic trash bag for disposal

For Large Glutaraldehyde Spills (One Gallon or More)

1. Breathing mask equipped with an organic vapour filter
2. Rubber boots or shoe protection
3. Squeegee
4. Plastic dust pan

5. Plastic scoop to disperse ammonium carbonate

For small spills (less than one gallon): Mix eight ounces of household ammonia cleaning solution with eight ounces of water. With a mop, sponge or squeegee, blend the diluted ammonia solution into the spilled glutaraldehyde for one to two minutes until the glutaraldehyde odour is 'neutralized'.

For large spills: Using a plastic scoop, sprinkle sufficient ammonium carbonate powder to cover most of the surface of the spilled glutaraldehyde. This may require up to 500 grams of ammonium carbonate per gallon of glutaraldehde estimated to be spilled. Allow about five minutes for the ammonium carbonate to begin to dissolve and 'neutralize' the glutaraldehyde. Collect the liquid slurry with a mop, sponge, towel, squeegee and/or plastic dust pan and flush it down the drain, with large amounts of water. Rinse the cleaning utensils, and immediately discard the rinse water down the drain with large amounts of water. Thoroughly rinse any sponges or towels with water and immediately discard in a tighlty closed plastic trash bag.

Latex

Though latex gloves are worn as a personal protective equipment, healthcare workers can become allergic to them. There has been an increase in latex allergies varying from contact dermatitis, to systemic reactions.

REFERENCES

1) Farrington M, Pascoe G. Risk Management and Infection Control – Time to get our priorities right in the UK. J Hosp Infect. 2001; 47: 15-24

2) Updated U S Public Health Service Guidelines for the Management of Occupational Exposures to HBV, HCV, and HIV and Recommendations for Post-exposure Prophylaxis. In Recommendations and Reports. Morbidity and Mortality Weekly Report. U S Department of Health and Human Services. Centre for Disease Control and Prevention (CDC), Atlanta, GA 30333. 2001.Vol 50 / No. RR – 11; 43

3) Castillo DN, Pizatetla TJ, Stout N. Injuries. In: Levy BS, Wegman DH (Eds). Occupational Health; recognizing and preventing work related disease and injury. 4th edn. Philadelphia, Lippincott, Williams and Wilkins. 2000: 461-476.

4) Spencer EM, Mills AE, Rorty MV and Werhane PH. Compliance, Risk management and Quality improvement programmes (Chap 10). In Organization Ethics in Health Care. Oxford University Press. New York 2000:171-185

5) Sutton PM, Nicas M, Harrison RJ. Implementing a Quality assurance Program for Tuberculosis Control. In Handbook of modern hospital safety Ed. Charney W. Lewis Publishers. Boca Raton. 1999; 246-252.

6) Charney W, Fisher J and Ishida C. The inefficiency of Surgical Masks for Protection against Droplet Nuclei TB. In: Handbook of modern hospital safety. Ed. Charney W. Lewis Publishers. Boca Raton. 1999; 222-237.

7) Pipin J. Efficiency of face masks in preventing inhalation of airborne contaminants. Oral Maxillofac. Surg. 1987; 45: 319- 323

8) O'Grady NP, Gerberding JL, Weinstein RA et al. Patient safety and the science of prevention:

The time for implementing the Guidelines for the Prevention of Intravascular Catheter-related infections is now. Crit Care Med. 2003; 31(1) 291-21.

9) Schwab SJ et al. Multicenter clinical trial results with the LifeSite hemodialysis access system. Kidney Int. 2002; 62(3): 1026-33.

10) Gellin B. Prevention and chemoprophylaxis. In Infection diseases Eds. Armstrong D, Cohen J. Mosby Publishers. 1999; 1: 4.1-4.19

11) Practice recommendation for Health-care Facilities Implementing the US Public Health Service Guidelines for Management of Occupational Exposures to Blood-borne Pathogens.Morbidity and Mortality Weekly Report (MMWR) Recommendations and Reports. June 29, 2001 / Volume 50 / No.RR-11

12) CH Collins Laboratory Acquired infections 3rd edn. Butterworth & Heinemann 1993; 28-40.

13) Girard R, Perraud M, Pruss A et al. In: Ducel G, Fabry J, Nicolle L. Prevention of hospital-acquired infections – A practical guide. 2nd edn. WHO 2002: 47-54

14) Cheeseman D. Intravenous care: the benefits of closed-system connectors. Br J Nurs. 2001; 10(5): 287-95.

15) Jagger J, Hunt E, Pearsons RD. Estimated cost of needlestick injuries for six major needled devices. Infect Control Hosp Epidemiol. 1990. 11(11): 584-588.

16) Bently M, Jagger J. Surveillance of percutaneous injuries in a 77-hospital network. Part I. In: Handbook of modern hospital safety. Ed. Charney W. Lewis Publishers. Boca Raton. 1999; 251-56.

17) World Health Organization Communications Office. Injection Safety. Tropical Doctor. 2003 33(1): 48-9

18) Wugofski L. Needlestick Prevention Devices: A pointed Discussion. In Handbook of modern hospital safety Ed. Charney W. Lewis Publishers. Boca Raton. 1999; 321-325

Chapter 22

Experts Speak

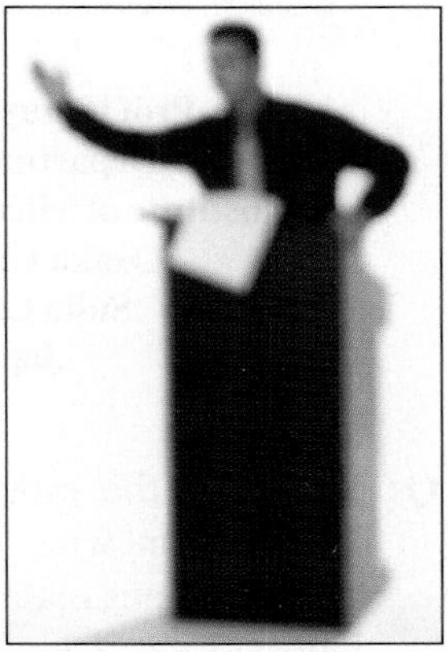

Believe one who has proved it. Believe an expert.

—Virgil, in *Aeneid*

Highlights

Prof Kazuyoshi Ikuta

Dr Ashok Rattan

Dr Hema Kapoor

Dr Sridhara Iyengar

Dr Aman Mahajan

Dr Mala Chhabra

Ms Anjali Bagati

Peter Laser

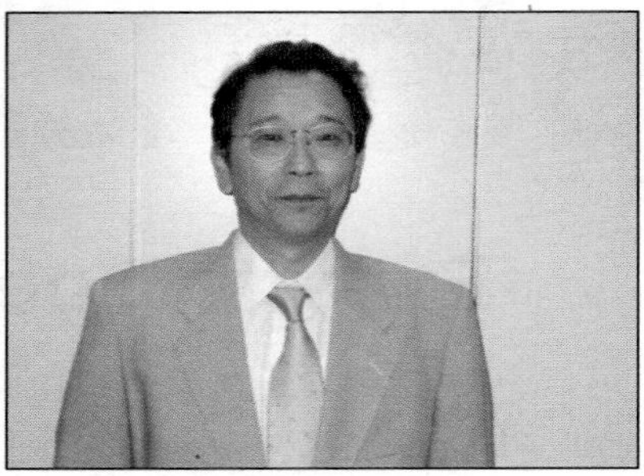

Prof Kazuyoshi Ikuta
Head, Department of Virology
Institute of Microbial Diseases
Osaka University
Suita Campus
Japan

Q: What are the most important points to keep in mind when handling biohazardous and infectious material, like HIV, in the P3 laboratory in your set-up?

A: It is very important that general housekeeping in the P3 biohazard laboratory is of a very high standard. All users must do their best to keep the laboratory tidy. Before entering the P3 level laboratory, all users must wear lab-coats, rubber boots, gloves, N-95 masks and goggles. Before starting work, the levels of air pressure in the room must be checked. Essentially, users must pay attention to the possibility of infection with the experimental materials in the laboratory. While working with HIV, one must consider its tropism to T-lymphocytes as susceptible host cells. HIV-2 is not as active a virus for transmission. Experiments using needles for HIV injection into animals or obtaining blood from HIV infected model animals are very dangerous to work with and must be disposed of appropriately.

Q: How do your laboratory personnel protect themselves from infections while working in the laboratory? Do they receive any specific training in handling biohazardous material?

A: It is compulsory for every prospective P3 laboratory user to attend the orientation seminar on handling biohazardous material, which is held every year. The Biosafety Committee then authorizes members to use such laboratories after ascertaining their identities and the kind of organisms they propose to work with. We have a Manual on the use of a P3 laboratory. Personnel handling or working with hazardous microorganisms like SARS virus, take adequate precautions—wearing lab-coats and two pairs of gloves (inner white and outer blue gloves). The outer blue gloves are used only when working with the organisms at the safety bench. They are removed when the worker leaves the bench. This is to prevent contamination of door knobs and other apparatus.

Beginners must always work with an expert or supervisor for at least a year. Sera samples from all users of laboratory are collected after informed consent and stored in a freezer for future use if necessary. In the event of an emergency, such as a fire alarm, all infectious materials are placed in an incubator or a freezer as quickly as possible before fleeing the place. If it is not possible to exit via the doors, the window panes must be smashed (with the hatchet kept for the purpose).

Strict instructions are given to all users to report any actual or potential exposure to infection, to a responsible person such as project leader or supervisor or professor.

Q: How is the infectious material disposed of in your laboratory?

A: Nothing can be taken out of the P3 laboratory without sterilization. Users must dispose of every biohazardous material only after autoclaving. This includes needles, syringes, tubes, pipettes used for blood from patients (or even apparently healthy individuals), etc.

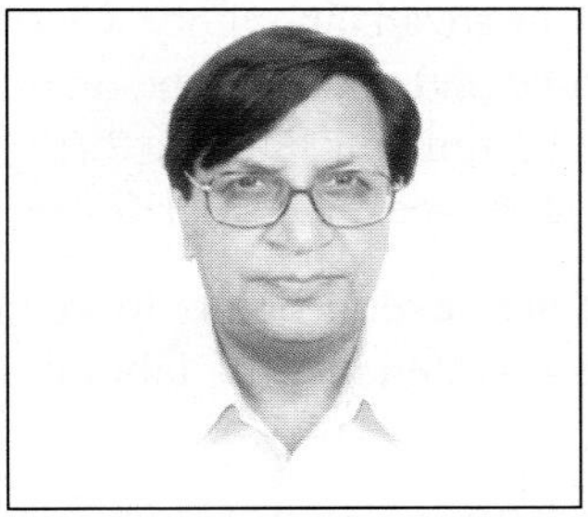

Dr Ashok Rattan
Medical Microbiologist & Laboratory Director
Caribbean Epidemiology Centre (CAREC)
Pan American Health Organization
World Health Organization

Q: What in your opinion is the role of the pharmaceutical industry in developing newer antimicrobials ?

A: The idea underpinning discovery of an antibiotic usually emanates from academia, but almost all drugs are developed by the pharmaceutical industry at high financial risk. Although industrial research and development teams are motivated by scientific and medical concerns, funds are usually provided on the expectations of profit.

Antibacterials have a worldwide market of US$ 24 billion, but the growth rate is projected to be flat for the next decade. Consequently, in research and development groups of many companies, resources are being reallocated to other chronic disease therapeutic areas that promise greater commercial opportunities.

Q: What is the present/future scenario of antimicrobial agents? Will they deliver the goods? Will they succeed in the race against resistant microorganisms?

A: Historically, antibiotic resistance has been the driving force for the discovery and development of new antimicrobial agents since the late 1950s. Throughout the past five decades, new resistance mechanisms have continued to appear and new agents have, in turn, been introduced to meet the challenge. Examples include the development of new penicillins and cephalosporins to avoid hydrolysis by newly identified β lactamases, the development of telithromycin to treat macrolide-resistant Streptococcus infection, the development of oxazolidinones for MRSA and VISA and daptomycin and oritavancin to address vancomycin resistant enterococci.

The knowledge base concerning bacterial physiology and genetics was extremely limited during 1940s to 1960s, the period during which the progenitors of all the antibiotics in clinical use today were identified by simple growth inhibition tests. Today complete genome sequences of more than 140 bacteria are publicly available. Functional genome technologies have evolved which allow the study of transcriptional and translational activity of a given bacteria on a genome wide scale by transcriptional profiling and proteomic analysis. We know more now about causative agents and how to control them. So, the future seems to be promising. Even so, the battle won't be easy unless practitioners exercise extreme caution and control in prescribing drugs and play their cards right to hold out against resistant organisms.

Q: What are your suggestions/opinions/experiences as to how to combat the problem of drug resistance?

A: The Center for Disease control, Atlanta has developed a four step, 12 point programme shown to be effective in prevention and control of infections, clinicians hold the key in this activity, which includes:

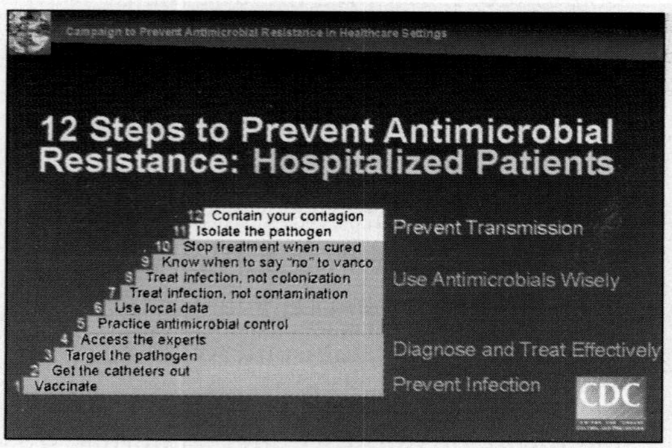

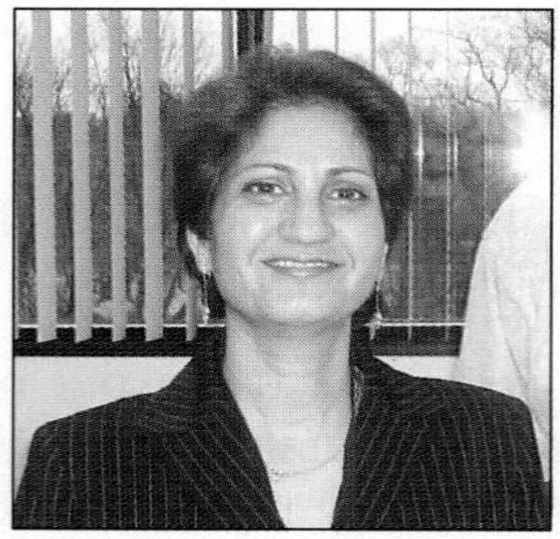

Dr Hema Kapoor
Technical Director
Infectious Diseases
Quest Diagnostics Incorporated
Philadelphia Business Unit
USA

Q: How do you maintain the quality control of your laboratory equipment? Is any specific person appointed to look into these issues, or are all laboratory workers trained to handle and maintain the quality control of the equipment they use? (E.g. incubators, deep freezers, centrifuges, etc.)

A: There are several points to keep in mind in the maintenance of laboratory equipment:

1. The status of Laboratory equipment, instruments and test systems are monitored under a preventive maintenance programme based on manufacturer's operating manuals.

   All records are documented in the equipment maintenance logbook or an equivalent.

2. Equipment will not be used unless it is in a safe and reliable operating state.

3. Operating manuals and preventive maintenance schedules are readily available to testing personnel.

4. The incubator, refrigerator and freezer temperatures are monitored and recorded daily with a certified or calibrated thermometer. Calibrated (non-certified) thermometers are checked against a certified one (NBS traceable), annually to establish precision of non-certified thermometers in daily use. An outside calibration and maintenance organization can provide this function and furnish documentation, which is dated and signed by the person performing the calibration.
5. Only staff with documented training operates the equipment.
6. Calibration verification must be performed on equipment used for moderately complex or highly complex analyses where appropriate, unless specified otherwise by the manufacturer, every six months or:
   a. More frequently if specified by the manufacturer
   b. When reagent manufacturers are changed
   c. When control values begin to reflect an unusual trend or are outside acceptable limits (+/- 2 standard deviations from the mean)
7. All records of corrective action taken and repairs are documented in the individual units'equipment maintenance log or suitable ledger maintained by testing site personnel.
8. Equipment monitoring records are regularly reviewed, dated and signed by Laboratory Director.

Q: How are your SOPs designed? Do they include only procedures or other aspects like risks and hazards and how to handle these? How often are the SOPs updated? Who are they targeted against?

A: All diagnostic work done on a clinical specimen is accomplished according to a written procedure selected, developed and optimized for each situation in advance of the actual test done for a patient. Procedures used are equivalent to or exceed requirements recognized by existing state or federal regulations. For clinical testing procedures we usually follow National Committee for Clinical Laboratory Standards, Approved Guideline, Volume 4, Number 2, Clinical Laboratory Procedure Manuals. The procedures include the following criteria as applicable:

a. Qualifications for acceptance and rejection of samples
b. Safety concerns unique to a particular procedure
c. Testing procedure (analytical methodology and principles) including limitations of procedures, reagents and calculation explanation
d. Quality control and calibration requirements
e. Corrective action guidelines
f. Report handling procedures and instructions on reporting results, reportable ranges, test values outside of reportable ranges and critical or panic values
g. Disposal of specimens and related by-products is performed in accordance with local health department's 'Waste Handling and Disposal Policy'.

h. Reference materials pertinent to specific procedures

i. Appropriate criteria for specimen storage and preservation to ensure specimen integrity until testing is completed

j. Criteria for the course of action to be taken in the event that a test system becomes inoperable

k. Criteria for referral of specimens, including procedures for specimen submission and handling

l. Procedures for microscopic examination, including the detection of inadequately prepared slides

m. Preparation of slides, solution, calibrators, controls, reagents, stains and other materials used in testing

These procedures are written by the supervisors of the laboratory but initiated by the testing personnel and approved, dated and signed for use at least annually by the Laboratory Director. Changes in the procedures must also be approved, signed and dated by the Laboratory Director or designated technical consultant.

Procedures must be re-approved, signed and dated if the directorship of the laboratory changes.

The laboratory must maintain a copy of each procedure with the dates of initial use and discontinuance every two years.

Q: How do you manage laboratory accidents? What are the methods of waste disposal followed?

A: There is a Safety Officer who is responsible for writing Health and Safety Manual which consists of the following:

a. Safety of employees

b. Training

c. Emergency first aid assistance procedure

d. Laboratory chemical fume hood and biological safety procedures

e. Building ventilation

f. Occupational exposure handling

g. Personal protective equipment

h. Disposal of wastes

i. Chemical hygiene plan

j. Chemical spill plan

k. Radiation safety programme

Every new employee undergoes health and safety, blood-borne pathogens and waste disposal training. People who use Biological Safety Cabinets and level 3 laboratories have special training on these, plus for the use of N-95 respirators when necessary.

Vaccination is given for respective disease organisms on a regular basis and blood testing is done for antibody titres on a regular basis.

Mantoux test and x-ray chest evaluations are performed for every new employee and annually for employees who work with TB agents or if anyone shows signs or symptoms.

If any laboratory accident occurs, the employee completes accident/injury report, if able; otherwise, the supervisor or the attending physician fills the accident report.

First Aid providers receive training annually and a list is maintained in the safety manual.

Waste disposal is by chemical disinfection, autoclave and incineration. Sharps are discarded in special puncture-proof containers.

Q: Are there any measures of assessing performance of laboratory personnel? In other words, their performance management.

A: External Proficiency Testing: Each laboratory performing moderate complexity or high complexity laboratory procedures participates in an external proficiency testing programme that is approved by Health Care Fed Accreditation CLIA (Clinical Laboratory Improvement Amendments) programme.

1. Each test in the moderate or high complexity category must be tested with three challenge sets containing up to five specimens per year.
2. The samples must be examined or tested with the laboratory's regular patient workload by personnel who routinely perform the testing in the laboratory, using the laboratory's routine methods.
3. Proficiency test results must be completed and mailed within the time period specified by the suppliers. Normally, this is 10 working days. Results received after the cut-off date are scored as zero, regardless of the answer reported.
4. Each laboratory performing external proficiency testing is required to maintain a proficiency test score of 80% or better on repeat challenges. Failure to maintain a score of 80% requires withdrawal of the test from clinical use by the laboratory for 6 months and until competency is demonstrated. Laboratories that fail a particular analyte two times consecutively have to submit a corrective action plan.
5. Records of external proficiency testing must be maintained on site or in the health district's central office for two years.
6. Records of external proficiency testing results must be reviewed and signed by the Laboratory Director or Technical Consultant.

Internal Proficiency Testing: The CLIA'88 legislation requires that each laboratory, regardless of complexity level, must demonstrate that tests performed in different sites yield equivalent results for the same analytes. The laboratory maintains its own internal proficiency testing system, using reagents purchased from an external vendor and evaluating the results.

Review of Proficiency Testing: All testing personnel review and initial the final proficiency testing reports which discuss results. The objective is to instruct testing personnel with regard to procedures and potential sources of error, testing problems or variation in testing results.

Competency Evaluation of Personnel: The CLIA'88 legislation requires a mechanism to evaluate competency in test performance for each person who performs a clinical diagnostic test.

1. The laboratory director, site coordinator or other designated person critically observes the individual being

checked to determine that procedural methods and protocols are followed correctly, the technique is adequate and that safety guidelines are followed.

2. Each new person performing testing is checked initially prior to performing a test for clinical purposes, again after six months and yearly thereafter.
3. Records of competency evaluation are maintained on site for two years. The competency evaluation form for individuals is kept with their personal records. A summary form listing each employee and the tests for which they have been checked are also maintained.

Training: Ongoing training is an essential quality assurance event. HCFA and other accrediting agencies require that training take place and that attendance is documented. It does not matter whether an individual receives training on site or off site, or whether it is a short 15 minute 'consulting' session or an all day programme; it still must be documented. A training schedule for each person performing testing is maintained by the supervisor.

Q: How do you approach the investigation of an outbreak of infection in a healthcare set-up?

A: In a hospital setting, infection-control Team (IC practitioner or infection-control officer/nurse and laboratorian, etc.) meet regularly and any outbreak is notified to them, and they do the investigation and institute interventions if any are needed. If the outbreak is of a reportable disease, ICT will notify the health department. Interventions are based on the CDC guidelines, e.g. for Salmonella, Listeria, Staphylococcus, Hepatitis, etc. IC team regularly reviews their policies.

If it is in more than one hospital and public is involved, local health department does the investigations and it is reported to the State health department. State health department helps do the investigation and forward data and laboratory reports or specimens to CDC for federal records like pulse net for food-borne outbreaks, arbonet for arboviral, flu surveillance for flu, etc.

The State Health Department (SHD) carries out the disease surveillance programmes with the help of epidemiologists. Every SHD has divisions like communicable diseases, infectious diseases, immunization, chronic disease etc. Attending physicians, hospitals and laboratories have to follow the protocols of reportable diseases as per the state rules.

The reporting protocols vary with the diseases:

a. Within 24 hours, e.g. Tuberculosis, Yellow fever, Botulism, Nosocomial infections
b. Within 7 days. E.g. Most diseases fall in this category
c. Only total number of cases are required to be reported. E.g. flu, chicken pox
d. Animal bites should be reported to local health department only

All laboratories are equipped with laboratory information systems. Three categories of tests are performed—waived complexity tests, moderate complexity tests and high complexity tests.

Physician office laboratories perform only the waived tests (Hb, glucose, etc.).

Clinical hospital laboratories perform moderate complexity tests and the Reference laboratories perform high complexity tests as also the other varieties. Most big laboratories have a bar code reading system, which can read demographic data from the bar code of the specimen tube.

Reporting is done electronically through Laboratory Information System (LIS), which can either throw out a fax report or electronic report to the physician office or the submitting laboratory.

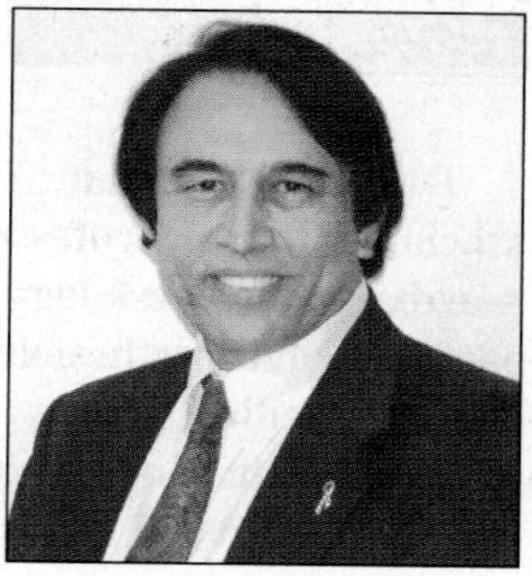

Dr Sridhara Iyengar, Bsc, MD, FRCSC, FACS, DABS, DABTS
Cardiovascular and Thoracic Surgeon
Los Angeles, USA

Q: As a practitioner in a high risk area of medical care, what are your views on HAI and ways to control it in your area of expertise?

A: Hospital Acquired infections result in increased morbidity, mortality and expenditure. The infecting organisms are transmitted either by hospital personnel, physicians, other patients or from endogenous flora. The inappropriate use of antibiotics produces resistant bacteria and fungi, which are unresponsive to routine antibiotics. These patients require stronger, more toxic and more expensive antibiotics to combat the infection. In general, debilitated patients (due to surgery, serious illness, or on antineoplastic agents) are more susceptible to nosocomial infections. The duration of cardiac surgery, the use of cardiopulmonary bypass machine and intra cardiac surgical procedures make the patient more susceptible for infections with grave consequences.

The common pathogens in cardiac surgery include *Staphylococcus aureus, E.coli, Pseudomonas,* other Enterobacteriaceae organisms, fungi and viruses.

Prophylactic antibiotic is used routinely in cardiac surgery. The most important fact that one must be aware of is that the tissues must be bathed in the drug before the skin incision is made. This is accomplished by giving the antibiotic intravenously at least two hours before the start of surgery. In the current practice, commonly, the antibiotic is given just before the skin incision is made. This will only increase the plasma concentration and does not ensure tissue concentration. If the length of surgery extends beyond four hours, another dose of antibiotic should be given intraoperatively.

Avenues of infection are: 1) surgical incisions, 2) indwelling intravenous and bladder catheters, 3) endotracheal tube, 4) intravenous fluid access and use of multi-dose saline vials, 5) endogenous flora, which invades the compromised individual.

There is a direct correlation between the length of stay in the hospital, duration of surgery and the acquisition of nosocomial infection. Patients who spend more than five days in the hospital prior to surgery have a greater likelihood of developing the nosocomial infection. The length of the surgery and exposure of the wound also tend to subject the patient to higher risk.

The surgical wound infection increases the morbidity and mortality rate, as well as prolongs hospital stay and increases medical cost. Preventive measures rather than post-infection treatments should be the main goal in reducing complications.

A full course of appropriate antibiotics should be used only when indicated. Strict hygienic principles must be observed before examining or coming in contact with each patient. Any patient who has persistent fever, elevated white cell count after two to three days following surgery or who is in a debilitated state of health should have careful evaluation of all possible sources of infection.

Before making the decision to change or continue with an antibiotic, a systematic evaluation of the patient must be undertaken. This includes a complete physical examination with particular attention paid to all surgical wound sites, vascular access sites and catheter sites. When indicated, these catheters should be replaced with new ones and the catheter tip should be sent for a complete bacteriological examination. Chest x-rays, laboratory tests for CBC, urine culture, sputum culture, blood culture and sensitivity tests must be routine.

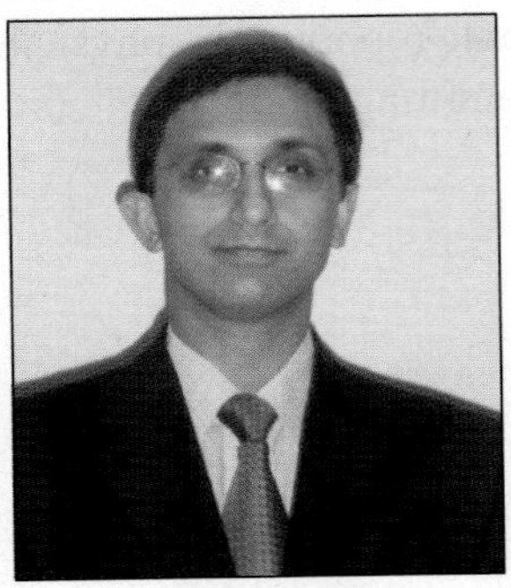

Dr Aman Mahajan
Associate Clinical Professor
Cardiac Anaesthesiology
Department of Anaesthesiology,
UCLA Medical Center,
UCLA School of Medicine and Health Sciences,
USA

Q: Please give us an insight as to how you deal with the cleaning, maintenance and upkeep of TEE (Trans Esophageal Endoscopy) transducers in your institution.

A: TEE transducers are extremely fragile pieces of equipment in an echocardiography system and come in frequent contact with patient's body fluids such as saliva, gastric juices and blood (due to mucosal injuries). To allow for repeated use of the transducers for patient care, it is imperative that high level disinfection be employed to prevent spread of pathogens.

At UCLA, TEE transducers are initially exposed to precleaners (soapy water) to remove mucus or bioburden. High level disinfection is then performed by soaking the TEE transducers in glutaraldehyde 2.4% solutions for a period of 45 minutes. Ortho-phthalaldehyde 0.55% (non-glutaraldehyde) solutions can also serve as an alternative for achieving this goal. Soaking of the probes in isopropyl alcohol or bleach is not recommended as these agents can cause lens delamination and material degradation. Transducers are then thoroughly rinsed with water before patient use. Care should be taken to shield the transducer electronics from the wet solutions. An electrical leak test is routinely performed on each transducer before patient use. Attention should also be given to the transport and storage containers, ensuring adequate disinfection of these as well.

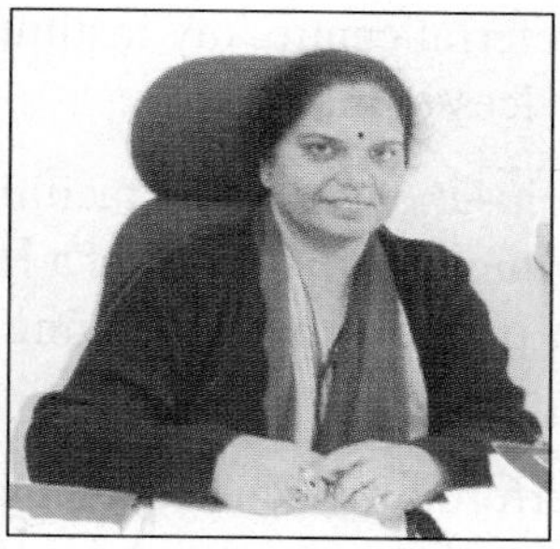

Dr Mala Chhabra
Deputy Director
Zoonosis Division
National Institute of Communicable Diseases
Delhi

Q. As one of the country's top referral and surveillance centres for community acquired infections, what role does your institution have in the surveillance and investigation of hospital acquired infections?

A. In the 21st century, with continuously changing medical environment, increasing use of intricate medical procedures, increasing number of immunocompromised patients and ever-increasing emergence of antibiotic resistant microorganisms, the biggest challenge faced by medical practitioners is to prevent healthcare facility associated infections.

Every healthcare facility must equip itself for this challenge by a two-pronged approach:

1. Constitution of an efficient infection-control unit and 2. Continuous surveillance for HAI with validated methods and timely feedback to the healthcare practitioners.

As a referral centre, my institution offers its services in many ways:

- Helps the healthcare facilities in confirming the diagnosis of a HAI during an outbreak by identifying causative microorganisms
- Performs molecular surveillance of the organism involved in HAI, thus tracing the source of infection in an outbreak
- Provides adequate training of personnel in the diagnosis and management of HAI outbreaks
- Trains personnel in active surveillance measures during and between outbreaks of HAI by using validated methodologies
- Plays a supervisory role in the investigation of an outbreak of HAI, by directing infection-control practices in its control
- Plays an active role in arranging for individual hospital findings to be discussed in forum such as conferences/seminars to bring out inter hospital comparisons. This would help in continuously updating and modifying the guidelines for hospital infection control and need-based measures to be taken at local and national levels

Q. Is there an existing communicable disease surveillance network in India?

A. Every country has its own internal network of surveillance. The National network then coordinates with the WHO global network as follows:

The Epidemiological and Laboratory units of District hospitals report to the respective units of the State hospitals.

The State hospitals, ESI hospitals, Railway Hospitals, Armed Forces hospitals and Private hospitals seek the services of the epidemiological and laboratory wings of the National Institute of Communicable Diseases (NICD), for confirmation and reference regarding outbreaks and epidemics.

The National Reference Centres, including both ICMR and NICD report to the regional office of WHO, which in turn, conveys its data to the WHO global coordinator.

Thus, there is a hierarchy of referral services to handle outbreaks and epidemics in the community as well as in hospitals.

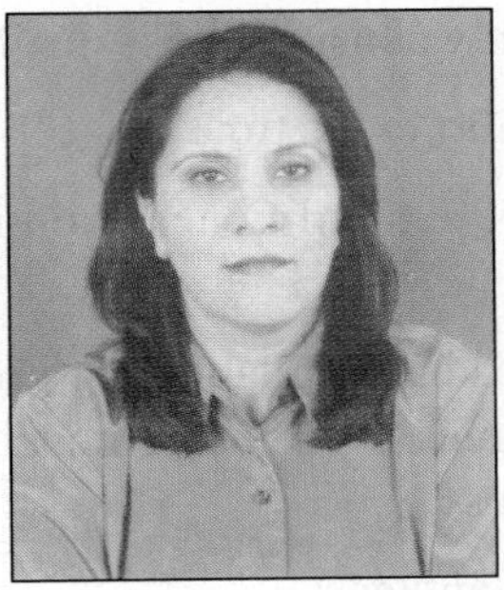

Ms Anjali Bagati
Head-Technical Medical Division
Healthcare Markets Group
3M India Ltd.

Q: As an expert in sterilization processes, please comment on the adequacies/inadequacies of these processes in the healthcare settings.

A: Necessity is the mother of invention. Before 1865, when the germ theory was unknown and unproven, there was no felt-need for sterilization of instruments, for special operating room attire or packaged sterile items. Lord Lister, the Father of Antiseptic surgery, once remarked that healthcare personnel must be able to see specific microorganisms with their mental eye, as distinctly as they see flies with their corporal eye. Yes, each situation must be evaluated on its own merits. Any item coming in contact with the patient or patient's body fluids is potentially infectious. Application of principles and techniques of quality management are of utmost importance. The quality and standards must be measurable at each process level in order to evaluate their end result in any healthcare setting.

By and large, areas like CSSD, laundry, house-keeping, etc. are considered as non-revenue generating disciplines. Hence, investments in terms of setting standards or the compliance to those also fall short. But one must realize the long-term benefits of such investments.

Medical devices being used for invasive procedures should be subjected to thorough cleaning/ disinfecting/sterilizing processes to remove accumulated deposits of biosoils. This is most effectively achieved by use of multi-enzymatic liquid cleaning agents. Multi-enzymatic refers to the presence of proteases, lipases, amylases and cellulases.

These agents assist in the breakdown of organic soils and thereby reduce microbial contamination. Reduction of bioburden is a key step for sterilization and disinfection.

Biological monitors are recognized by most international authorities as being closest to the ideal monitors for sterilization processes. Yet, chemical indicators must be used in conjunction with biological and mechanical indicators to monitor whether or not all the parameters required for sterilization are met with in each load (time, temperature, quality of steam, pH and gas concentration in case of ETO process).

Compliance to these practices holds great importance and cost benefit for any healthcare facility. In other words, it is directly proportional to the reputation of the hospital/healthcare institution.

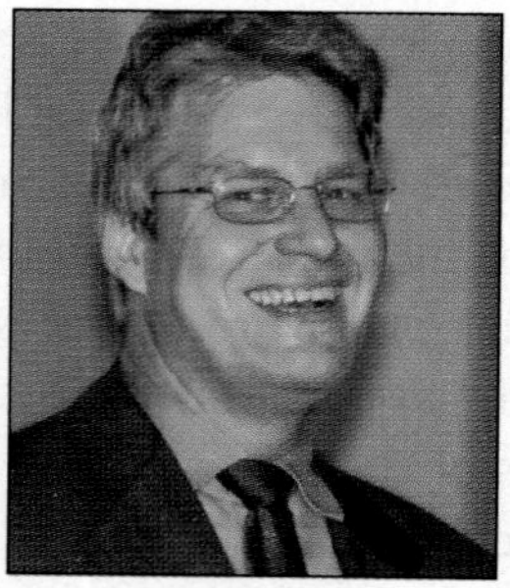

Peter Laser
Executive Director
Business Development
Karl Storz Endoscopy India Pvt. Ltd.

Q: Kindly share your expertise and comment on the benefits and fallacies of the commonly used sterilization processes.

A: Since the discovery of microorganisms as the source of infections, it has been the ultimate target of doctors to keep their equipment free from these disease-causing organisms. The rampant development and application of endoscopes presents a new challenge to everyone concerned, and often it is required that even tiny and sophisticated electronic parts need to be sterilized and not merely disinfected.

The industry offers, basically, two different types of sterilization—thermal and chemical.

Both of these have advantages and disadvantages as can be summarized as under.

Thermal (e.g. Autoclaving):

Advantages:

1. Very simple
2. Only consumable is distilled water
3. Short cycle time
4. 100% sterility achieved in 7 minutes at 137°C
5. Readily available from reputed companies even in the developing countries

Disadvantages:

1. Not suitable for all types of equipment
2. The process puts a thermal stress on equipment.

Chemical (Liquid)

Advantages:

1. Suitable for almost all types of equipment.
2. It is a cold process with no thermal stress.
3. Liquid has some dissolving effect too on protein residues.

Disadvantages:

1. Chemicals may be aggressive and lead to corrosion of instruments.
2. Solution once activated has a limited efficiency time.
3. Sterility is achieved only after several hours.
4. Residues of the solutions may cause irritation and adverse effects on patients.
5. High recurring costs after expiry of shelf life

Chemical (ETO Gas)

Advantages:

1. Practically no corrosive effects
2. Very high efficiency
3. Suitable for all types of equipment

Disadvantages:

1. Long cycle time, upto 72 hours
2. Expensive

From the above, it is evident that there is no ideal method of sterilization that can be applied to all types of equipment and under all conditions. But it is possible to achieve sterility by opting for the appropriate method for each equipment and following prescribed methods meticulously.

It is often tempting to opt for disposable items in order to circumvent all these problems of sterilization. However, there is often a temptation to reuse disposable items due to cost constraints (especially in the developing countries), and this can be even more dangerous than the use of inappropriately sterilized reusable items. This is a serious point to be noted.

INDEX

A

B

C

D

E

F

G

H

I

J

K

L

M

N

O

P

Q

R

S

T

U

V

W